Inflammation Protocols

METHODS IN MOLECULAR BIOLOGY™

John M. Walker, SERIES EDITOR

240. **Mammalian Artificial Chromosomes:** *Methods and Protocols*, edited by *Vittorio Sgaramella and Sandro Eridani, 2003*
239. **Cell Migration in Inflammation and Immunity:** *Methods and Protocols*, edited by *Daniele D'Ambrosio and Francesco Sinigaglia, 2003*
238. **Biopolymer Methods in Tissue Engineering,** edited by *Anthony P. Hollander and Paul V. Hatton, 2003*
237. **G Protein Signaling:** *Methods and Protocols,* edited by *Alan V. Smrcka, 2003*
236. **Plant Functional Genomics**: *Methods and Protocols*, edited by *Erich Grotewold, 2003*
235. ***E. coli* Plasmid Vectors**: *Methods and Applications*, edited by *Nicola Casali and Andrew Preston, 2003*
234. **p53 Protocols,** edited by *Sumitra Deb and Swati Palit Deb, 2003*
233. **Protein Kinase C Protocols**, edited by *Alexandra C. Newton, 2003*
232. **Protein Misfolding and Disease:** *Principles and Protocols*, edited by *Peter Bross and Niels Gregersen, 2003*
231. **Directed Evolution Library Creation**: *Methods and Protocols*, edited by *Frances H. Arnold and George Georgiou, 2003*
230. **Directed Enzyme Evolution**: *Screening and Selection Methods*, edited by *Frances H. Arnold and George Georgiou, 2003*
229. **Lentivirus Gene Engineering Protocols**, edited by *Maurizio Federico, 2003*
228. **Membrane Protein Protocols**: *Expression, Purification, and Characterization*, edited by *Barry S. Selinsky, 2003*
227. **Membrane Transporters:** *Methods and Protocols,* edited by *Qing Yan, 2003*
226. **PCR Protocols, Second Edition,** edited by *John M. S. Bartlett and David Stirling, 2003*
225. **Inflammation Protocols,** edited by *Paul G. Winyard and Derek A. Willoughby, 2003*
224. **Functional Genomics:** *Methods and Protocols*, edited by *Michael J. Brownstein and Arkady B. Khodursky, 2003*
223. **Tumor Suppressor Genes:** *Volume 2: Regulation, Function, and Medicinal Applications*, edited by *Wafik S. El-Deiry, 2003*
222. **Tumor Suppressor Genes:** *Volume 1: Pathways and Isolation Strategies*, edited by *Wafik S. El-Deiry, 2003*
221. **Generation of cDNA Libraries:** *Methods and Protocols*, edited by *Shao-Yao Ying, 2003*
220. **Cancer Cytogenetics:** *Methods and Protocols*, edited by *John Swansbury, 2003*
219. **Cardiac Cell and Gene Transfer:** *Principles, Protocols, and Applications*, edited by *Joseph M. Metzger, 2003*
218. **Cancer Cell Signaling:** *Methods and Protocols*, edited by *David M. Terrian, 2003*
217. **Neurogenetics:** *Methods and Protocols*, edited by *Nicholas T. Potter, 2003*
216. **PCR Detection of Microbial Pathogens:** *Methods and Protocols*, edited by *Konrad Sachse and Joachim Frey, 2003*
215. **Cytokines and Colony Stimulating Factors:** *Methods and Protocols*, edited by *Dieter Körholz and Wieland Kiess, 2003*
214. **Superantigen Protocols,** edited by *Teresa Krakauer, 2003*
213. **Capillary Electrophoresis of Carbohydrates,** edited by *Pierre Thibault and Susumu Honda, 2003*
212. **Single Nucleotide Polymorphisms:** *Methods and Protocols*, edited by *Pui-Yan Kwok, 2003*
211. **Protein Sequencing Protocols, 2nd ed.,** edited by *Bryan John Smith, 2003*
210. **MHC Protocols,** edited by *Stephen H. Powis and Robert W. Vaughan, 2003*
209. **Transgenic Mouse Methods and Protocols,** edited by *Marten Hofker and Jan van Deursen, 2003*
208. **Peptide Nucleic Acids:** *Methods and Protocols,* edited by *Peter E. Nielsen, 2002*
207. **Recombinant Antibodies for Cancer Therapy:** *Methods and Protocols.* edited by *Martin Welschof and Jürgen Krauss, 2002*
206. **Endothelin Protocols,** edited by *Janet J. Maguire and Anthony P. Davenport, 2002*
205. ***E. coli* Gene Expression Protocols,** edited by *Peter E. Vaillancourt, 2002*
204. **Molecular Cytogenetics:** *Protocols and Applications,* edited by *Yao-Shan Fan, 2002*
203. ***In Situ* Detection of DNA Damage:** *Methods and Protocols,* edited by *Vladimir V. Didenko, 2002*
202. **Thyroid Hormone Receptors:** *Methods and Protocols,* edited by *Aria Baniahmad, 2002*
201. **Combinatorial Library Methods and Protocols,** edited by *Lisa B. English, 2002*
200. **DNA Methylation Protocols,** edited by *Ken I. Mills and Bernie H. Ramsahoye, 2002*
199. **Liposome Methods and Protocols,** edited by *Subhash C. Basu and Manju Basu, 2002*
198. **Neural Stem Cells:** *Methods and Protocols,* edited by *Tanja Zigova, Juan R. Sanchez-Ramos, and Paul R. Sanberg, 2002*
197. **Mitochondrial DNA:** *Methods and Protocols,* edited by *William C. Copeland, 2002*
196. **Oxidants and Antioxidants:** *Ultrastructure and Molecular Biology Protocols,* edited by *Donald Armstrong, 2002*
195. **Quantitative Trait Loci:** *Methods and Protocols,* edited by *Nicola J. Camp and Angela Cox, 2002*
194. **Posttranslational Modifications of Proteins:** *Tools for Functional Proteomics,* edited by *Christoph Kannicht, 2002*
193. **RT-PCR Protocols,** edited by *Joe O'Connell, 2002*
192. **PCR Cloning Protocols, 2nd ed.,** edited by *Bing-Yuan Chen and Harry W. Janes, 2002*
191. **Telomeres and Telomerase:** *Methods and Protocols,* edited by *John A. Double and Michael J. Thompson, 2002*
190. **High Throughput Screening:** *Methods and Protocols,* edited by *William P. Janzen, 2002*
189. **GTPase Protocols:** *The RAS Superfamily,* edited by *Edward J. Manser and Thomas Leung, 2002*
188. **Epithelial Cell Culture Protocols,** edited by *Clare Wise, 2002*
187. **PCR Mutation Detection Protocols,** edited by *Bimal D. M. Theophilus and Ralph Rapley, 2002*
186. **Oxidative Stress Biomarkers and Antioxidant Protocols,** edited by *Donald Armstrong, 2002*

METHODS IN MOLECULAR BIOLOGY™

Inflammation Protocols

Edited by

Paul G. Winyard

and

Derek A. Willoughby

*William Harvey Research Institute,
London, UK*

Humana Press ✳ Totowa, New Jersey

©2003 Humana Press Inc.
999 Riverview Drive, Suite 208
Totowa, New Jersey 07512

www.humanapress.com

All rights reserved. No part of this book may be reproduced, stored in a retrieval system, or transmitted in any form or by any means, electronic, mechanical, photocopying, microfilming, recording, or otherwise without written permission from the Publisher. Methods in Molecular Biology™ is a trademark of The Humana Press Inc.

All papers, comments, opinions, conclusions, or recommendations are those of the author(s), and do not necessarily reflect the views of the publisher.

This publication is printed on acid-free paper. ∞
ANSI Z39.48-1984 (American Standards Institute)
Permanence of Paper for Printed Library Materials.

Production Editor: Mark J. Breaugh.

Cover Illustration: Background: Indirect immunoperoxidase staining of frozen ST. *See* Fig. 1 on p. 285. Inset: Histopathological evaluation of arthritis. *See* Fig. 2 on p. 154.

Cover design by Patricia F. Cleary.

For additional copies, pricing for bulk purchases, and/or information about other Humana titles, contact Humana at the above address or at any of the following numbers: Tel.: 973-256-1699; Fax: 973-256-8341; E-mail: humana@humanapr.com or visit our Website: www.humanapress.com

Photocopy Authorization Policy:
Authorization to photocopy items for internal or personal use, or the internal or personal use of specific clients, is granted by Humana Press Inc., provided that the base fee of US $20.00 per copy is paid directly to the Copyright Clearance Center at 222 Rosewood Drive, Danvers, MA 01923. For those organizations that have been granted a photocopy license from the CCC, a separate system of payment has been arranged and is acceptable to Humana Press Inc. The fee code for users of the Transactional Reporting Service is: [0-89603-970-6/03 $20.00].

Printed in the United States of America. 10 9 8 7 6 5 4 3 2 1

Library of Congress Cataloging in Publication Data

Inflammation protocols / edited by Paul G. Winyard and Derek A. Willoughby.
    p. cm. -- (Methods in molecular biology ; v. 225)
  Includes bibliographical references and index.
  ISBN 0-89603-970-6 (alk. paper)   1-59259-374-7 (E-ISBN)
   1. Inflammation--Laboratory manuals. 2. Inflammation--Mediators--Laboratory manuals. 3. Anti-inflammatory agents--Laboratory manuals. I. Winyard, Paul G., 1959- II. Willoughby, D. A. III. Series.

RB131 .I537 2003
616'.0473--dc21

2002033398

Preface

Inflammation has been described as the basis of many pathologies of human disease. When one considers the updated signs of inflammation, they would be vasodilation, cell migration, and, in the case of chronic inflammation, cell proliferation, often with an underlying autoimmune basis. Generally, inflammation may be divided into acute, chronic, and autoimmune, although the editors believe that most, if not all, chronic states are often the result of an autoimmune response to an endogenous antigen. Thus, a proper understanding of the inflammatory basis may provide clues to new therapeutic targets not only in classical inflammatory diseases, but atherosclerosis, cancer, and ischemic heart disease as well.

The lack of advances in classical inflammatory diseases, such as rheumatoid arthritis, may in part arise from a failure to classify the disease into different forms. That different forms exist is exemplified in patients with differing responses to existing antiinflammatory drugs, ranging from nonresponders to very positive responders for a particular nonsteroidal antiinflammatory drug (NSAID). Though researchers have progressively unraveled the mechanisms, the story is far from complete. It should also be noted that the inflammatory response is part of the innate immune response, or to use John Hunter's words in 1795, "inflammation is a salutary response." That may be applied in particular to the defensive response to invading microorganisms.

Because of the large multidisciplinary scope of inflammation research, it is inevitable that a protocols collection such as *Inflammation Protocols* will represent a limited selection of the more important tools for studying inflammation. The editors have therefore focused this volume on those methods that they believe are most likely to be applicable to investigations of potential new antiinflammatory drugs in active target areas for R&D such as transcription factors, adhesion molecules, cyclooxygenase-2 (COX-2) inhibitors, nitric oxide synthases, and metalloproteinases. Some of the experimental protocols (especially the in vitro ones) described in this book are generic, in the sense that they are applicable to the study of many different inflammatory diseases, whereas others attempt to model particular human inflammatory diseases or particular aspects of inflammation.

Inflammation Protocols has been divided into three sections: (1) in vitro systems for studying aspects of inflammation, (2) in vivo models, and (3) relevant pharmacodynamic measurements for the assessment of antiinflammatory compounds. Each section opens with one or two introductory chapters that attempt to provide an overview, or at least viewpoints, of the significance of the methods in that section of the book.

There is no doubt that we will have introduced a particular "flavor" to the book that might not be to everyone's taste–inflammation researchers are of course notorious for having their own favorite cell or inflammatory cascade. Perhaps a second volume will eventually be needed to produce a wider coverage of inflammation protocols, but the editors must recoup their energies before contemplating that prospect. Despite this, we hope that the present volume will provide a unique and contemporary collection of methods that will be useful to both the established experimenter and newcomers to the field of inflammation.

Finally, we are very grateful indeed to the contributing authors, all of them leading researchers within their respective fields. We would also like to thank the series editor, John M. Walker, for his efficient help in reviewing the manuscripts. Most of all, we would like to express our appreciation to Lin Wells, who has somehow managed to maintain a high level of administrative organization within the project, despite the disruptive behavior of the Editors and some of the Contributors!

Paul G. Winyard
Derek A. Willoughby

Contents

Preface v
Contributors xi

PART I. IN VITRO SYSTEMS FOR STUDYING ASPECTS OF THE INFLAMMATORY RESPONSE AND TESTING ANTIINFLAMMATORY DRUGS

1. Key Stages in the Acute Inflammatory Response and Their Relevance as Therapeutic Targets: *Introduction to Part 1*
   Paul G. Winyard 3
2. IκB Kinase and NF-κB Signaling in Response to Pro-Inflammatory Cytokines
   Mireille Delhase 7
3. Screening for Inhibitors of Transcription Factors Using Luciferase Reporter Gene Expression in Transfected Cells
   Deborah Phippard and Anthony M. Manning 19
4. Adhesion Molecule Expression on Cytokine-Stimulated Human Endothelial Cells
   Susan L. Cuvelier and Kamala D. Patel 25
5. Phagocytosis by Inflammatory Phagocytes: *Experimental Strategies for Stimulation and Quantification*
   M. Rachel Morris, Sharon Dewitt, Iraj Laffafian, and Maurice B. Hallett 35
6. Cytosolic Ca^{2+} Measurement and Imaging in Inflammatory Cells
   Sharon Dewitt, Iraj Laffafian, M. Rachel Morris, and Maurice B. Hallett 47
7. Detection and Visualization of Oxidase Activity in Phagocytes
   Maurice B. Hallett, Caroline Cole, and Sharon Dewitt 61
8. Measurement of Complement Activation
   Tom Eirik Mollnes 69
9. Measurement of Matrix Metalloproteinase Activities in the Medium of Cultured Synoviocytes Using Zymography
   Linda Troeberg and Hideaki Nagase 77

10. Measurement of Aggrecanase-Generated Interglobular Domain Catabolites in the Medium and Extracts of Cartilage Explants Using Western Blot Analysis
   Clare E. Hughes, Christopher B. Little, and Bruce Caterson 89
11. In Vitro Model of Human Articular Cartilage Degradation
   William D. Shingleton 99

PART II. IN VIVO MODELS OF INFLAMMATION

12. In Vivo Models of Inflammation: *Introduction to Part 2*
   Derek A. Willoughby 109
13. Carrageenan-Induced Paw Edema in the Rat and Mouse
   Christopher J. Morris 115
14. Pleural Models of Inflammation: *Immune and Nonimmune*
   Adrian R. Moore 123
15. Models of Acute Inflammation in the Ear
   Miklós Gábor 129
16. Migration of Specific Leukocyte Subsets in Response to Cytokine or Chemokine Application In Vivo
   Mauro Perretti and Stephen J. Getting 139
17. Inflammatory Joint Disease: *Clinical, Histological, and Molecular Parameters of Acute and Chronic Inflammation and Tissue Destruction*
   Nancy L. McCartney-Francis, James Chan, and Sharon M. Wahl 147
18. The Assessment of Inflammation, Cartilage Matrix, and Bone Loss in Experimental Monoarticular Arthritis of the Rat
   Michael P. Seed 161
19. Collagen-Induced Arthritis
   Adrian R. Moore 175
20. Air-Pouch Models of Inflammation and Modifications for the Study of Granuloma-Mediated Cartilage Degradation
   Paul Colville-Nash and Toby Lawrence 181
21. Quantitative Analysis of Angiogenesis Using the Murine Chronic Granulomatous Air Pouch
   Chandan A. S. Alam 191

22. Models of Coronary Artery Occlusion and Reperfusion
    for the Discovery of Novel Antiischemic
    and Antiinflammatory Drugs for the Heart
    **Nicole S. Wayman, Michelle C. McDonald,
    Prabal K. Chatterjee, and Christoph Thiemermann** 199
23. Assessment of Anticolitic Drugs in the Trinitrobenzene
    Sulfonic Acid (TNBS) Rat Model of Inflammatory Bowel Disease
    **Brendan J. R. Whittle, Maryan Cavicchi,
    and Dominique Lamarque** 209
24. An In Vivo Model of Ischemia/Reperfusion and Inflammation
    of the Kidneys of the Rat
    Prabal K. Chatterjee and Christoph Thiemermann 223
25. In Vivo Models of Inflammation:
    Immune Rejection and Skin Transplantation In Vivo
    Isabelle Binet and Kathryn J. Wood 239
26. Wound Healing: *A Model of Dermal Wound Repair*
    Annette Tomlinson and Mark W. J. Ferguson 249

PART III. PHARMACODYNAMIC ENDPOINTS IN EXPERIMENTAL MODELS
AND IN CLINICAL STUDIES IN HUMANS

27. An Iconoclastic Approach to Pharmacodynamics in Model Systems:
    Their Relevance to Humans: *Introduction to Part 3*
    David R. Blake and Gordon J. Taylor 263
28. A Reply to "An Iconoclastic Approach to Pharmacodynamics
    in Model Systems: Their Relevance to Humans"
    Derek A. Willoughby 269
29. Quantifying Inflammation In Vivo
    Using Radiolabeled Antibodies and Leukocytes
    Diane Marshall and Dorian O. Haskard 273
30. Immunoperoxidase Histochemistry
    for the Detection of Cellular Adhesion Molecule,
    Cytokine, and Chemokine Expression in the Arthritic Synovium
    Zoltan Szekanecz and Alisa E. Koch 283
31. Roles of Nitric Oxide and Superoxide in Inflammation
    **Daniela Salvemini, Harry Ischiropoulos,
    and Salvatore Cuzzocrea** 291
32. Analysis of Nitrite and Nitrate in the Study of Inflammation
    **Claire A. Davies, Sophie A. Rocks, Meg C. O'Shaughnessy,
    David Perrett, and Paul G. Winyard** 305

33. In Vivo Assays for COX-2
   Chi-Chung Chan 321
34. Measurement of 8-epi-PGF$_{2\alpha}$ as a Marker of Lipid Peroxidation
   In Vivo by Immunoaffinity Extraction
   and Gas Chromatography-Mass Spectrometry
   Nitin K. Gopaul and Erik E. Änggård 329
35. Laboratory Assessment of the Acute Phase Response:
   Using CRP as a Model
   Robert F. Ritchie and Thomas B. Ledue 343
36. Assays of Matrix Metalloproteinases (MMPs) and MMP Inhibitors:
   Bioassays and Immunoassays
   Applicable to Cell Culture Medium, Serum, and Synovial Fluid
   Jon B. Catterall and Tim E. Cawston 353

Index 365

Contributors

CHANDAN A. S. ALAM • *The William Harvey Research Institute, London, UK*
ERIK E. ÄNGGÅRD • *The William Harvey Research Institute, London, UK*
ISABELLE BINET • *University Hospital of Geneva, Geneva, Switzerland*
DAVID R. BLAKE • *University of Bath, Bath, UK*
BRUCE CATERSON • *University of Cardiff, Cardiff, UK*
JON B. CATTERALL • *University of Newcastle, UK*
MARYAN CAVICCHI • *Hospitalier Universitaire Henri Mondor, Paris, France*
TIM E. CAWSTON • *University of Newcastle, Newcastle, UK*
CHI-CHUNG CHAN • *Merck Frosst Centre for Therapeutic Research, Quebec, Canada*
JAMES CHAN • *NIDCR, NIH, Bethesda, MD*
PRABAL K. CHATTERJEE • *The William Harvey Research Institute, London, UK*
CAROLINE COLE • *University of Wales College of Medicine, Cardiff, UK*
PAUL COLVILLE-NASH • *The William Harvey Research Institute, London, UK*
SUSAN L. CUVELIER • *University of Calgary, Calgary, Alberta, Canada*
SALVATORE CUZZOCREA • *University of Messina, Italy*
CLAIRE A. DAVIES • *The William Harvey Research Institute, London, UK*
MIREILLE DELHASE • *University of California at San Diego, La Jolla, CA*
SHARON DEWITT • *University of Wales College of Medicine, Cardiff, UK*
MARK W. J. FERGUSON • *University of Manchester, Manchester, UK*
MIKLÓS GÁBOR • *University of Szeged, Szeged, Hungary*
STEPHEN J. GETTING • *The William Harvey Research Institute, London, UK*
NITIN K. GOPAUL • *The William Harvey Research Institute, London, UK*
MAURICE B. HALLETT • *University of Wales College of Medicine, Cardiff, UK*
DORIAN O. HASKARD • *Imperial College School of Medicine, London, UK*
CLARE E. HUGHES • *University of Cardiff, Cardiff, UK*
HARRY ISCHIROPOULOS • *University of Pennsylvania, Philadelphia, PA*
ALISA E. KOCH • *Northwestern University Medical School and Department of Veterans Affairs, Chicago, IL*
IRAJ LAFFAFIAN • *University of Wales College of Medicine, Cardiff, UK*
DOMINIQUE LAMARQUE • *Hospitalier Universitaire Henri Mondor, Paris, France*
TOBY LAWRENCE • *The William Harvey Research Institute, London, UK*
THOMAS B. LEDUE • *Foundation for Blood Research, Scarborough, ME*

CHRISTOPHER B. LITTLE • *Cell and Matrix Biology Research Unit, University of Melbourne, Melbourne, Australia*
NANCY L. MCCARTNEY-FRANCIS • *NIDCR, NIH, Bethesda, MD*
MICHELLE C. MCDONALD • *The William Harvey Research Institute, London, UK*
ANTHONY M. MANNING • *Roche Pharmaceuticals, Palo Alto, CA*
DIANE MARSHALL • *Celltech, Slough, UK*
TOM EIRIK MOLLNES • *University of Oslo, Oslo, Norway*
ADRIAN R. MOORE • *Celltech, Slough, UK*
CHRISTOPHER J. MORRIS • *University of Bath, Bath, UK*
M. RACHEL MORRIS • *University of Wales College of Medicine, Cardiff, UK*
HIDEAKI NAGASE • *Imperial College, London, UK*
MEG C. O'SHAUGHNESSY • *The William Harvey Research Institute, London, UK*
KAMALA D. PATEL • *University of Calgary, Calgary, Alberta, Canada*
DAVID PERRETT • *Barts and The London School of Medicine and Dentistry, London, UK*
MAURO PERRETTI • *The William Harvey Research Institute, London, UK*
DEBORAH PHIPPARD • *Roche Pharmaceuticals, Palo Alto, CA*
ROBERT F. RITCHIE • *Foundation for Blood Research, Scarborough, ME*
SOPHIE A. ROCKS • *The William Harvey Research Institute, London, UK*
DANIELA SALVEMINI • *Metaphore Pharmaceuticals, St. Louis, MO*
MICHAEL P. SEED • *The William Harvey Research Institute, London, UK*
WILLIAM D. SHINGLETON • *University of Newcastle, Newcastle, UK*
ZOLTAN SZEKANECZ • *University of Debrecen, Debrecen, Hungary*
GORDON J. TAYLOR • *University of Bath, Bath, UK*
CHRISTOPH THIEMERMANN • *The William Harvey Research Institute, London, UK*
ANNETTE TOMLINSON • *University of Manchester, Manchester, UK*
LINDA TROEBERG • *Imperial College, London, UK*
SHARON M. WAHL • *NIDCR, NIH, Bethesda, MD*
NICOLE S. WAYMAN • *The William Harvey Research Institute, London, UK*
BRENDAN J. R. WHITTLE • *The William Harvey Research Institute, London, UK*
DEREK A. WILLOUGHBY • *The William Harvey Research Institute, London, UK*
PAUL G. WINYARD • *Peninsula Medical School, St. Luke's Campus, Universities of Exeter and Plymouth, Exeter, UK*
KATHRYN J. WOOD • *University of Oxford, Oxford, UK*

I

In Vitro Systems for Studying Aspects of the Inflammatory Response and Testing Antiinflammatory Drugs

1

Key Stages in the Acute Inflammatory Response and Their Relevance as Therapeutic Targets

Introduction to Part 1

Paul G. Winyard

1. Introduction

Inflammation, in its broadest sense, is a host response to tissue injury. The four ancient, cardinal, signs of inflammation are redness, heat, swelling, and pain. These clinical signs of inflammation are, of course, the macroscopic culmination of molecular and cellular processes, many of which have become well defined over the last 120 years, and many of which may be reproduced in convenient experimental systems in vitro. In collecting the chapters for this section of the book, our aim is to provide a repository for experimental protocols for the in vitro study of key stages of the inflammatory response. For the reader who is unfamiliar with the field of inflammation, it is perhaps helpful to summarize and contextualize some of the key events of the inflammatory response, as it is these that may be reproduced in the form of in vitro model systems by using the protocols that follow.

Within the vast array of interdigitating and iterative molecular and cellular pathways that constitute inflammation, there are certain linear pathways that have recently received great attention as, perhaps, the "main highways" of the inflammatory response. By way of indicating the significance of some of the experimental protocols in this section, it is convenient to refer to one of these pathways (*see* **Fig. 1**), which begins (at least for the purposes of this discussion) with the stimulation of vascular endothelial cells by key "pro-inflammatory" cytokines such as tumor necrosis factor-α (TNF-α) and interleukin-1β (IL-1β). The importance of this pathway described later is validated, at least in part, by the promise of the therapeutic targets that have been defined at the different stages along its route, although there are numerous bifurcations away from this path

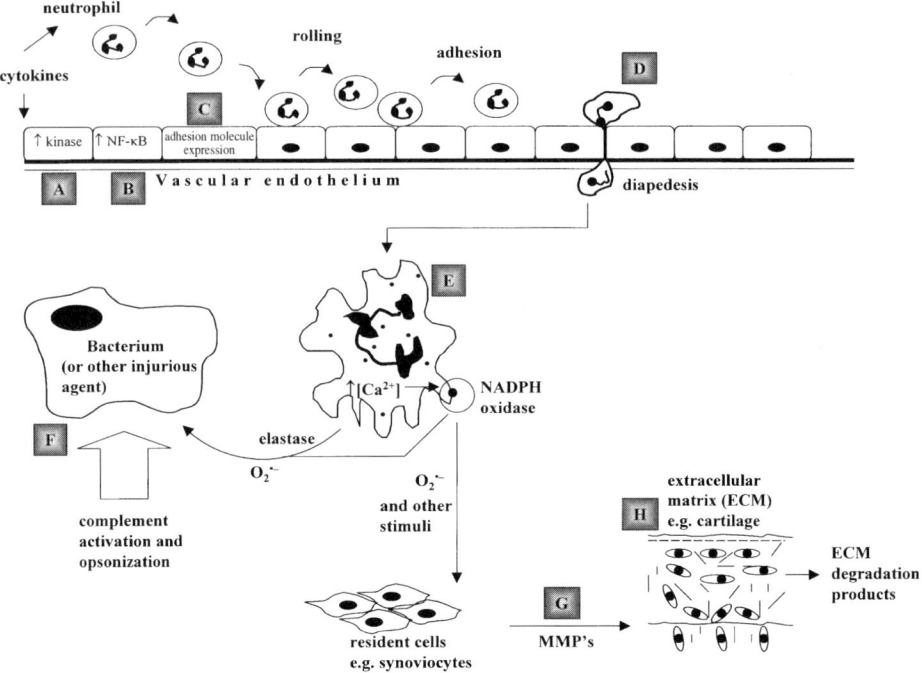

Fig. 1. Grossly simplified schematic diagram representing some of the key events of the inflammatory response. The letters correspond to some of the processes that can be investigated using protocols described within this first section of the book (or, if in brackets, elsewhere in this book). A, intracellular kinase activation by cytokines; B, activation of NF-κB; C, adhesion molecule expression; D, migration (of specific leukocyte subsets); E, stimulation of inflammatory phagocytes, including changes in cytosolic Ca^{2+} and plasma membrane NADPH oxidase; F, opsonisation involving activation of the complement cascade; G, release and activation of MMPs within the extracellular matrix; H, breakdown of the extracellular matrix by proteinases—e.g., degradation of cartilage by a MMPs and aggrecanase.

that are not discussed here. In many cases, the individual protocols described in this section will allow the in vitro screening of candidate therapeutic compounds.

Returning to a description of our illustrative "main highway" of inflammation, the binding of pro-inflammatory cytokines to their cognate plasma membrane receptors results in the activation of intracellular kinases that catalyze a cascade of phosphorylation events, including the phosphorylation (catalyzed by the IKK complex) of IκB, an inhibitory protein subunit bound to the transcription factor NF-κB. The control of gene transcription by specific proteins—

transcription factors—involves the binding of these proteins to short DNA sequence elements located adjacent to the promotor or in the enhancer regions of genes. The phosphorylation of IκB targets it for proteolytic degradation by the 26S proteasome, leaving the active NF-κB complex to be translocated to the nucleus, where it binds to a specific DNA motif and is thereby involved, together with other transcription factors, in controlling the transcription of an array of inflammation-associated genes. Indeed, a key feature of inflammatory diseases such as rheumatoid arthritis (RA) is the increased expression of certain genes that encode "inflammatory" proteins. These include a variety of adhesion molecules, as well as TNFα, IL-1β, and inducible nitric oxide synthase (iNOS) among many others.

Dr. Mireille Delhase describes methods for measuring cytokine-induced IKK activity and NF-κB activation in cultured cells. By stably transfecting cells with a construct containing the NF-κB-binding motif upstream of the luciferase gene, a convenient system for screening potential inhibitors of NF-κB may be created, as described by Dr. Deborah Phippard and Dr. Tony Manning. Recently, there has been considerable interest in the idea that transcription factors may be useful targets for novel therapeutic strategies in the treatment of human diseases, including inflammatory diseases.

As aforementioned, induction of the expression of several adhesion molecules, such as intercellular adhesion molecule-1 (ICAM-1), and E-selectin vascular cell adhesion molecule-1 (VCAM-1), represents a significant inflammatory event and a potential therapeutic target. The increased transcription of these proteins ultimately results in their upregulation on the plasma membrane surface of endothelial cells, and the levels of adhesion molecules may be measured using the techniques described by Dr. Susan Cuvelier and Dr. Kamala Patel. The increased expression of adhesion molecules, in turn, facilitates the "rolling" and adhesion to the vascular endothelium of inflammatory phagocytic cells at vessel sites adjacent to the site of inflammation. The phagocytic cells, such as neutrophils, then migrate through the vessel wall, via the process of diapedesis, and arrive at the focus of "acute" inflammation. The reader is referred to the second section of this book for a description of an in vivo technique for the study of this process, as provided by Professor Mauro Perretti and Dr. Stephen Getting. Later, in the "chronic" phase of inflammation, other cell types (e.g., macrophages and lymphocytes) will be recruited to the site of inflammation by an analogous process. As part of the classic, acute inflammatory response, neutrophils are activated by immune complexes, the complement system and/or pathogens to produce both free radicals (such as superoxide) and proteinases (such as elastase and cathepsin G) which act in concert to kill invading fungi or bacteria, but which may also cause tissue damage. This stimulation of neutrophils can be reproduced in vitro using isolated cells and the extent of the response in the presence of putative antiinflammatory compounds may be tested using the methods described by Dr. Maurice Hallett et al. This group also describes specific methods for the measurement of neutrophil intracellular Ca^{2+} fluxes and $O_2^{\bullet-}$ production by a plasma membrane NADPH oxidase. The killing of bacteria by neutrophils involves their opsonization by plasma proteins, including various components of the complement cascade. Furthermore, certain components of the complement cascade are chemotactic for neutrophils. A protocol by which the extent of complement activation may be determined is described by Professor Tom Eirik Mollnes.

Phagocytic cells, and sometimes resident cells at the site of inflammation, are also stimulated by cytokines such as TNF and IL-1 to release matrix metalloproteinases (MMPs). In respect of the inflamed joint, the resident cells of the synovial membrane—the so-called type B synoviocytes—are activated by cytokines to release MMPs. The MMPs involved in inflammatory tissue destruction include collagenases, gelatinases, and stromelysins. The activities of these proteinases may be determined, again in an in vitro system, according to the zymographic technique detailed by Dr. Linda Troeberg and Professor Hideaki Nagase. Among the expressed metalloproteinases is aggrecanase, which plays an important role in the degradation of cartilage within the rheumatoid joint. Professor Bruce Caterson et al. describe a protocol for the measurement of aggrecanase activity, whereas Dr. Bill Shingleton describes an in vitro model of articular cartilage degradation.

In finishing this introduction to in vitro protocols for the study of inflammation it should be stressed again that, for the sake of simplicity, the description above refers to one of many pathways of acute inflammation. Many of the experimental systems described in this section of the book are relevant to more than one stage or type of inflammation, e.g., acute versus chronic, immune vs nonimmune, and so on. Although, for convenience, the inflammation protocols in this book have been divided between in vitro and in vivo methods, it is vital to have both. It is, of course, impossible to reproduce inflammation in vitro. In vivo, the environment at the site of inflammation changes millisecond by millisecond—this can never be reproduced in a test tube. However, the complementary use of both in vitro and in vivo techniques is a powerful strategy in the study of inflammation and antiinflammatory drug development: For example, the cytokines can be identified in vivo, whereas the signal transduction pathways leading to the production of such cytokines can be characterized in vitro. The combination of the outputs from these two approaches may then allow the demonstration of the importance of a particular pathway by the in vivo testing of selective inhibitors.

2

IκB Kinase and NF-κB Signaling in Response to Pro-Inflammatory Cytokines

Mireille Delhase

1. Introduction

Exposure to pro-inflammatory cytokines (TNFα and IL-1) results in activation of signaling cascades that lead to stimulation of activity of the transcription factors AP-1 and NF-κB and induction of genes that are controlled by these transcription factors. Such genes code for cytokines (TNFα, IL-1, IL-2, IL-6, and GM-CSF), chemokines, adhesion molecules, and enzymes (iNOS and X-2) that produce secondary inflammatory mediators *(1)*.

Transcription factors of the Rel/NF-κB family function as heterodimers and in mammals include RelA (p65), RelB, c-Rel, NF-κB1 (p50), and NF-κB2 (p52). Unlike the Rel proteins, which are synthesized in their functional forms, NF-κB1 and NF-κB2 are synthesized as large precursors, p105 and p100, respectively, that require proteolytic processing to produce the mature p50 and p52 subunits *(2,3)*. In nonstimulated cells, NF-κB dimers are kept inactive in the cytoplasm through interaction with inhibitory proteins, the IκBs. In response to cell stimulation by a variety of stimuli including cytokines, endotoxin (LPS), dsRNA, oxidants and ionizing radiation, a multisubunit complex, the IκB kinase complex (IKK) is rapidly activated and phosphorylates two critical serines (e.g., Ser-32 and Ser-36 in IκBα) in the N-terminal regulatory domain of the IκBs *(4,5)*. Phosphorylated IκBs are recognized by a specific E3 ubiquitin ligase complex and undergo polyubiquitination, which targets them for rapid degradation by the 26S proteasome *(6)*. NF-κB dimers, freed from the IκBs, translocate to the nucleus and activate the transcription of specific target genes.

The IKK complex is composed of three subunits: two highly homologous catalytic subunits, IKKα and IKKβ and a regulatory subunit, IKKγ (or NEMO) *(4)*. Biochemical studies and analysis of knockout mice indicate that the catalytic subunit IKKβ and the regulatory subunit IKKγ but not the catalytic subunit IKKα, are absolutely required for IκB phosphorylation and NF-κB activation in response to pro-inflammatory stimuli *(7–14)*. IKK activation by such stimuli depends on phosphorylation of the IKKβ subunit at two serine residues (Ser-177 and Ser-181) within its activation loop *(7)*. Despite the conservation of these serines in the IKKα subunit, IKKα does not play an essential role in IKK and NF-κB activation by all major stimuli *(7)*. Instead, IKKα plays a critical role in developmental processes, in particular terminal differentiation of keratinocytes during formation of the epidermis *(13,14)*. Recently, IKKα has been found to be involved in activation of a second NF-κB pathway involving processing of NF-κB2 *(15)*. This pathway is particularly important for B-cell maturation and secondary lymphoid organ formation, key events in the development of adaptive immunity.

This chapter focuses on the basic techniques allowing the study of IKK and NF-κB activation in response to cell stimulation by pro-inflammatory cytokines.

2. Materials
2.1. Stock Solutions

1. Stocks of the reagents are prepared and stored as follows and are stable for at least 6 mo.
   a. Dithiothreitol (DTT) (1 M) in 10 mM sodium acetate, stored at –80°C.
   b. Phenylmethylsulfonide fluoride (PMSF) (100 mM) in ethanol, stored at room temperature.
   c. p-nitrophenyl phosphate (pNPP) (1 M) in H_2O, stored at –20°C.
   d. Na_3VO_4 (100 mM) in H_2O, stored at 4°C.
   e. Aprotinin (10 mg/mL) in 10 mM HEPES, pH 8.0, stored at –80°C.
   f. Bestatin (10 mg/mL) in H_2O, stored at –80°C.
   g. Leupeptin (10 mg/mL) in H_2O, stored at –80°C.
   h. Pepstatin (10 mg/mL) in ethanol, stored at –80°C.
   i. All protease inhibitors are available from Sigma and Calbiochem (San Diego, CA).
2. Sterile penicillin/streptomycin stock solution and 200 mM L-glutamine stock solution are kept at –20°C in 10-mL aliquots. These reagents, as well as Dulbecco's modified Eagle's medium (DMEM), may be obtained from Gibco BRL, Life Technologies, Rockville, MD.
3. Recombinant mouse and human TNFα and IL-1 are available from several commercial sources (BioSource International, Camarillo, CA or R&D Systems, Minneapolis, MN). The lyophilized cytokines are reconstituted at 10 µg/mL in PBS

plus 0.1% bovine serum albumin (BSA, tissue culture grade) and stored at –80°C in 100-µL aliquots.
4. ATP stock solution: 100 mM in H$_2$O, stored at –80°C in 50-µL aliquots.
5. ^{32}P-orthophosphate (cat. no. Nex-53C) is from NEN Life Science Products, Boston, MA).
6. [γ-^{32}P]ATP is from Amersham Pharmacia Biotech, Piscataway, NJ.

2.2. Cell Lysis Buffers

1. Lysis buffer: 50 mM Tris-HCl, pH 7.6, 250 mM sodium chloride (NaCl), 3 mM ethylenediamine tetraacetic acid (EDTA), 3 mM ethyleneglycol tetraacetic acid (EGTA), 1% (v/v) Triton X-100, 0.5% (v/v) Nonidet (P-40) (NP40), 10% glycerol, 20 mM sodium fluoride (NaF), 40 mM β-glycero-3-phosphate. This buffer is prepared as a stock solution, filtered through a 0.45-µm filter unit, and stored at 4°C. Before use, the following should be added: 2 mM DTT, 1 mM PMSF, 2 mM pNPP, 1 mM sodium orthovanadate (Na$_3$VO$_4$), and 10 µg/mL each of aprotinin, bestatin, leupeptin, and pepstatin (*see* **Subheading 2.1.**).
2. RIPA buffer: 20 mM Tris-HCl, pH 7.6, 150 mM NaCl, 1 mM EDTA, 1 mM EGTA, 1% NP40, 0.5% (w/v) sodium deoxycholate (DOC), 0.05% sodium dodecyl sulfate (SDS), 10% glycerol, 20 mM NaF, 40 mM β-glycero-3-phosphate, 2.5 mM sodium metabisulfite, 5 mM benzamidine, 2 mM DTT, 1 mM PMSF, 20 mM pNPP, 1 mM Na$_3$VO$_4$, and 10 µg/mL each of aprotinin, bestatin, leupeptin, and pepstatin (*see* **Subheading 2.1.**).

2.3. Bacterial Culture Medium and Bacteria Lysis Buffers

1. Lbroth: bacto-tryptone 10 g/L, bacto-yeast extract 5 g/L, NaCl 5 g/L, adjusted to pH 7.5 with NaOH. 100 µg/mL ampicillin and 2% glucose are added.
2. Base buffer: PBS, pH 8.0, 1 mM EDTA, 0.5% (v/v) Triton X-100, 5 mM DTT, store at 4°C. This buffer is stable for several months if prepared without DTT. DTT can be added just before use (*see* **Subheading 2.1.**).
3. Buffer I : Base buffer containing 0.3 M ammonium sulfate [(NH$_4$)$_2$SO$_4$].
4. Lysis buffer: Buffer I supplemented with 1 mM PMSF and 10 µg/mL of protease inhibitors (aprotinin, bestatin, leupeptin, and pepstatin) (*see* **Subheading 2.1.**).
5. Elution buffer: 100 mM Tris-HCl, pH 8.0, 20 mM glutathione.
6. Dialysis buffer: 20 mM Tris-HCl, pH 8.0, 100 mM NaCl, 0.2 mM EDTA, 10 mM β-glycero-3-phosphate and 10% glycerol.

2.4. Kinase Assay

1. Kinase buffer (10X): 200 mM HEPES, pH 7.5, 100 mM magnesium chloride (MgCl$_2$).
2. Reaction buffer: kinase buffer [1X] supplemented with 20 mM β-glycero-3-phosphate, 10 mM pNPP, 1 mM DTT, and 20 µM "unlabeled" ATP. This buffer should be prepared just before use.

2.5. Reagents for Electrophoretic Mobility Shift Assay

1. Oligonucleotide probes:
   NF-κB:5'-GGATCCTCAACAGAGGGGACTTTCCGAGGCCA-3'
   3'- AGTTGTCTCCCCTGAAAGGCTCCGGTCCTAGG-5'
   NF-Y:5'-GTAGGAACCAATGAAATGCGAGG-3'
   3'- TTGGTTACTTTACGCTCCGGATG-5'
   Consensus oligonucleotide sequences for binding of transcription factors are also available from Promega (Madison, WI). The oligonucleotides are diluted at 1 µg/µL in TE buffer (10 mM Tris-HCl, pH 8.0, 1 mM EDTA) and stored at –20°C.
2. Klenow buffer (1X): 10 mM Tris-HCl, pH 7.9, 50 mM NaCl, 10 mM MgCl$_2$, and 1 mM DTT).
3. EMSA buffer (10X): 100 mM Tris, pH 7.6, 500 mM potassium chloride (KCl), 10 mM EDTA, and 50% glycerol, stored at –20°C.
4. Nu-Clean D25 spin columns for probe purification are available from Eastman Kodak Company, Rochester, NY.
5. Poly(dI.dC) is from Amersham Pharmacia Biotech.
6. Gel loading buffer (10X): 250 mM Tris-HCl, pH 7.6, 40% glycerol, and 0.2% (w/v) bromophenol blue, stored at 4°C.
7. Acrylamide stock solution (40%): Dissolve 38.71 g of acrylamide and 1.29 g of bis-acrylamide in 100 mL H$_2$O. Solution is filtered and kept at 4°C.
8. TBE (10X): Dissolve 121.1 g of Tris base, 55 g of boric acid, and 7.4 g of EDTA into 1 L of H$_2$O. Adjust the pH to 8.3 with solid boric acid.
9. Nondenaturing gel: Mix 36 mL of H$_2$O, 4.5 mL of acrylamide stock solution, 4.5 mL of TBE 10X, 450 µL of a 10% (w/v) solution of ammonium persulfate (APS) in H$_2$O, and 45 µL of TEMED.

3. Methods
3.1. Cell Culture and Cytokine Stimulation

1. Adherent cells (HeLa, HEK295, 3T3 fibroblasts) are cultured in DMEM high glucose supplemented with 10% fetal bovine serum (FBS), 2 mM L-glutamine, and 1% (v/v) penicillin/streptomycin stock solution at 37°C in a 5% CO$_2$ atmosphere.
2. Tumor necrosis factor α (TNFα) and interleukin-1 (IL-1) stocks solutions are diluted, respectively, at 20 ng/mL and 10 ng/mL final concentration in pre-warmed serum-free medium, then added to the cells. Stimulation is performed at 37°C for various periods of time.
3. After stimulation, the cells are placed on ice, medium is removed and the cells are washed twice with ice-cold phosphate-buffered saline (PBS). Cells are harvested in 1 mL PBS/100-mm dish using a cell lifter and pelleted by centrifugation for 5 min at 4°C at 2000 g.
4. Cell pellets are kept frozen at –80°C or directly lysed by resuspension in lysis buffer (400 µL per cell pellet from a 100-mm dish) with incubation on ice for 10–15 min. The lysate is centrifuged at 13,000g for 10 min at 4°C.

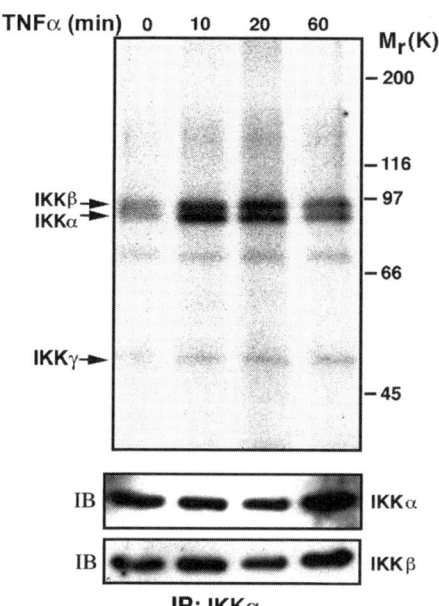

Fig. 1. Cytokine-induced IKK phosphorylation. HeLa cells incubated for 5 h with [^{32}P]orthophosphate were stimulated with TNFα (20 ng/mL) for the indicated times, then lysed. The IKK complex was immunoprecipitated (IP) with an antibody to IKKα (clone # B78-1 from PharMingen), resolved by gel electrophoresis and transferred onto a PVDF membrane. Phosphoproteins were detected by autoradiography. IKKα and IKKβ were identified by immunoblotting (IB) using specific antibodies (anti-IKKα, clone # B78-1 from PharMingen and anti-IKKβ H470 from Santa Cruz Biotechnology).

5. The supernatant is transferred to a clean tube and the protein concentration is determined by Bradford assay *(17)*.
6. The lysates (WCE, whole cell extracts) are stored at −80°C until use. WCEs can be used for analysis of protein composition by western blotting, immune-complex kinase assay and electrophoretic mobility shift assay (EMSA).

3.2. Detection of IKK Phosphorylation by ^{32}P Metabolic Labeling (see **Note 1**)

1. Cells at subconfluence (70–80%) (one 60-mm dish per assay) are washed twice in phosphate-free DMEM and incubated for 1 h in the same medium.
2. The medium is then replaced by labeling medium (4 mL per dish) consisting of phosphate-free DMEM supplemented with 10% dialyzed FBS and 1–2 mCi/mL ^{32}P-orthophosphate. Cells are labeled for 4–5 h at 37°C.
3. TNFα or IL-1 stimulation of the cells is performed as described in **Subheading**

3.1. Cytokines are diluted directly into the labeling medium (20 ng/mL for TNFα and 10 ng/mL for IL-1) and stimulation is performed for 5 to 15 min.
4. Bulk IKK phosphorylation is observed after 5 min following cytokine stimulation (see **ref. 7** and **Fig. 1**). Labeling medium is removed, cells are placed on ice, and washed twice with ice-cold PBS.
5. Cells are lysed by addition of 1 mL of lysis buffer directly to the culture dish. Cells are scraped using a cell lifter, transferred to a microcentrifuge tube and lysed on ice for 10 min. Cellular debris are pelleted by centrifugation at 13,000g for 10 min at 4°C.
6. Supernatants are transferred to clean tubes. Cell lysates are clarified by incubation for 1–2 h at 4°C on a rotator in the presence of 10 µL of preimmune serum (if available) or 10 µg of nonspecific control IgG and 50 µL of 50% slurry of protein A/G-Sepharose beads. Beads are pelleted by centrifugation at 13,000g for 5 min at 4°C and supernatants are transferred to clean tubes.
7. Immunoprecipitation of the IKK complex is performed by rotating the cell lysate overnight at 4°C after addition of 1–5 µg of anti-IKK antibody (see **Note 2**) and 25 µL of 50% of slurry of protein A/G-Sepharose beads. The immune-complexes are collected by centrifugation for 1 min at 13,000g, then washed once in lysis buffer containing 300 mM NaCl, once in the same buffer supplemented with 2 M urea and twice in RIPA buffer. The supernatants are discarded and the immune complexes are resuspended in SDS-loading buffer.
8. The IKK subunits are resolved on a 7.5% SDS-PAGE gel (12X 16 cm) according to a standard procedure *(17)*. The proteins are transferred onto a nitrocellulose or Immobilon-P polyvinylidene fluoride membrane. The phosphoproteins are detected by exposure of the membrane to Kodak, Biomax-MR film for 2–12 h at –80°C. After exposure, the membrane can be used to detect protein levels by immunoblotting.

3.3. Measurement of IKK Activity by An Immune-Complex Kinase Assay

Rapid and transient activation of the IKK complex in response to cell stimulation by pro-inflammatory cytokines (TNFα and IL-1) can be best measured and quantified by an immune-complex kinase assay using GST-IκBα (1–54) as a substrate (see **Fig. 2A**).

Fig. 2. *(opposite page)* IKK and NF-κB activation by TNFα and IL-1. (**A**) HeLa cells (left panel) and LL-2 cells (lung carcinoma cell line, right panel) were stimulated with TNFα and IL-1 for the indicated times. IKK was isolated by immunoprecipitation with anti-IKKα (clone # B78-1, PharMingen) or anti-IKKγ(clone 73-764, PharMingen) and its activity was measured by phosphorylation of GST-IκBα (1-54) as described in **Subheading 3.3**. (**B**) IκBα degradation was analyzed by immunoblotting. IκBα phosphorylation (middle panel) was detected using an antibody directed against P-Ser-32 of IκBα (#9241, New England Biolabs, Beverly, MA). IκBα (bottom panel) was detected by immunoblotting using an anti-IκBα antibody (#IMG-127, Imgenex or # C-21, Santa

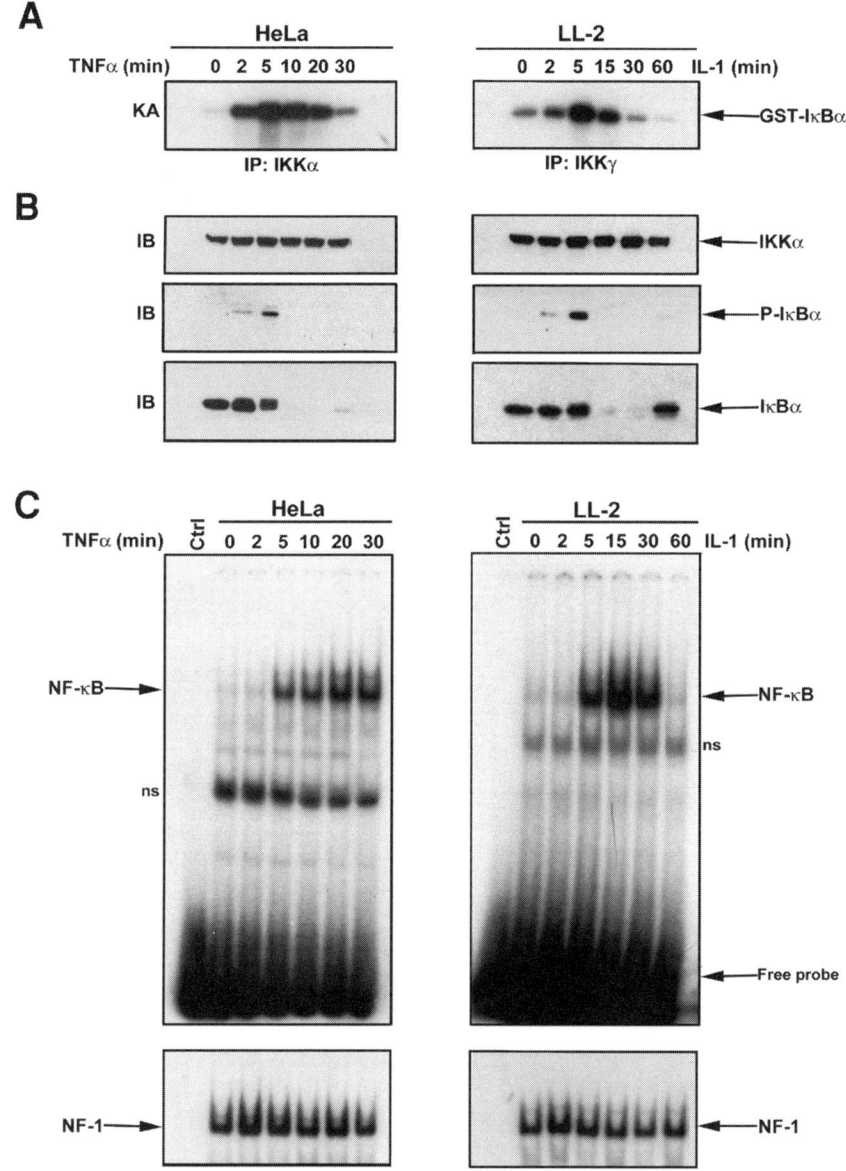

Fig. 2. *(continued)* Cruz Biotechnology). IKKα expression (top panel), used as control for equal protein loading, was determined by immunoblotting using an anti-IKKα antibody (#IMG-136, Imgenex). (**C**) NF-κB DNA-binding activity was measured by electrophoretic mobility shift assay (EMSA). Cells were left untreated or were stimulated with TNFα (left panel) or IL-1 (right panel) for the indicated times, after which WCEs were prepared and NF-κB and NF-Y DNA-binding activities were measured by EMSA as described in **Subheading 3.4.** ns = nonspecific.

3.3.1. Expression and Purification of GST-IkBa (1–54) Fusion Protein in Escherichia coli

1. A cDNA fragment encoding the first 54 N-terminal amino acids (including Ser 32 and Ser 36) of human IκBα was inserted in frame at the 3' end of the GST sequence of a pGEX expression vector (Amersham Pharmacia Biotech) (*see* **Note 3**).
2. BL21 bacteria transformed with this recombinant plasmid are grown at 37°C in 500 mL Lbroth containing 100 µg/mL ampicillin and 2% glucose until the absorbance at 600 nm measured in a 1-cm pathlength cuvet is between 0.4 and 0.5.
3. Protein expression is induced by addition of 2 mM isopropyl-β-thiogalactopyranoside (IPTG) for 3 h at 37°C.
4. Bacteria are collected by centrifugation and resuspended on ice in 30 mL of ice-cold bacteria lysis buffer. Lysozyme is added to a final concentration of 1 mg/mL and bacteria are lysed by sonication (Virsonic 600 sonicator). Bacterial debris are removed by centrifugation at 20,000g for 20 min at 4°C.
5. The supernatant is transferred to a clean tube and incubated for 1 h at 4°C with 500 µL of 50% slurry of glutathione Sepharose 4B equilibrated with PBS.
6. The beads are collected by centrifugation at 500g for 5 min and washed twice with buffer I containing 1 mM PMSF, twice with base buffer containing 1 mM PMSF and once with PBS (10 bed volumes for each wash). The beads are then transferred to a microcentrifuge tube.
7. The GST fusion protein is eluted by incubation of the beads with two bed volumes of elution buffer for 1 h at 4°C on a rotator. After centrifugation, the supernatant is collected and the beads are subjected to a second 1-h elution step. The supernatants from the two elution steps are combined and dialyzed at 4°C against 2 L of dialysis buffer.
8. The quality and quantity of fusion protein is evaluated by SDS-PAGE followed by Coomassie blue staining *(17)* using known amounts of BSA as standard. GST-IκBα (1–54) protein solution is stored at –80°C in 100 µL aliquots.

3.3.2. IKK Immune-Complex Kinase Assay

1. To determine whether IKK activity is induced by a given stimulus, cells are left untreated or are treated for various periods of times with a specific activator (for example TNFα or IL-1) as described in **Subheading 3.1.** WCEs are prepared as described in **Subheading 3.1.**
2. WCEs containing equal amounts of proteins (typically 20–100 µg) from nonstimulated and stimulated cells are aliquoted into prechilled microcentrifuge tubes. The volume is adjusted to 300 µL with cell lysis buffer.
3. Anti-IKK antibody (1 to 2 µg per reaction) (*see* **Note 2**) or control serum (pre-immune serum or control IgG) and 20 µL of 50% slurry of protein A/G-Sepharose are added to the lysates. Immunoprecipitation is performed for a minimum of 2 h at 4°C on a rotator.
4. The immune-complexes bound to the beads are collected by centrifugation at 2000g for 1 min at 4°C. The supernatants are discarded and the beads are washed once with lysis buffer containing 400 mM NaCl, once with the same buffer containing 2 M urea and twice with 1X kinase buffer.

5. The immune-complexes are resuspended in a 30-μL reaction buffer as described in **Subheading 2.4.** containing 5μCi of [γ-^{32}P]ATP (6000 Ci/mmole) and 1 μg of GST-IκBα(1–54) substrate (*see* **Subheading 3.3.1**). The kinase reaction is allowed to proceed for 30 min at 30°C.
6. The reactions are stopped by addition of SDS sample loading buffer *(16)*. The samples are heated at 100°C for 5 min to denature the proteins and then analyzed by SDS-PAGE (10% gel). Electrophoresis is stopped before the free isotope (which migrates on the gel together with the yellow *p*NPP band) runs off the gel.
7. The bottom of the gel containing the free isotope is cut off and discarded. The gel is stained with Coomassie blue *(17)*, destained in 10% acetic acid, 10% methanol in H$_2$O and dried. This step allows visualization of the substrate to verify equal loading.
8. The dried gel is exposed to Kodak X-OMAT-AR films. Alternatively, the kinase assay gel can be directly transferred to a PVDF membrane, which is then exposed to film. This allows further detection of IKK in the immune-complexes by immunoblotting.
9. The IKK activity is determined by the amount of radioactive ^{32}P incorporated into the GST-IκBα(1-54) substrate. Quantification can be performed on a phosphoimager (preferred) or by densitometric scanning of the films.

3.4. Measurement of NF-κB Activation by Electrophoretic Mobility Shift Assay

3.4.1. Oligonucleotide Probe Labeling

1. Complementary oligonucleotides are synthesized according to consensus sequences for binding of transcription factors (*see* **Subheading 2.5.**).
2. 10 μL of both oligonucleotide stock solutions (at 1 μg/μL) are diluted into 100 μL of TE in a microcentrifuge tube. The tube is heated at 80°C for 10 min in a beaker of water, then slowly cooled down to room temperature (about 1 h) to allow annealing of the oligonucleotides. The double-stranded (ds) oligonucleotide stock solution is stored at –20°C.
3. The EMSA probe is prepared by incubation for 20 min at room temperature of 1 μL of ds oligonucleotide stock solution in a 20-μL reaction mixture containing 1X Klenow buffer (*see* **Subheading 2.5.**). 25 μ*M* of each dATP, dTTP, and dGTP, 50 μCi [α-^{32}P]dCTP and 5 units of Klenow enzyme (*see* **Note 4**).
4. The labeling reaction is stopped by addition of 25 μ*M* of unlabelled dCTP and incubation is continued for 5 min at room temperature.
5. The probe is purified on a Nu-Clean D25 spin column (*see* **Note 5**) and stored at –20°C.

3.4.2. Electrophoretic Mobility Shift Assay

1. Aliquots of WCEs containing 10 μg of protein (adjusted to 10 μL with cell lysis buffer) are incubated for 30 min at room temperature in a 20-μL volume reaction containing 2 μL of 10X EMSA buffer (*see* **Subheading 2.5.**), 1 μL of 20 m*M* DTT, 2 μg of poly(dI.dC) and 15,000–30,000 cpm of probe. H$_2$O is added to bring the volume to 20 μL.

2. The reactions are stopped by addition of 2 μL of 10X gel loading buffer (*see* **Subheading 2.5.**) and the samples are run on a 4% nondenaturing polyacrylamide gel (20 × 20 cm).
3. Electrophoresis is stopped when the free probe (which migrates together with the bromophenol blue band) is 2.5 cm from the bottom of the gel. The gel is fixed (optional) for 15 min in a solution of 10% acetic acid, 10% methanol in H_2O, then dried and exposed to Kodak X-OMAT-AR film for autoradiography (*see* **Fig. 2C**).

4. Notes

1. Precautions must be taken when performing metabolic labeling with ^{32}P-orthophosphate. Work must be carried out behind a 2.5-cm-thick acrylic shield. A thick layer of lead can be attached to the outside of the shield to provide additional protection against radiation. A 1-cm-thick acrylic cell house should be used to provide shielding when the cell dishes are in the incubator or when they are moved in the laboratory. Researchers should wear two layers of gloves during all steps of the labeling procedure.
2. Immunoprecipitation of the entire IKK complex can be performed using an antibody against any of the IKK subunits. Several commercial antibodies have been tested and found to quantitatively immunoprecipitate the IKK complex. We currently use anti-IKKα [clone # B78-1, PharMingen (San Diego, CA), this monoclonal antibody recognizes the human IKKα but not the mouse IKKα], anti-IKKα M280 [Santa Cruz Biotechnology (Santa Cruz, CA)], anti-IKKγ (clones # C73-764 and C73-1794, PharMingen) and anti-IKKβ H470 (Santa Cruz Biotechnology) *(7,13)*. Intensive washings of the immunoprecipitates in RIPA buffer may disrupt interaction between IKKγ and the IKKα/IKKβ dimers. Therefore, to examine IKKγ phosphorylation, we recommend immunoprecipitating the IKK complex using an antibody against IKKγ.
3. This recombinant plasmid as well as a mutant version in which Ser 32 and Ser 36 have been replaced by Ala (GST-IκBα(1-54)AA) are available from the author's laboratory upon request.
4. If the annealed oligonucleotides do not contain 5' protruding ends, but instead are blunt ended, labeling cannot be performed using Klenow enzyme. Instead T_4 polynucleotide kinase in the presence of [γ-^{32}P] ATP should be used *(17)*.
5. Unincorporated nucleotides can also be removed by centrifugation through a "self made" 1-mL Sephadex G25 column.

Acknowledgment

The author would like to thank D. Rothwarf for helpful discussions and critical reading of the manuscript. This work was supported by the Sontag Foundation Fellowship of the Arthritis National Research Foundation and a research grant from the San Diego Chapter of the Arthritis Foundation.

References

1. Barnes, P. J. and Karin, M. (1997) Nuclear factor-κB - A pivotal transcription factor in chronic inflammatory diseases. *N. Engl. J. Med.* **15,** 1066–1071.
2. Baeuerle, P. A. and Baltimore, D. (1996) NF-kappa B: ten years after. *Cell* **87,** 13–20.
3. Ghosh, S., May, M. J., and Kopp, E. B. (1998) NF-kappa B and Rel proteins: evolutionarily conserved mediators of immune responses. *Ann. Rev. Immunol.* **16,** 225–260.
4. Rothwarf, D. M. and Karin, M. (1999) The NF-κB activation pathway: a paradigm in information transfer from the membrane to the nucleus. Science's STKE. www.stke.org/cgi/content/full/OC_sigtrans;1999/5/re1.
5. Karin, M. and Delhase, M. (2000) The IκB kinase (IKK) and NF-κB: key elements of proinflammatory signalling. *Sem. Immunol.* **12,** 85–98.
6. Karin, M. and Ben-Neriah, Y. (2000) Phosphorylation meets ubiquitination: the control of NF-κB activity. *Ann. Rev. Immunol.* **18,** 621–663.
7. Delhase, M., Hayakawa, M., Chen, Y., and Karin, M. (1999) Positive and negative regulation of IκB kinase activity through IKKβ subunit phosphorylation. *Science* **284,** 309–313.
8. Li, Q., Van Antwerp, D., Mercurio, F., Lee, K.-F., and Verma, I. M. (1999) Severe liver degeneration in mice lacking the IκB kinase 2 gene. Science 284, 321-325.
9. Li, Z.-W., Chu, W., Hu, Y., Delhase, M., Deerinck, T., Ellisman, M., Johnson, R. and Karin, M. (1999) The IKKβ subunit of IκB kinase (IKK) is essential for NF-κB activation and prevention of apoptosis. *J. Exp. Med.* **189,** 1839–1845.
10. Yamaoka, S., Courtois, G., Bessia, C., Whiteside, S. T., Weil, R., Agou, F., et al. (1998) Complementation cloning of NEMO, a component of the IκB kinase complex essential for NF-κB activation. *Cell* **93,** 1231–1240.
11. Rothwarf, D. M., Zandi, E., Natoli, G., and Karin, M. (1998) IKKγ is an essential regulatory subunit of the I_B kinase complex. *Nature* **395,** 297–300.
12. Makris, C., Godfrey, V. L., Krahn-Senftleben, G., Takahashi, T., Roberts, J. L., Schwarz, T., et al. (2000) Female mice heterozygous for IKKγ/NEMO deficiencies develop a dermatopathy similar to the human X-linked disorder incontinentia pigmenti. *Mol. Cell* **5,** 969–979.
13. Hu, Y., Baud, V., Delhase, M., Zhang, P., Deerinck, T., Ellisman, M., et al. (1999) Abnormal morphogenesis but intact IKK activation in mice lacking the IKKα subunit of the IκB kinase. *Science* **284,** 316–320.
14. Takeda, K., Takeuchi, O., Tsujimura, T., Itami, S., Adachi, O., Kawai, T., et al. (1999) Limb and skin abnormalities in mice lacking IKKα. *Science* **284,** 313–316.
15. Senftleben, U., Cao, Y., Xiao, G., Greten, F. R., Krahn, G., Bonizzi, G., et al. (2001). Activation by IKKα of a second evolutionary conserved, NF-κB signaling pathway. *Science* **293,** 1495–1499.
16. Mercurio, F., DiDonato, J., Rosette, C., and Karin, M. (1992) Molecular cloning and characterization of a novel Rel/NF-κB family member displaying structural and functional homology to NF-κB p50/p105. *DNA Cell Biol.* **11,** 523–537.
17. Ausubel, F., Brent, R., Kingston, R.E., Moore, D. D., Smith, J. A., Seidman, J. G., et al., Eds. (1991) *Current Protocols in Molecular Biology,* Wiley, New York.

3

Screening for Inhibitors of Transcription Factors Using Luciferase Reporter Gene Expression in Transfected Cells

Deborah Phippard and Anthony M. Manning

1. Introduction

Nuclear transcription factors (TF) regulate tissue- and stimulus-specific gene expression through their ability to integrate extracellular signals at the level of the nucleus (1). Multiple human diseases, including cancer, cardiovascular disease, neurologic and autoimmune disorders, result from aberrations in the expression of genes regulated by these transcription factors (2). Interest in the exploitation of transcription factors for the development of gene-regulating therapeutics has grown steadily over the past few years. The ability to modulate abnormal gene expression through manipulation of TF function offers an innovative approach to disease therapies. TF modulation holds particular promise in diseases where several proteins contribute simultaneously to the pathology, such as in autoimmune disease, where a plethora of cytokines, destructive enzymes, and cell-adhesion molecules combine to enhance disease progression.

A key technology for assaying TF function utilizes the assessment of activity of an enzyme whose expression is directed from a synthetic DNA construct introduced by transfection into the cell. The synthetic construct is regulated by the presence of distinct TF binding elements in its proximal promoter. Each synthetic reporter construct contains a selectable marker gene, and cells can be transiently or stably transfected with such constructs to facilitate high-throughput drug screening assays.

In a robotics-based high-throughput drug screening assay using human Jurkat T cells stably transfected with promoter-reporter constructs utilizing the firefly luciferase gene as a reporter and canonical AP-1 or NF-κB binding sites as promoter elements, we identified a series of compounds from a diversity library that inhibited both AP-1 and NF-κB mediated transcriptional activation without blocking basal transcription driven by the β-actin promoter *(3)*. The most potent of these compounds, SP-100030, inhibited Phorbol 12-myristate-13 acetate (PMA)-induced AP-1 or NF-κB-dependent luciferase activity with an IC50 of 30 nM *(4)*.

IL-2, IL-8, and TNF-α production by the PMA-stimulated Jurkat cells was similarly inhibited. Treatment with SP100030 (10 mg/kg/d.i.p.) decreased arthritis severity in a mouse model of collagen-induced arthritis *(5)*. Analysis of arthritic joints from these animals demonstrated that SP100030 decreased NF-κB binding and IL-2 gene expression. Promoter-reporter assays are therefore valuable tools in the drug discovery and research settings. This chapter provides a detailed methodology for screening for transcription factor inhibitors using promoter-reporter constructs in transfected cell cultures.

2. Materials
2.1. Cells and Culture Conditions

1. Human Jurkat T-cell lymphoma cells obtained from the ATCC (American Type Culture Collection, Manassas, VA) were expanded to give aliquots stored in liquid nitrogen until use.
2. Cells were cultured under sterile conditions in RPMI-1640 (Gibco Laboratories, Grand Island, NY) supplemented with 10% fetal calf serum (FCS) in the presence of 100 µg/mL penicillin and streptomycin and 2 m*M* L-glutamine.

2.2. Plasmid DNA Constructs

1. Firefly luciferase reporter plasmid; p(κB)$_4$LUC which contains four NF-κB sites (from the MHC promoter) cloned upstream of the minimal SV40 promoter in the pGL2 vector which is available from Promega Corp., Madison, WI.
2. The AP-1-LUC plasmid, contains an AP-1 binding site from the collagenase promoter driving luciferase expression in the pGL2 vector.
3. β-Actin-LUC. A reporter construct where luciferase expression is driven by the β-actin promoter.
4. Positive control plasmid; phRL-CMV which provides constitutive expression of *Renilla* luciferase under the control of the cytomegalovirus (CMV) promoter is available from Promega Corp.

2.3. Transfection Reagents

1. DEAE-dextran is available from Pharmacia Biotech, Piscataway, NJ.
2. Sterile phosphate-buffered saline (PBS) is available from Invitrogen Corp., Carlsbad, CA, and contains 1.04 m*M* KH$_2$PO$_4$, 155.17 m*M* NaCl, and 2.96 m*M* Na$_2$HPO$_4$. Store at room temperature.
3. Sterile STBS; 25 m*M* Tris-HCl, pH 7.4, 5 m*M* KCl, 0.7 m*M* CaCl$_2$, 137 m*M* NaCl, 0.6 m*M* Na$_2$HPO$_4$, 0.5 m*M* MgCl$_2$ is also available from Invitrogen.

2.4. Luciferase Detection

1. Luciferase cell culture lysis buffer; 25 mM Tris-phosphate (pH 7.8), 2 mM dithiothreitol (DTT), 2 mM 1,2-diaminocyclohexane-N,N,N',N'-tetraacetic acid, 10% glycerol, and 1% Triton X-100. Supplied with the Luciferase Assay System Kit (Promega Corp.). Stored at –20°C.
2. Lyophilized lysosyme, supplied with Promega's Luciferase Assay System. Prepare a fresh 5 mg/mL working stock for each use. Add 1 volume of 1 M K_2HPO_4 (pH 7.8), 20 mM ethylenediamine tetraacetic acid (EDTA) to 9 volumes of sterile distilled water. Add lysosyme to a final concentration of 5 mg/mL and vortex until dissolved.
3. Luciferase assay reagent is a component of Promega's Luciferase Assay System. Dispense reconstituted reagent into aliquots to avoid freeze/thaw cycles. Stored at –70°C and equilibrated to room temperature before use.
4. Packard TopCount luminometer (Perkin Elmer Life Sciences, Meriden, CT).

2.5. Compounds

1. SP100030 was obtained from Signal Pharmaceuticals, Inc. (San Diego, CA). The chemical formula is 2-chloro-4-(trifluoromethyl)pyrimidine-5-N-(3',5'-*bis*(trifluoromethyl)phenyl)-carboxamide.
2. PMA and phytohemagglutin (PHA) were obtained from Sigma (St. Louis, MO).

3. Methods
3.1. DEAE-Dextran Transfection

1. Count the cells and resuspend them in fresh medium containing 10% FCS at a density of 1× 10^6 cells/mL. Plate in 96-well round-bottom plates (200 µL per well) 18 h prior to transfection.
2. Resuspend cells in 1 mL of STBS containing 2–10 µg of the appropriate plasmid DNA and 100–500 µg/mL of DEAE-dextran in PBS. The optimal amount of DNA and DEAE-dextran should be determined for each cell line used. Each experiment should utilize appropriate controls, including cells transfected with target construct (e.g., NF-κB LUC), with control construct (e.g., β-actin or Renilla luciferase), and mock-transfected cells (DEAE-dextran but no DNA) (*see* **Notes 1–3**).
3. Incubate for 15 min at 37°C.
4. Wash cells with sterile PBS and resuspend in complete media. Divide each transfection into two equal pools, plate cells in 96-well round bottom plates and cultivate for approx 48 h.

3.2. Compound Preparation and Cell Treatment

1. Add compounds (e.g., SP100030 and analogs), dissolved in 0.2% dimethyl sulfoxide/H_2O, at the appropriate concentrations (3.30, 0.33, and 0.03 mg/µL for initial evaluation of screening libraries) to the microtiter plates containing the cells.

Incubate the plates at 37°C for 30 min prior to stimulation with PMA and PHA.
2. To induce transcriptional activation, 50 ng/mL of PMA and 1 μg/mL of PHA are added to each well, and the cells incubated for an additional 5 h at 37°C.
3. Note that for cells transfected with the AP-1-LUC construct, only 5 ng/mL of PMA should be added with the PHA to induce transcriptional activation. Cells transfected with the β-actin-LUC are not induced with PMA and PHA.

3.3. Detection of Luciferase Activity

1. Centrifuge the plates at 2200 rpm for 1 min at room temperature followed by removal of the media. 60 μL of luciferase cell lysis buffer, equilibrated at room temperature, should be added to each well, and cells lysed for 15 min.
2. For each cell lysate, transfer 40 μL to a black 96-well microtiter plate, and add 50 μL of luciferase substrate buffer. Meausure the luminescence immediately using a Packard TopCount luminometer (Perkin Elmer Life Sciences, Meriden, CT) (*see* **Note 4**).
3. The results are expressed as IC_{50} values, where the IC_{50} value is defined as the concentration of compound required to reduce cytokine levels to 50% of control values.

4. Notes

1. Standard transfection protocols concurrently expose cells to DEAE-dextran and DNA with short (approx 15 min incubation times) as long exposures to DEAE-dextran may be toxic to some cell lines. For maximal DNA uptake the protocol can be modified such that the cells are pretreated with DEAE-dextran, followed by a longer DNA incubation (*6*). The best protocol for a particular cell line should be determined experimentally. The addition of 80 μ*M* chloroquine together with the DNA is an option for both protocols and may dramatically improve transfection efficiency depending on the cell type.
2. For good transfection efficiency it is crucial that the plasmid DNA is of high quality, the A_{260}/A_{280} ratio should be ≥1.8. Transfection efficiency may also be low if cells at high passage number are used. Also, lymphocytes, in particular, will exhibit variability in transfection efficiency if they are left in culture beyond 1–2 wk.
3. The optimal amount of DNA to use for cell transfection will vary with the type of reporter construct and the cell line used. Generally, 2–6 μg of DNA will be sufficient for a 60-mm plate and 4–10 μg for a 100-mm plate. A dose response curve should be established to determine the optimal DNA concentration to use.
4. Luciferase reporter activity is detectable immediately upon translation as the protein does not require posttranslational modification. Additionally, the assay is rapid and sensitive as fluorescence is produced with a high quantum efficiency and there is no background luminescence in the host cells or the assay chemistry. Using current technology such as Promega's Luciferase Assay System it is possible to obtain 100-fold greater sensitivity over the chloramphenicol acetyltransferase (CAT) assay.

References

1. Tijan, R. and Maniatis, T. (1994) Transcriptional activation: a complex puzzle with few easy pieces. *Cell* **77,** 5–8.
2. Manning, A. M. (1996) Transcription factors: a new frontier for drug discovery. *Drug Discovery Today* **1,** 151–160.
3. Palanki, M. S. S., Erdman, P. E., Gayo-Fung, L. J., Shevlin, G. I., Sullivan, R. W., Suto, M. J., et al. (2000) Inhibitors of NF-κB and AP-1 gene expression: SAR studies on the pyrimidine portion of 2-chloro-4-trifluoromethylpyrimidine-5-[N-(3',5'-*bis*(trifluoromethyl)phenyl carboxamide. *J. Med. Chem.* **43(21),** 3995–4004.
4. Palanki, M. S. S., Erdman, P. E., Manning, A. M., Ow, A., Ransone, L. J., Spooner, C. et al. (2000) Novel inhibitors of AP-1 and NF-κB mediated gene expression. Structure-activity relationship studies of ethyl-[(methyl-2,5-dioxo(3-pyrrolinyl))amino]-2-(trifluoromethyl)pyrimidine-5-carboxylate. *Bioorg. Med. Chem. Lett.* **10,** 1645–1648.
5. Gerlag, D. M., Ransone-Fong, L., Palanki, M., Han, Z., Tak, P. P., Manning, A. M., et al. (2000) The effect of a T cell-specific NF-κB inhibitor on cytokine production in vitro and on murine collagen induced arthritis. *J. Immunol.* **165,** 1652–1658.
6. Al-Moslih, M. I. and Dubes, G. R. (1973) The kinetics of DEAE-dextran-induced cell sensitization to transfection. *J. Gen. Virol.* **18,** 189.

4

Adhesion Molecule Expression on Cytokine-Stimulated Human Endothelial Cells

Susan L. Cuvelier and Kamala D. Patel

1. Introduction

Leukocyte adhesion to vascular endothelial cells is central in regulating inflammatory responses. Endothelial cells line the vasculature and cover over 1000 m^2 in the average adult *(1)*. These cells were long thought to be inert, acting only to contain the blood. This view began to change when Waller in 1846, and then Cohnheim in 1867, made observations suggesting that molecular changes in the endothelium could regulate leukocyte adhesion *(2)*.

The development of culturing techniques that maintain endothelial cells in their differentiated state has greatly enhanced our understanding of the role that endothelial cells play in leukocyte recruitment *(3)*. Both in vitro and in vivo data show that activated endothelial cells present a proadhesive surface to unstimulated leukocytes, promoting leukocyte recruitment during an inflammatory response *(4–6)*.

Leukocyte adhesion to activated endothelial cells is a sequential, multistep process consisting of tethering, rolling, firm adhesion, and transmigration *(7)*. Each of these steps requires interactions between leukocytes and distinct adhesion molecules expressed on the endothelial cell surface. The series of protocols described in this paper can be used to measure and characterize adhesion molecule expression on cytokine-activated endothelial cells. Although these protocols were developed for use with Human Umbilical Vein Endothelial Cells (HUVEC), they are generally applicable to endothelial cells from different vascular beds, as well as different species. These protocols can also be used to examine adhesion molecule expression on other types of adherent cells and have been used successfully by our lab to detect ICAM-1 and VCAM-1 on breast carcinoma epithelial cells *(8)*.

From: *Methods in Molecular Biology, vol. 225: Inflammation Protocols*
Edited by: P. G. Winyard and D. A. Willoughby © Humana Press Inc., Totowa, NJ

2. Materials
2.1. Endothelial Cell Stimulation

1. Cultured human endothelial cells.
2. Appropriate serum-free medium. Stored at 4°C. Heated to 37°C before use.
3. Hanks Balanced Salt Solution (HBSS) with calcium chloride, magnesium chloride, and magnesium sulfate; without sodium bicarbonate and phenol red (Gibco BRL, Grand Island, NY), stored at 4°C. Heated to 37°C before use.
4. 25% human serum albumin (HSA) (Bayer Corporation, Elkhart, IN), stored at 4°C.
5. Recombinant human cytokines: IL-1β, TNF, IL-4, and Oncostatin M (R&D Systems, Minneapolis, MN). Stored in aliquots at –20°C and transferred to storage at 4°C as needed.

2.2. RNA Isolation

1. TRIzol Reagent (Gibco BRL), stored at 4°C.
2. Chloroform and isopropanol. Nucleic acid grade, stored at room temperature.
3. 75% ethanol made from three parts 100% ethanol and one part distilled water (Gibco BRL), stored at room temperature.
4. Distilled pathogen-free water (Gibco BRL), stored at room temperature.

2.3. Reverse Transcriptase Polymerase Chain Reaction (RT-PCR)

1. RNA samples, stored at –70°C.
2. Oligo (dT) 12-18 primer (Gibco BRL), stored at –20°C.
3. Ultrapure dNTP set 2'-deoxynucleoside 5'-triphosphate (Amersham Pharmacia Biotech, Little Chalfont, UK), stored at –20°C.
4. 0.1 M dithiothreitol (DTT) (Gibco BRL), stored at –20°C.
5. 5X first strand buffer (Gibco BRL), stored at –20°C.
6. SuperScript II RNase H$^-$ Reverse Transcriptase (Gibco BRL), stored at –20°C.
7. *Taq* PCR Master Mix Kit (Qiagen, Valencia, CA), stored at –20°C.
8. Forward and reverse primers.
9. 2% agarose gel containing 0.5 µg/mL ethidium bromide.
10. 1 Kb Plus DNA Ladder (Gibco BRL).

2.4. Western Blotting

1. 1X phosphate-buffered saline (PBS), pH 7.4 (Gibco BRL), stored at 4°C.
2. Lysis buffer: 1% Triton X-100, 5 mM sodium vanadate, 5 mM sodium ethylenediamine tetraacetic acid (EDTA), 1 mM phenylmethyl sulfonyl fluoride (PMSF), 10 µM pepstatin A, 50 mU/mL aprotinin, 10 µg/mL leupeptin, 1X MES-buffered saline (MBS), pH 7.4. Prepared immediately before use and kept on ice.
3. 5X Laemmli's buffer: 0.28 M Tris-HCl, pH 6.8, 44% glycerol, 0.09 g/mL sodium dodecyl sulfate (SDS), 0.3 mg/mL bromophenol blue, stored at room temperature, heated to 37°C before use. One part 1.0 M DTT is added to 10 parts 5X Laemmli's buffer before use.
4. 7.5% SDS-polyacrylamide gel electrophoresis (PAGE) gel.

5. Prestained Protein Marker, Broad Range (New England Biolabs, Beverly, MA), stored at –20°C, heated to 95–100°C for 3–5 min before use.
6. Immobilon-P Transfer membrane (PVDF) (Millipore Corporation, Bedford, MA).
7. Human adhesion molecule-specific antibodies (see **Note 1**), stored in aliquots at –20°C and transferred to storage at 4°C as needed.
8. Horseradish peroxidase (HRP)-conjugated sheep anti-mouse antibody (Amersham Pharmacia Biotech), stored at 4°C.
9. SuperSignal West Pico Chemiluminescent Substrate (Pierce, Rockford, IL), stored at room temperature or 4°C for up to 1 yr.
10. Hyperfilm (Amersham Pharmacia Biotech).

2.5. Cell Surface ELISA

1. HBSS, HSA, human adhesion molecule-specific antibodies, and HRP-conjugated sheep anti-mouse antibody (as described in **Subheadings 2.1.** and **2.4.**).
2. Mouse IgG isotype-matched control (non-immune control) (R & D Systems, Minneapolis, MN), stored at 4°C.
3. TMB-ELISA (Gibco BRL), stored at 4°C in light-proof container for up to 1 yr, warmed to room temperature before use.
4. 1.0 M phosphoric acid, stored at room temperature.

2.6. Flow Cytometry

1. 1X Trypsin-EDTA in HBSS (Gibco BRL), stored at 4°C, warmed to 37°C before use.
2. 1X PBS (Gibco BRL), stored at 4°C, warmed to 37°C before use.
3. Human adhesion molecule-specific antibodies and mouse IgG isotype-matched control (as described in **Subheadings 2.4.** and **2.5.**).
4. FITC- or PE-conjugated sheep anti-mouse antibody (Amersham Pharmacia Biotech), stored at 4°C.

3. Methods
3.1. Endothelial Cell Stimulation

1. Culture endothelial cells as described for HUVEC *(3,4)*, human pulmonary microvascular endothelial cells (HPMEC) *(9)*, and human dermal microvascular endothelial cells (HDMEC) *(10–12)* (see **Note 2**). Endothelial cells are also available commercially from companies such as Cambrex (East Rutherford, NJ). Grow to tight confluence.
2. Remove the medium and wash cells once with fresh serum-free medium.
3. Stimulate cells in serum-free medium with 0.5% HSA containing cytokine(s) of interest (see **Table 1**) at 37°C and 5% CO_2. If the stimulation time is 4 h or less, cells may be stimulated in HBSS with 0.5% HSA instead of medium.

3.2. RNA Isolation

1. Stimulate 35-mm diameter culture dish of endothelial cells as described. Remove the medium (see **Note 3**).

Table 1
Upregulation of Adhesion Molecule Expression in HUVEC by Various Stimuli

Stimulus	Stimulation Time	Expected Adhesion Molecule Upregulation
IL-1β, TNF	4 h	E-selectin *(13)*, ICAM-1 *(14,15)*, VCAM-1 *(16,17)*
	24 h	E-selectin *(13)*, ICAM-1 *(14)*, VCAM-1 *(16,17)*
IL-4	24 h	P-selectin *(18)*, VCAM-1 *(18,19)*
Oncostatin M	15 min	P-selectin *(20)*
	4 h	E-selectin *(20)*, ICAM-1 *(20)*, VCAM-1 *(20)*
	24 h	P-selectin *(18)*

2. Homogenize the cells in TRIzol reagent (1.0 mL per dish) by pipetting the solution up and down 2–3 times. Transfer the homogenate to a clean 1.7 mL Eppendorf tube. Incubate at room temperature for 5 min (*see* **Note 4**).
3. Add 200 µL of chloroform and mix by shaking vigorously. Incubate at room temperature for 3 min.
4. Centrifuge the samples at 12,000g for 15 min at 4°C. Carefully remove the upper aqueous phase and transfer to a clean 1.7 mL Eppendorf tube.
5. Add 500 µL of isopropanol to each tube and mix by inverting. Incubate at room temperature for 3 min.
6. Pellet the RNA by centrifugation at 12,000g for 15 min at 4°C.
7. Wash the pellet in 1 mL of 75% ethanol and centrifuge at 7500g for 5 min at 4°C. Air-dry the pellet and dissolve in 10 µL of distilled water.
8. Quantitate the RNA by reading the absorbance at 280 nm and store at –70°C.

3.3. RT-PCR

1. Reverse transcription is performed in a volume of 20 µL containing 5 µg total RNA, 1 µL of 500 µg/mL Oligo (dT) 12–18 primer, 1 µL 10 m*M* Ultrapure dNTP set (10 m*M* each of dATP, dGTP, dCTP, and dTTP), 2 µL 0.1 *M* DTT, 4 µL 5X first strand buffer, and 1 µL SuperScript II reverse transcriptase.
2. Incubate the RT mixture at 21°C for 10 min and then at 42°C for 50 min. Stop the reaction by heating the RT mixture to 70°C and holding for 15 min. Place the RT mixture on ice for PCR, or store at –20°C for later use.
3. Prepare the mixture for PCR by adding, in order, 19 µL *Taq* PCR Master Mix Kit distilled water, 2 µL 10 µ*M* forward primer (*see* **Table 2**), 2 µL 10 µ*M* reverse primer, 2 µL cDNA (from RT reaction) and 25 µL 2X *Taq* PCR Master Mix. Perform PCR for 35 cycles as follows: 1 min at 94°C for denaturing, 1 min at 55°C for annealing and 1 min at 72°C for elongation. Finish with one cycle of 5 min at 72°C for elongation. Hold at 4°C.
4. Separate the PCR products on a 2% agarose gel containing 0.5 µg/mL ethidium

Table 2
Primers for RT-PCR Detection of Adhesion Molecule Expression by Endothelial Cells

Adhesion Molecule	Forward Primer	Reverse Primer	Expected Size (basepairs)
E-selectin (21)	5'-AACGAGAAGC CAACGTGTAA-3'	5'-CTTTTGGTAG CTTCCGTCTG-3'	872
P-selectin (21)	5'-TGAAGAAAAA GCACGCATTG-3'	5'-AGCGGCTCAC ACGAAATAG-3'	714
ICAM-1 (8)	5'-GGCAAGAACC TTACCCTACG-3'	5'-GAGACCTCTG GCTTCGTCAG-3'	586
VCAM-1 (8)	5'-AGGGGACCA CATCTACGCT-3'	5'-ACAGAGCTC CCATTCACGA-3'	1043
β-actin (positive control) (8)	5'-CATGGATGAT GATATCGCCG-3'	5'-ACAGCCTGGA TAGCAACGTA-3'	417

bromide and visualize bands using UV light. Run molecular weight marker on gel for determination of band size.

3.4. Western Blotting

1. Stimulate 35-mm-diameter culture dish of endothelial cells as described. Place dish on ice. Remove the medium and add 1 mL 1X PBS to dish.
2. Scrape dish with cell scraper and transfer cells to 1.7-mL Eppendorf tube. Rinse dish with 500 µL 1X PBS and add wash to Eppendorf tube.
3. Pellet cells by centrifugation for 5 min at 300g at 4°C. Remove supernatant.
4. Resuspend pellet in 100 µL cold lysis buffer. Lyse cells on ice for a minimum of 30 min.
5. Centrifuge lysate for 10 min at 20,000g at 4°C. Transfer supernatant to clean tube.
6. Add 25 µL of 5X Laemmli's buffer with 0.1 M DTT to supernatant (*see* **Note 5**). Heat to 95–100°C and hold for 5 min.
7. Separate the proteins on a 7.5% SDS-PAGE gel. Run molecular weight markers on gel for determination of band size.
8. Transfer proteins to PVDF membrane.
9. Block membrane, and probe with primary antibody followed by HRP-conjugated secondary antibody according to the instructions of the antibody manufacturer. Incubate membrane in SuperSignal for 5 min and visualize bands using photographic film (*see* **Fig. 1**).

3.5. Cell Surface ELISA

1. Stimulate 24-well culture plate with 16-mm diameter wells of endothelial cells as described. Place dish on ice. Remove the medium and add 1 mL HBSS to dish. Allow cells to cool on ice for 5 min.

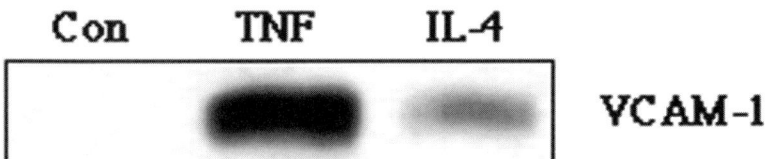

Fig. 1. Detection of VCAM-1 protein by Western Blotting. HUVEC were stimulated for 24 h at 37°C and 5% CO_2 in M199/A alone (Con) or M199/A with 20 ng/mL of TNF (TNF) or IL-4 (IL-4). Cells were lysed in a Triton X-100-containing buffer and separated on a 7.5% SDS-PAGE gel. Proteins were transferred to PVDF and the membrane was probed with an anti-VCAM-1 antibody. The figure shown is representative of at least three experiments.

2. Remove supernatant and add 250 μL of primary antibody (2 μg/mL) in HBSS with 1% HSA (see **Notes 6** and **7**). Incubate on ice for 1 h.
3. Wash wells three times with 500 μL of 4°C HBSS (see **Note 8**).
4. Add 250 μL of appropriate HRP-conjugated secondary antibody (1:1000 dilution) in HBSS with 1% HSA (see **Note 9**). Incubate on ice for 1 h.
5. Wash wells three times with 500 μL of 4°C HBSS.
6. Add 200 μL of TMB-ELISA. Incubate at room temperature until blue color has developed (see **Note 10**). Add 200 μL of 1 M phosphoric acid to wells to stop color development.
7. Read absorbance of duplicate points at 450 nm (see **Fig. 2**).

3.6. Flow Cytometry

1. Stimulate T_{75} flask of endothelial cells as described. Remove the medium and add 5 mL of trypsin-EDTA (see **Note 11**). Incubate at room temperature for approx 1 min. Harvest cells by pipetting the suspension up and down 2–3 times with an automatic pipettor. Transfer suspension to a 50-mL Falcon tube containing 5 mL of medium.
2. Rinse flask two times with 1X PBS. Transfer rinses to Falcon tube.
3. Pellet cells by centrifugation for 5 min at 300g. Wash cells by resuspending pellet in 20 mL 1X PBS and centrifuging for 5 min at 300g.
4. Discard supernatant and resuspend pellet in 600 μL 1X PBS. Divide into six equal aliquots. Each aliquot can be stained with a different antibody (see **Note 12**).
5. Add 1 μg of primary antibody to each tube. Incubate at room temperature for 30 min.
6. Pellet cells by centrifugation for 5 min at 300g. Wash cells by resuspending pellet in 3 mL 1X PBS and centrifuging for 5 min at 300g.
7. Aspirate off the supernatant. Resuspend cells in 90 μL of 1X PBS and add 10 μL of FITC- or PE-conjugated secondary antibody. Incubate at room temperature, shielded from light, for 30 min.

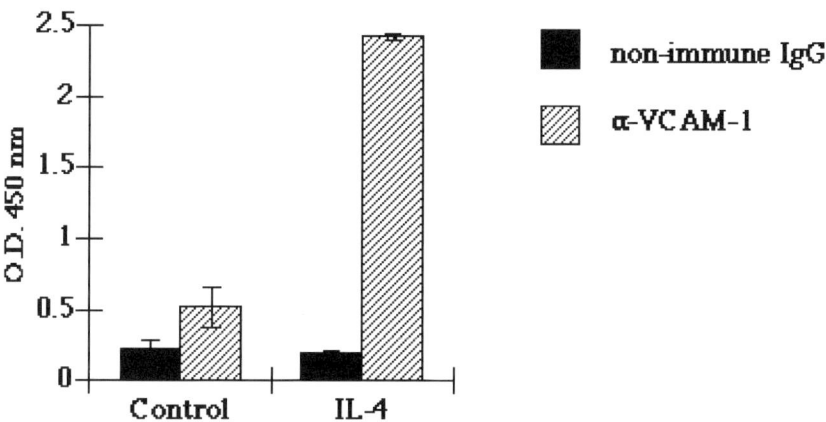

Fig. 2. Detection of surface-associated VCAM-1 protein by ELISA. HUVEC were stimulated for 24 h at 37°C and 5% CO_2 in M199/A alone (Control) or M199/A with 20 ng/mL of IL-4 (IL-4). Cells were labeled with nonimmune mouse IgG_1 or an α-VCAM-1 antibody. After 1 h at 4°C, the monolayers were washed and HRP-conjugated sheep α-mouse secondary antibody was added. After 1 h at 4°C, the monolayers were washed and TMB-ELISA substrate was added. The reaction was stopped after 3 min by the addition of 1.0 M phosphoric acid. Antibody binding was determined by measuring absorbance at 450 nm. Data shown are mean ± deviation and are from a representative experiment.

8. Wash cells by resuspending pellet in 3 mL 1X PBS and centrifuging for 5 min at 300g.
9. Resuspend cells by adding 0.2–0.3 mL of 1X PBS and vortexing gently. Measure FITC- or PE-labeled cells using flow cytometry.

4. Notes

1. We frequently obtain adhesion molecule-specific antibodies directly from principle investigators. However, antibodies against most adhesion molecules are commercially available from companies such as R & D Systems (Minneapolis, MN), Coulter-Immunotech (Miami, FL), and Cedarlane Laboratories (Hornby, ON).
2. Many protocols for culturing endothelial cells recommend using fetal bovine serum (FBS) in the culture medium. Our laboratory, however, has found that endothelial cells grow better in medium containing human serum than in medium containing fetal bovine serum. Human serum can be isolated from normal donors and pooled as described *(4)*.
3. RNA is extremely sensitive to digestion by RNases, which are present on skin and most workspaces. To prevent loss of RNA samples due to RNase digestion, use extreme care when working with RNA. Wear gloves, use only RNase- and DNase-free Eppendorf tubes and pipet tips and keep the work area clean.

4. During the RNA isolation, there are a number of steps at which the procedure can be stopped and samples can be stored. Samples in TRIzol may be stored at –70°C for up to 1 wk and defrosted prior to continuing. Samples in 75% ethanol may be stored at –70°C for up to 1 wk and used immediately upon removal from the freezer.
5. Cell lysates may be frozen after the addition of 5X Laemmli's buffer and separated by SDS-PAGE at a later date.
6. To measure background binding, label a well of cells with an isotype-matched, non-immune primary antibody as a negative control.
7. P-selectin levels on endothelial cells are generally very low, making detection difficult. Multiple primary antibodies that recognize different epitopes on P-selectin can be used in the cell surface enzyme-linked immunoabsorbent assay (ELISA) to increase the sensitivity of detection.
8. Endothelial cell monolayers tend to be very delicate. Add HBSS washes slowly to the centre of the wells using an automatic pipettor to prevent lifting of the cells. Examine the cells using a microscope following the surface ELISA procedure to ensure that cells have not been lost.
9. The amount of secondary antibody used may need to be titrated to achieve an optimal signal to background ratio.
10. For comparison, all wells in a single experiment should be incubated in TMB-ELISA for the same amount of time. Color development should be allowed to occur until the absorbance of all samples falls within the linear range of the spectrophotometer used to measure absorbance. Data from samples whose absorbance falls outside of the linear range of the spectrophotometer should not be used.
11. Surface expression of P-selectin is often difficult to detect and the trypsin-EDTA digestion required to detach endothelial cells from culture dishes may cleave adhesion molecules making detection more difficult. Surface ELISA is generally a preferable method to flow cytometry, especially for detecting P-selectin.
12. To measure background binding, label a tube of cells with an isotype-matched, non-immune primary antibody as a negative control.

References

1. Silverstein, E. A. (1999) The vascular endothelium, in: *Inflammation: Basic Principles and Clinical Correlates.* (Gallin, J. I., Snyderman, R., Fearon, D. T., Haynes, B. F., and Nathan, C., eds.), Lippincott Williams and Wilkins, Philadelphia, PA, pp. 207–226.
2. Cohnheim, J. (1889) *Lectures on General Pathology. A Handbook for Practitioners and Students.* The New Syndenham Society, London, UK.
3. Jaffe, E. A., Nachman, R. L., Becker, C. G., and Minick, C. R. (1973) Culture of human endothelial cells derived from umbilical veins: Identification by morphologic and immunologic criteria. *J. Clin. Invest.* **52,** 2745–2756.
4. Zimmerman, G. A., McIntyre, T. M., and Prescott, S. M. (1985) Thrombin stimulates the adherence of neutrophils to human endothelial cells in vitro. *J. Clin. Invest.* **76,** 2235–2246.

5. McIntyre, T. M., Zimmerman, G. A., and Prescott, S. M. (1986) Leukotrienes C4 and D4 stimulate human endothelial cells to synthesize platelet-activating factor and bind neutrophils. *Proc. Natl. Acad. Sci. USA* **83**, 2204–2208.
6. Bevilacqua, M. P., Pober, J. S., Mendrick, D. L., Cotran, R. S., and Gimbrone, M. A. Jr. (1987) Identification of an inducible endothelial-leukocyte adhesion molecule. *Proc. Natl. Acad. Sci. USA* **84**, 9238–9242.
7. Springer, T. A. (1994) Traffic signals for lymphocyte recirculation and leukocyte emigration: The multistep paradigm. *Cell* **76**, 301–314.
8. Ali, S., Kaur, J., and Patel, K. D. (2000) Intercellular cell adhesion molecule-1, vascular cell adhesion molecule-1, and regulated on activation normal T cell expressed and secreted are expressed by human breast carcinoma cells and support eosinophil adhesion and activation. Am. J. Pathol. 157, 313–321.
9. Hewett, P. W. and Murray, J. C. (1993) Human lung microvessel endothelial cells: Isolation, culture and characterization. *Microvasc. Res.* **46**, 89–102.
10. Marks, R. M., Czerniecki, M., and Penny, R. (1985) Human dermal microvascular endothelial cells: An improved method for tissue culture and a description of some singular properties in culture. *In Vitro Cell. Dev. Biol.* **21**, 627–635.
11. Gupta, K., Ramakrishnan, S., Browne, P. V., Solovey, A., and Hebbel, R. P. (1997) A novel technique for culture of human dermal microvascular endothelial cells under either serum-free or serum-supplemented conditions: Isolation by panning and stimulation with vascular endothelial growth factor. *Exp. Cell Res.* **230**, 244–251.
12. Richard, L., Velasco, P., and Detmar, M. (1998) A simple immunomagnetic protocol for the selective isolation and long-term culture of human dermal microvascular endothelial cells. *Exp. Cell Res.* **240**, 1–6.
13. Bevilacqua, M. P., Stengelin, S., Gimbrone, M. A., Jr., and Seed, B. (1989) Endothelial leukocyte adhesion molecule 1: An inducible receptor for neutrophils related to complement regulatory proteins and lectins. *Science* **243**, 1160–1165.
14. Pober, J. S., Gimbrone, M. A., Jr., Lapierre, L. A., Mendrick, D. L., Fiers, W., Rothlein, R., et al. (1986) Overlapping patterns of activation of human endothelial cells by interleukin 1, tumor necrosis factor, and immune interferon. *J. Immunol.* **137**, 1893–1896.
15. Buzby, J. S., Knoppel, E. M., and Cairo, M. S. (1994) Coordinate regulation of steel factor, its receptor (kit), and cytoadhesion molecule (ICAM-1 and ELAM-1) mRNA expression in human vascular endothelial cells of differing origins. *Exp. Hematol.* **22**, 122–129.
16. Osborn, L., Hession, C., Tizard, R., Vassallo, C., Luhowskyj, S., Chi-Rosso, G., et al. (1989) Direct expression cloning of vascular cell adhesion molecule 1, a cytokine-induced endothelial protein that binds to lymphocytes. *Cell* **59**, 1203–1211.
17. Carlos, T. M., Schwartz, B. R., Kovach, N. L., Yee, E., Rosso, M., Osborn, L., et al. (1990) Vascular cell adhesion molecule-1 mediates lymphocyte adherence to cytokine-activated cultured human endothelial cells. *Blood* **76**, 965–970.
18. Yao, L., Pan, J., Setiadi, H., Patel, K. D., and McEver, R. P. (1996) Interleukin 4 or oncostatin M induces a prolonged increase in P-selectin mRNA and protein in human endothelial cells. *J. Exp. Med.* **184**, 81–92.

19. Schleimer, R. P., Sterbinsky, S. A., Kaiser, J., Bickel, C. A., Klunk, D. A., Tomioka, K., et al. (1992) IL-4 induces adherence of human eosinophils and basophils but not neutrophils to endothelium: Association with expression of VCAM-1. *J. Immunol.* **148,** 1086–1092.
20. Modur, V., Feldhaus, M. J., Weyrich, A. S., Jicha, D. L., Prescott, S. M., Zimmerman, G. A., et al. (1997) Oncostatin M is a proinflammatory mediator: In vivo effects correlate with endothelial cell expression of inflammatory cytokines and adhesion molecules. *J. Clin. Invest.* **100,** 158–168.
21. Ali, S. and Patel, K. D. Unpublished observations.

5

Phagocytosis by Inflammatory Phagocytes

Experimental Strategies for Stimulation and Quantification

M. Rachel Morris, Sharon Dewitt, Iraj Laffafian, and Maurice B. Hallett

1. Introduction

Phagocytosis is perhaps the key goal to which the activity of myeloid cells such as neutrophils and macrophages is directed. In vivo, neutrophils triggered to leave the blood stream, migrate through the extracellular matrix (ECM) and are guided to sources of microbes in order to kill them after phagocytosis. Methods for quantifying this event in vitro are therefore useful in the experimental assessment of agents and conditions that may modify the phagocytic ability of the phagocyte.

Although a number of cell types can undertake phagocytosis, the neutrophil, the first line of antimicrobial defence, is probably the most efficient cell-type at phagocytosis (*1*). It is important to distinguish the three mechanisms by which neutrophils undertake phagocytosis. One route for phagocytosis does not require opsonization, and the other two do. A number of particles of various surface chemistries are readily phagocytosed by neutrophils without opsonization. However, i) the rate at which particles are taken up by this route is submaximal and can be potentiated by opsonization, and ii) the relevance of the uptake of nonopsonized particles to the situation in vivo is unclear. Within the body, particles rarely exist for long without becoming opsonized (i.e., coated) with either complement component C3bi, antibody or possibly both. Many microbial surfaces activate the complement system (*see* **Chapter 8**), which results in the adsorption of the C3bi fragment of the third complement component (C3) to the activating surface to produce C3bi opsonized particle. Later in the inflammatory response, when antibodies are produced, these bind

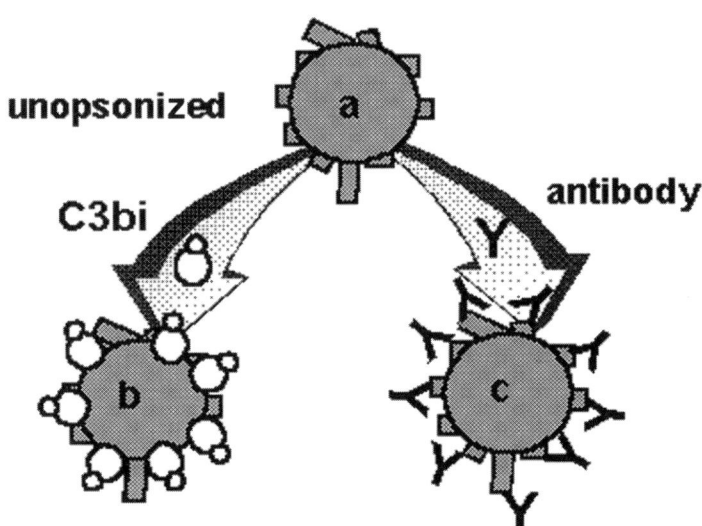

Fig. 1. The biological particle (**a**) presents a surface composed on various proteins, which after opsonization by C3bi (**b**) or antibody (**c**) presents either C3bi or the F_c portion of antibody.

to antigens on the surface of the microbe through the F_{ab} portion of the antibody, leaving the F_c regions free. Adhesion of antibodies to microbial surfaces, soluble antigens or each other (to form immune complexes) can also cause activation of complement and the deposition of C3bi on the surface or complex. Thus, by either opsonising the surface of the microbe or particle with C3bi or antibody, the surface is transformed from presenting as one of a large number of possible varieties into just two possible presentations, i.e., either C3bi or F_c portion of antibody (*see* **Fig. 1**).

Neutrophils have receptors for C3bi, called CR3 (complement receptor 3), β2 integrin, and CD11b/CD18 (*2*), and also have a variety of receptors for the F_c portion of (IgG) antibody, F_c receptors labelled CD16, CD32, and CD64 (reviewed in detail in **ref. 3**). These two receptor types bind their counter-ligand either C3bi or antibody and signal the neutrophil to undergo a program of activity, which leads to a more rapid internalization of the particle than would occur otherwise.

In this chapter, the use of test particles for quantifying phagocytosis in vitro is presented, along with methods for their in vitro opsonization and for their fluorescent labeling to permit their tracking microscopically or by flow cytometry. Methods are also given for quantifying the number of particles within neutrophils and for presenting the resultant data. Finally, a method for presenting particles for phagocytosis is given that is applicable to individual

Table 1
Experimentally Useful Phagocystic Stimuli

Particle	Size	Uniformity	Labels	Detection
1. Zymosan	2–3 µm	+	FITC/RITC, and so on	Fluorescent and brightfield microscopy; Flow cytometry
2. Oil droplets	various	–	Oil Red O	Microscopy or flotation
	0.5–5 µm	+++	FITC/RITC, and so on	Fluorescent microscopy; Flow cytometry
3. Latex beads	various	+	FITC/RITC/ acridine orange, and so on	Fluorescent microscopy; Flow cytometry
4. Bacteria				

neutrophils and can be coupled to fluorescent measurement from the same cell to correlate phagocytosis with cytosolic free Ca^{2+} measurement (*see* **Chapter 6**) and oxidase activity (*see* **Chapter 7**).

2. Materials

1. Krebs buffer medium: 120 mM NaCl, 4.8 mM KCl, 1.2 mM KH_2PO_4, 1.2 mM $MgSO_4$, 1.3 mM $CaCl_2$, 25 mM HEPES, and 0.1% bovine serum albumin (BSA), adjusted to pH 7.4 with NaOH (*see* **Note 1**)
2. Fluorescent latex particles, labelled zymosan, *Escherichia coli* and *Staphylococcus aureus* particles can be purchased from Molecular Probes and elsewhere.
3. Fluorescein-isothiocyanate and rhodamine-isothiocyanate are available commercially from Sigma-Aldrich and elsewhere.
4. Opsonization kits, including polyclonal antidodies to zymosan, *E. coli* or *S. aureus* are also comercially available (as "opsonizing reagent").

3. Methods
3.1. Phagocytosable Particles

A number of experimental test particles have been used. Perhaps the most widely used experimental targets for phagocytosis are zymosan (yeast), oil droplets and commercially available latex "beads." The sizes (*see* **Note 2**) of these particles is given in **Table 1** together with reference to their use.

3.2. Opsonization

Antibody opsonization is achieved by incubation with antibody to the particles or the use of an opsonization kit . Opsonization kits, including polyclonal antidodies to zymosan, *E. coli* or *S. aureus* are also comercially available (as "opsonizing reagent"). Zymosan particles can also be readily opsonized with human C3bi. The procedure has two parts: i) producing human serum with complement, and ii) the opsonization process.

3.2.1. Production of Human Serum

1. Take 10–20mL of blood (human) into a glass container (universal tube) **without** heparin or other anticoagulant.
2. Leave for several hours (preferably overnight) at 4°C to clot and for the clot to contract. It is often useful to release the clot from the sides of the glass tube as this allows clot contraction to occur. Centrifuge the tube to sediment free red blood cells.
3. Remove the serum with a plastic pipete trying to avoid collecting free red blood cells. Do not attempt to recover more serum than about half the original blood volume.
4. Centrifuge the serum to sediment any contaminating red blood cells. The serum should be clear and "straw" colored. If the serum remains red after centrifugation, it should be discarded as this indicates that haemolysis has occurred (possibly as a result of complement activation).
5. The serum can be aliquotted and stored at –20°C until required.

3.2.2. C3bi Opsonization of Particles

1. Zymosan (10 mg) is suspended in Krebs medium (0.5 mL).
2. This is added to 0.5 mL of fresh or thawed stored human serum.
3. The suspension is incubated at 37°C for 30 min (keeping the zymosan in suspension if possible).
4. The zymosan is washed in PBS by centrifugation (300g, 2 min) and resuspension (*see* **Note 3**)
5. The suspension can be stored at 4°C for short periods. However, sterile conditions or storage at –20°C is required for longer periods.

3.2.3. Characterization of Opsonized Particles

It is important to confirm that opsonisation has been correctly performed by i) comparison with nonopsonized particles of their uptake by neutrophils, and ii) showing that blockade of CR3 (β2-integrin) by pretreatment of the neutrophils with antibody to CD18 or CD11b reduces the phagocytic uptake to the nonopsonized level.

3.3. Fluorescent Labeling

There are a number ways by which a fluor can be covalently coupled to a protein. Although kits are available for some linkages, one of the simplest and most effective is to employ the reaction between the protein and isothiocyanate. The fluorescein and rhodamine isothiocyanate-conjugates are commercially available from a number of sources (FITC and RITC). Also, fluorescently labeled antibody preparations are commercially available. In order to label zymosan particles with the probe, there are essentially two steps: i) establishing the reaction, which occurs at high pH, and ii) removal of the reactant, high pH, and separation of the labeled zymosan from the free fluor.

1. High pH bicarbonate reaction buffer (0.25 M) is made from Na_2CO_3 (1 M) and $NaHCO_3$ (1 M) stocks mixed in a ratio of 1:9 and diluted in water 1:4, pH adjusted to pH 9.0.
2. Zymosan (10 mg) is suspended in 900 µL of reaction buffer.
3. 100 µL of FITC (5 mg/mL **dissolved in the NaHCO3 buffer**) is added to the reaction buffer containing zymosan.
4. The reactants are incubated at 4°C overnight (being kept suspended if possible).
5. The zymosan is removed from the reaction mixture by centrifugation at 300g for 5 min (*see* **Note 2**).
6. The zymosan is resuspended in PBS and washed again by centrifugation.
7. **Steps 5** and **6** are repeated until the washing medium is free of fluorescent material (at least three times) and when viewed microscopically, the zymosan particles are observable against a black background which is no brighter than a control field with no fluor present.
8. The preparation can be stored at 4°C or opsonized. (*see* **Note 3**)

3.4. Presentation of Stimuli

The particulate stimuli can be presented to neutrophils in three ways: i) both cells and particles in suspension (suspension), ii) neutrophils adherent with particles in suspension "raining" down on the cells (sedimentation), and ii) neutrophils adherent and particles presented by micromanipulation. Each method of presentation is useful for different purposes.

3.4.1. Suspension Presentation

In this approach, a suspension of particles is added to a suspension of neutrophils. The method relies on the random contact between particles and cells in the suspension medium. Obviously, the number of random collisions between the two will depend upon the concentration of each. A common strategy is to ensure that the number of particles is in large excess to the number of cells. Neutrophils can internalise more than nine zymosan particles/cell, so it is clear that if the ratio of particles to cells is less than this, phagocytosis will be limited not by the capability of the cells, but by the availability of the particles. A typical protocol is given.

1. Follow protocol for opsonisation, or retrieve from storage.
2. Resuspend neutrophils in Krebs medium (*see* **Table 1**) to give 10^6 cells/mL, warm to 37°C

3. Add 10 µL of stock zymosan to give final conc of 1 mg/mL
4. Incubate at 37°C, keeping cells suspended.
5. Sample at 10, 15, 30, and 60 min for microscopic counting or flow cytometry.

3.4.2. Sedimentation Presentation

An important feature of the suspension method of presentation is that all surfaces of the neutrophil have an equal chance of encountering a particle (by random collision) and so cells can accumulate large numbers of particles. However, it is an unusual situation for neutrophils to encounter microbes in this way. Instead, neutrophils encounter microbes in the extravascular space after they have changed their morphology from spherical (as in the blood stream or in the suspension) to flattened and chemotactic. For this reason, another approach which may be used is to adhere the neutrophils to a surface and allow particles to contact them by sedimenting onto their exposed surface. With this approach, although the number of particles internalized may be less, the physiological process may be closer to that which occurs in vivo. There the surface to which the neutrophils are allowed to adhere is, however, a consideration. If one chooses an integrin engaging surface such as may be presented by a protein coating, this may reduce the availability of these receptors for phagocytosis. However, if one chooses a nonphysiological (and convenient) surface such as glass, the CR3 receptors may remain available but as the neutrophils have a tendency to become increasingly flattened onto the glass, this causes a limitation to the available plasma membrane to form phagosomes (i.e., the cells become so stretched that there is no possibility of the further "stretching" required for phagocytosis). A typical methodology is given in which glass is used as the substrate, but the time for adhesion is short to minimise this effect.

1. An area is marked on a clean (ethanol washed) glass slide.
2. Neutrophils (10^6/mL) are added to the marked area and allowed to sediment for 10 min at 37°C.
3. Nonadhered neutrophils are removed by washing the slide with Krebs medium.
4. Zymosan is diluted in Krebs medium (10 mg/mL) and 100 µL added to the marked area of the side.
5. This is transferred to a humid incubator chamber and maintained at 37°C for the required time (e.g., 10, 30, 60 min).
6. The excess, nonphagocytosed material is removed by washing and phagocytosis quantified by counting.

3.4.3. Micromanipulation

Another advantage of the sedimentation approach is that an individual living neutrophil can be observed before during and after phagocytosis. This would enable the time between contact, pseudopod formation, and so on to be determined. Also, if the neutrophil were loaded with an cytosolic free Ca^{2+} indicator (*see* **Chapter 6**), the Ca^{2+} signaling events accompanying phagocytosis would also be observable *(4)*. However, the sedimentation method provides a random distribution of particles as they sediment and it cannot be predicted when a particular cell will make contact with a particle. This can be frustrating as particles may sediment onto the focal plane but fail to contact the cell under observation. This problem is also compounded by local heating effects caused by the ullumination source. This can occur even with heated stages and cause conventional currents away from the source of observation which carry particles away from the cell under observation.

These problem are, however, overcome by a micromanipulation technique whereby the particle is fed to the neutrophil under observation (**Fig. 3**). Thus, the timing of contact can be precisely controlled. Also the position on the cell at which contact is made can be controlled and the same cell can be "fed" multiple times. The method relies on a micropipet attached to a micromaniupulator, through which a slight negative pressure is applied. A zymosan particle which has sedimented near the cell under observation is "picked up" by positioning the tip of the micropipete near by. This is then carried to the cell and presented. Once adherence between the particle and cell has occurred, the particle can be released and phagocytosis observed. The tip of the micropipet should be smaller than the particle, ideally 1–2 μm so that pressure control can be effective. The positioning of the micropipet is best achieved using a motorized microprocessor controlled manipulator. These are commercially available from Eppendorf, WPI, and others. It is not necessary to have the complicated electronic control required for microinjection (i.e., z stabbing) and less expensive micromanipulators are adequate for the task.

3.5. Microscopic and Flow Cytometric Detection of Phagocytosis

There are essentially two approaches for detecting phagocytosis: i) microscopic, in which individual neutrophils are observed and the number of particles phagocytosed per cell counted, and ii) the use of flow cytometry to quantify the fluorescence associated with each cell as it passes through the laser beam. Both approaches have advantages and disadvantages. The microscopic approach is not automated and requires observation of a large number of cells. This is obviously time consuming, but has the advantage i) that adherence of particles to cells is not taken as phagocytosis, and ii) that gross effects on cell morphology or the health of cells (if subjected to a pharmacological agent, for example) are apparent during the counting. In contrast, flow cytometry has the advantage that it is automated and quick, but the disadvantage that it is more difficult to distinguish adherence from internalisation, or have feedback on the health of the cells.

3.5.1. Fixing and Staining

Perhaps the simplest approach is to fix and stain the cells after the period of phagocytosis (**Fig. 2**). Once fixed, batches of slides can be stained together and counting performed independently of knowledge of the conditions (i.e., the counter can be blinded for the experiment). This approach is applicable to both adherent cells and to cell in suspension.

1. For adherent cell, proceed to **step 2**. For cells in suspension, a sample (50 µL) is centrifuged onto a glass slide (cytospin).
2. The cells are fixed by immersion of the slides in methanol 15 min at room temperature.
3. The slides are placed in May-Grunwald stain (Fisher Scientific) diluted 1:1 with PBS pH 6.8, 15 min at room temperature.
4. The slides are placed in Giemsa stain (Raymond A Lamb) diluted 1:10 in PBS pH 6.8, 15 min at room temperature.
5. Excess stain is removed by brief washing in PBS pH 6.8.
6. Allowed to air-dry before mounting fluid (Styrolite, BDH) is added.
7. Neutrophils and their internalized zymosan particles are counting microscopically (X40–100) *see* **Fig. 2**.

3.5.2. Fluorescence Microscopy

With stained slides, the zymosan particles are obvious as they are of a uniform size with a characteristic morphology. However, with smaller particles or less clearly defined particles (such as latex beads), the use of a fluorescent marker is useful to unambiguously identify an intracellular structure as resulting from the internalized particle rather than from some other source. By changing between bright field viewing (phase contrast, DIC, and so on) and fluorescence, the number of particles per cell can be quantified. Alternatively, it is often possible to balance the brightness of the two images to be observed together (especially if video or digital cameras are used). This permits easier counting as only one image is presented to the counter. Another approach is to stain the neutrophil nuclei with acridine orange so that the position of the cells (as marked by nucleus) and the number of associated fluorescent particles can again be counted from a single image.

3.5.3. Flow Cytometry

Flow cytometry provides a quick and effective way of quantifying fluorescence per cell. With fluorescent particles as the phagocytic stimulus, these can be accurately quantified. Although it is possible with precisely sized and uniformly labeled particles to obtain separate peaks corresponding to 1, 2, 3, and so on particles/cell *(5)*, often the spread of signal as a result of variation in particle size and fluorescent labeling prevents and only the average fluorescence per cell can be measured.

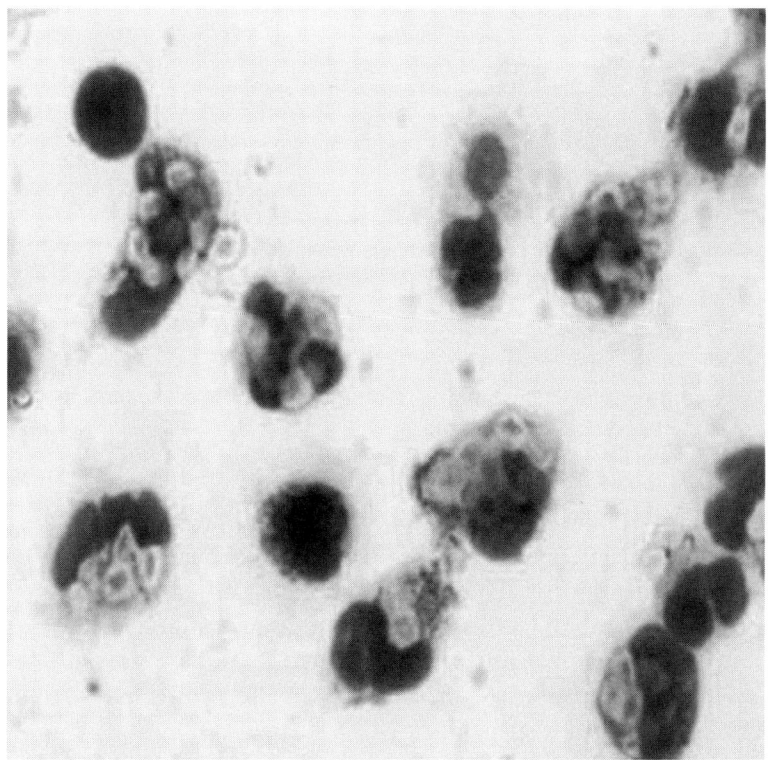

Fig. 2. A fixed and stained image of neutrophils with internalized zymosan particles. The particles are readily recognized within the cells and can be counted individually.

3.5.4. Adherence vs Internalization

One important consideration, is to ensure that association of the particle (or the particle marker) is the result of phagocytosis and not adherence. This is especially important if a pharmacological agent is added that prevents phagocytosis, but not adherence or one that promotes adhesion, but not phagocytosis. It is thus recommended that when an apparent difference in phagocytosis is identified that internalization and adhesion is clearly distinguished. It is unlikely to be achieved using flow cytometry, but there are a few approaches for use microscopically. One approach is to use trypan blue as a "quencher" of the fluorescein signal from adherent but noninternalized particles. As trypan blue cannot penetrate the plasma membrane of healthy cells, as fluorescent particles observed associated with the cell must be internalized (6). This discrimination in intensity between quenched external particles and non- quenched internalized particles should ideally be all-or-none, but in practice (depending on the number of fluors/particle, intensity of illumination, and so on in our hands) this is rarely the

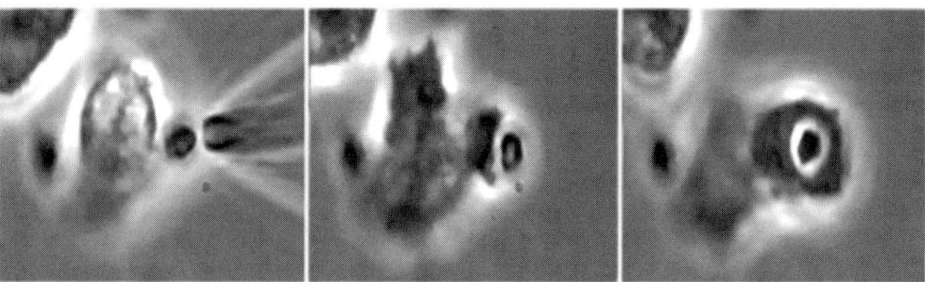

Fig. 3. Micromanipulation of zymosan as a technique for the study of phagocytosis. The sequence shows the presentation of a C3bi opsonised zymosan particle to a human neutrophil using a micropipet. The images are about 45 s apart. The process of phagocytosis is observable in real time.

case. An alternative method is to employ confocal imaging. Here, the position of the fluorescent particle within the cell (rather than on the cell) can be clearly made by optical sectioning. By combining other fluorescent markers such as acridine orange for the nucleus or plasma membrane markers, the position of the particle can be unambiguously established. Obviously, it would be impractical to use this as "work-horse" method, but can be confirmatory when differences in phagocytosis are suspected.

3.6. Parameters to Consider

With flow cytometry, several thousand cells can be interrogated easily. However, when microscopic counting, this number may be smaller. However, it is possible to count a minimum of 100 cells per slide and with at least three slides for a condition (or time-point) 300–500 cells can be counted. This is sufficient to give some statistical confidence.

There are several parameters which emerge when performing such a count, each of which carries different information. The first is the percentage of cells that have undergone phagocytosis (irrespective of the number of particles they then take up), given as $(N_p/N_t) \times 100\%$, where N_p is the number of cells with phagocytic particles within and N_t is the total number of cells observed. Obviously, when all cells within the population that are able to have undergone phagocytosis, this parameter is not a sensitive indicator of differences. Often, there is a fraction of the population that do not undergo phagocytosis (possibly these represent an immature or elderly subpopulation). The next parameter to consider is the mean number of particles/cell. Here, the information about particle number is retained and is given by n/N_t, where n is the total number of particles within N_t cells, or simply by noting separately the number of particles

Phagocytosis by Inflammatory Phagocytes

in each cell and taking the mean. As there may be a fraction of neutrophils which fail to undertake phagocytosis, this mean often underrepresents the mean uptake of those phagocytic-competent cells. In which case, it may be useful to report the mean number of particles/cell in the phagocytic cells only, i.e., n/N_p, or take the population mode rather than the mean. Kinetic analysis of uptake of live bacteria and their killing can also be achieved by determining the rate constants that describe the two steps *(7)*.

4. Notes

1. Unlike conventional Krebs medium, HEPES-buffered Krebs medium has no hydrogen-carbonate (bicarbonate) and the pH is maintained by HEPES. The medium also has no glucose added. As neutrophils are essentially anaerobic (with few, if any mitochondria), glucose is rapidly converted to lactic acid. Consequently, if neutrophils are kept at a high density, in the presence of glucose, there is an accumulating fall in pH (even with pH buffers such as HEPES, once the pH moves outside the effective range, it can fall surprisingly quickly). This is obviously undesirable as the extracellular environment is not held constant and so comparison of the cellular activity at different times is not possible. Also, the pH will eventually fall to a point where the cells lose there responsiveness.
2. An important consideration in choosing which test particle to use is consistency of size. There is evidence to suggest that neutrophils and macrophages are able to phagocytose particles within a certain size range, but that outside this range particles are either too small to present a sufficient phagocytic stimulus or are too large to be engulfed. It is, therefore, important i) that the population of particles to be presented to the phagocytes is reasonably uniform, i.e., does not have a large standard deviation of sizes about the mean, and ii) the mean size (and its standard deviation) is constant from preparation to preparation. One way to ensure this is to avoid comparing phagocytic measurements performed with different batches of phagocytic stimuli, and to only accept data in which all conditions and controls were performed using particles from the same batch of particles. Oil particles are generated by sonication of oil:water emulsions *(8)*.
3. After centrifugation, it is important that zymosan particles are resuspended correctly. A problem which can be encountered is the aggregation of individual zymosan particles into large conglomerates. It is important that these are dispersed as they will not be phagocytozed and, thus, reduce the available number of particles. As the number of conglomerates will be random, different cell samples may be exposed to differing numbers of particles. The problem is avoided by not centrifuging the zymosan suspension for too long or at too high a speed and by using plastic pipettes to thoroughly resuspend. This latter manoeuvre is best achieved by resuspending the zymosan in a small volume of medium and forcing the entire volume into an out of the pipette. Only when this has been repeated five times, or until the suspension looks microscopically homogeneous, is the remaining medium added to give the finally required density of particles.

References

1. Klebanoff, S. J. and Clark, R. A. (1978) *The Neutrophil: Function and Clinical Disorders.* North-Holland, Amsterdam.
2. Stewart, M., Theil, M., and Hogg, N. (1995) Leukocyte integrins. *Curr. Opin. Biol.* **7,** 690–696.
3. Daeron, M. (1997) Fc -receptor biology. *Ann. Rev. Immunol.* **15,** 203–234.
4. Dewitt, S. and Hallett, M. B. (2002) Cytosolic free Ca^{2+} changes and calpain are required for B2-integrin-accelerated phagocytosis by human neutrophils. *J. Cell. Biol.* **159**, 181–189.
5. Fredrickson, A. G., Hatzis, C., and Srienc, F. (1992) A statistical analysis of flow cytometric determinations of phagocytosis rates. *Cytometry* **13,** 423–431.
6. Hed, J. (1986) Methods for distinguishing ingested from adhering particles. *Methods Enzymol.* **132,** 198–203.
7. Hampton, M. B. and Winterbourn, C. C. (1999) Methods for quantifying phagocytosis and bacterial killing by human neutrophils. *J. Immunol. Methods* **232,** 15–22.
8. Stossel, T. P. (1986) Oil-droplet method for measuring phagocytosis. *Methods Enzymol.* **132,** 192–197.

6

Cytosolic Ca²⁺ Measurement and Imaging in Inflammatory Cells

Sharon Dewitt, Iraj Laffafian, M. Rachel Morris, and Maurice B. Hallett

1. Introduction

The ability to measure and manipulate cytosolic free Ca^{2+} concentration is important for understanding many aspects of the physiology of inflammatory cells. The evidence for the role of this ion in triggering and controlling neutrophils, monocytes, lymphocytes, and others cells relevant to inflammation is accumulating. Although each cell type may differ in the detail, there are some general principals for measuring cytosolic free Ca^{2+} that apply to all these cell types. The methods most applicable to inflammatory cells mainly revolve around the use of fluorescent indicators and photoactive reagents. These can be loaded into the cells as lipid-soluble esters or can be microinjected into the cell. In this chapter, we will outline some of the techniques that have been used to monitor, visualize, and manipulate Ca^{2+} in inflammatory cells. For specific details relating to neutrophils, *see* **ref. *1*** and for details of other methods, such as the expression of luminescent and fluorescent indicators of Ca^{2+}, *see* **ref. *2***.

1.1. Principle of Action

The fluorescent Ca^{2+} chelator probes have revolutionized the study of cytosolic free Ca^{2+} in small cells, including in inflammatory cells (*3,4*). The main advance with these indicators was the ester groups both "masked" the Ca^{2+} binding region of the molecule and made them lipid soluble. This means that the ester-derivative can cross the plasma membrane and enter the cytosol. Here, esterases cleave the ester bond to generate the acid form of the probe, which becomes entrapped within the cell as it is hydrophilic and thus unable to easily cross the plasma (or other) membrane. The acid form of the probe is also the

Ca^{2+} sensing form. Two problems are often associated with loading inflammatory cells from its acetoxymethyl ester; i) the accumulation of indicator into organelles, and ii) partial (rather than full) hydrolysis of fura2-AM within the cell, to generate products with increased hydrophilicity, but that are insensitive to Ca^{2+} *(5)*. However, awareness of the potential for such problems is often sufficient to detect and prevent them. It is also important to limit the amount of fura2, which is to be loaded into the cytosol because i) as the indicator is a Ca^{2+} chelator, it will buffer cytosolic free Ca^{2+} changes and "blunt" the response, and ii) this will reduce toxicity of de-esterification of the probe, which can cause a reduction in ATP levels *(6)* and may have other toxic effects on the cell, including stimulation of cell aggregation.

Recently, methods for microinjection of small cells have improved and it is possible to introduce the acid form of the Ca^{2+} probe indicator (e.g., fura2) directly into the cytosol *(1,7)* thereby circumventing the problems of location and toxicity associated with ester-loading. SLAM-injection (simple-lipid-assisted micro-injection) is easy to use on a number of inflammatory cell types, including neutrophils. This approach will not be described here, but it permits microinjection of cells difficult or impossible to microinject by conventional means without causing severe cell damage *(7,8)*.

2. Materials

The properties of fluorescent Ca^{2+} probes suitable for use in inflammatory cells is given in Table 1. These reagents and those for manipulation of cytosolic free Ca^{2+} are available from Molecular Probes, Sigma, Calbiochem, Teflabs, or their agents.

3. Methods

3.1. Choosing Which Fluorescent Ca^{2+} Probe to Use

3.1.1. Ca^{2+} Affinity

There are now many commercially available Ca^{2+} probes in which the "esterase-accumulation" principle is utilized (*see* **Table 1**). How is a probe chosen for use? It is important to remember that as in other cell types, inflammatory cells usually have resting cytosolic free Ca^{2+} concentrations of near 100 nM, and that on stimulation this rises transiently to near 1 µM. As the fluorescent signal depends upon the binding of Ca^{2+} to the probe, the Ca^{2+} dissociation constant, K_d, defines the range over which the probe can be usefully employed. A probe with a kd of 300 nM will be only approx 25% saturated in the resting cell, and thus, 75% of its dynamic range will be available to monitor a rise in cytosolic free Ca^{2+}. It will, however, be difficult to measure cytosolic free Ca^{2+} concentrations above 1–3 mM, as the probe will be more

Table 1
Fluorescent Chelator Probes for Cytosolic Free Ca^{2+} Measurement in Neutrophils

	K_d (Ca^{2+}) (nM)	Excitation Wavelength (nm)	Emission	Mode of Use
Calcium crimson	205	588	611	S
Calcium Green-1	189	506	534	S
Calcium Green-2	574	506	531	S
Calcium Green-5N	3300	506	531	S
Calcium Orange	328	554	575	S
Chlortetracycline*	400,000	380	410	S
FFP-18	400	340 and 380	505	R
Fluo3	864	506	526	S
Fluo3FF	62,000	506	526	S
Fura red	133	420 and 480	640	R
Fura2	224	340 and 380	505	R
FuraFF	38,000	340 and 380	504	R
Indo-1	250	340	410 and 485	R
Mag-fura-2	25,000	340 and 380	504	R
Mag-fura-5	28,000	340 and 380	504	R
Quin2	114	340	490	S
Rhod-2	1000	553	576	S

All these probes are available as cell permeant esters, except chlortetracycline, which is readily membrane permeant. The mode of use is given as single wavelength (S) or the ratio of two wavelengths (R)

than 90% saturated with Ca^{2+}. In contrast, a probe with a K_d of 1 mM would be more useful for higher Ca^{2+} changes. As the probe is also a chelator of Ca^{2+}, the K_d for Ca^{2+} will also determine its Ca^{2+} buffering effect in the cytosol. Fortunately, neutrophils and lymphocytes (and probably other inflammatory cells) have high endogenous Ca^{2+} buffering with estimates ranging from 1:1000–1:3000 (6,9). An intracellular fura2 concentration of 25–50 mM is estimated to increase the Ca^{2+} buffering only by about 10 %. With probes of higher K_d such as fluo3 the effect of artefactual buffer is even less.

3.1.2. Single or Dual Wavelength Ca^{2+} Probes

Fluorescent Ca^{2+} probes can be used that change their signal at two wavelengths, either on excitation or emission (ratiometric dyes), or at only one wavelength (see **Table 1**). The single wavelength, nonratiometric indicators, such as fluo3 and calcium green greatly increase in emission intensity on binding Ca^{2+} and can be excited at 488 nm, a wavelength produced by laser light (as used in confocal microscopy or flow cytometry). Techniques involving confocal microscopes are increasingly more powerful as they can provide precision in the locating of the Ca^{2+} change and also can give information on very fast time scales (1–10 ms). However, as the indicators produce only a single intensity change on binding Ca^{2+}, caution must be exercised in interpreting an increase in intensity as being solely because of an increase in cytosolic free Ca^{2+} concentration. For example, if a brightly loaded organelle moves into the confocal imaging plane, this would give an increased fluorescent signal unrelated to cytosolic free Ca^{2+} concentration. For this reason, it is recommended that Ca^{2+} measurements are initially performed using ratiometric measurement as it is certain that the ratio change is caused by a Ca^{2+} signal. With fura2, the excitation spectrum shifts on binding Ca^{2+}, so that there is significant fluorescence from both the Ca^{2+}-bound and the Ca^{2+}-free forms of the probe. This permits monitoring of both the Ca^{2+}-free and the Ca^{2+}-bound forms of the indicator. Conventionally, two wavelengths are chosen, one on either side of the isoemissive point (usually 340 nm and 380 nm). The signal at 340 nm will increase and the signal at 380 nm decrease as Ca^{2+} increases. This is the "Ca^{2+} signature" for these probes.

3.2. "Ester Loading" Procedure

There are several points at which variation can be made. For example, the steps below marked by an asterisk can be omitted. However, a crucial point of the loading procedure rests on using a cell suspension medium which contains Ca^{2+} (e.g., 1–2 mM). This is important (*see* **Note 1**) because as the Ca^{2+} chelator is generated within the cytosol it will bind Ca^{2+} (the extent depending on its K_d). Without additional extracellular Ca^{2+} to replace this, Ca^{2+} will be displaced from Ca^{2+} stores within the cell (or worse, not replaced at all). Another important point in the method is the 1000-fold dilution of the ester stock solution. This provides a suitable final concentration of the ester, but more importantly a suitable low concentration of its solvent dimethyl sulfoxide (DMSO). DMSO can have toxic effect on cells and it is therefore important that it is kept to a minimum. At 0.1% (i.e., 1/1000), the effects of DMSO are minimal.

1. Dissolve ester in dry DMSO (*see* **Note 1**) to give a stock (1–5 mg/mL). Store at −20°C.
2.* Mix 2.5 mL Pluronic (25%w/v in DMSO) with 5 mL of ester stock. This step may assist transfer into the cells, pluronic being a "dispersing agent," which assists in keeping the ester in solution.
3. Add 1 mL of ester (1–5 mg/mL ± pluronic) to 1 mL of cell suspension (*see* **Note 2**) of 1–50X 10^6 cell/mL in Ca^{2+} containing medium.
4. Incubate cells for 20–60 min (room temperature or 37°C).
5. Resuspend cells in fresh medium.

6.* Store cells on ice to reduce leakage of Ca^{2+} probe.

It is recommended that before accepting that loading has been successful for a given cell type, the following simple checks are made.

1. Check fluorescence at 360 nm excitation (505 nm emission) is significantly higher than in nonloaded cells. Record excitation or emission spectrum (quartz cuvet) of loaded cells to ensure that conversion of ester to its acid is complete. (For fura2, the ester and the acid have clearly different spectra, see e.g., Molecular Probes Handbook.)
2. Treat cells with either digitonin (150 mM) or Ca^{2+} ionophore (nonfluorescent ionomycin or Br A23187). Check the spectral change is consistent with Ca^{2+} saturation for the probe, e.g., for fura2 the excitation spectrum peaks at 340 nm. Add EGTA (20 mM) and check spectral change is consistent with zero saturation for the probe, e.g., for fura2 the excitation peak is shifted to approx 380 nm and the two spectra cross at approx 360 nm.
3. Observe the fluorescence microscopically (e.g., Zeiss filters LP420/G365 or similar) to check loading has no obvious nonuniformity (i.e., in granules or phagosomes).

3.3. Measurement of Cytosolic Free Ca^{2+}

For a single wavelength indicator, the cytosolic free Ca^{2+} concentration can be calculated from:

$$Ca^{2+} = K_d (F - F_{min})/(F_{max} - F)$$

where F is the fluorescent signal through the experiment, and F_{min} and F_{max} are the minimum and maximum obtainable signal from the indicator in the presence and absence of saturating amounts of Ca^{2+}. F_{max} and F_{min} are obtained at the end of the experiment by permeabilizing the cell (with ionophores) in the presence of Ca^{2+} and then chelating the Ca^{2+} with EGTA. The single wavelength approach may be used confocally or flow cytometrically, but is not advised for conventional fluorometry or imaging. For these latter procedures, ratio dyes is preferable. The ratio of the two signals will be independent of the concentration (or amount) of probe and the free Ca^{2+} required to give this signal ratio can be calculated

$$Ca^{2+} = K_d \cdot \beta \cdot (R - R_{min})/(R_{max} - R)$$

where $\beta = S_{f2}/S_{b2}$, where Sxy is the emission signal at wavelength y ($y=1$ for 340 nm and 2 for 380 nm) from the fully Ca^{2+} saturated indicator ($x=b$), totally Ca^{2+} free indicator ($x=f$) or variable Ca^{2+} saturation in the cell during the experiment ($x=v$), and $R = S_{v1}/S_{v2}$, $R_{max} = S_{b1}/S_{b2}$ and $R_{min} = S_{f1}/S_{f2}$.

The characteristic "Ca^{2+} signature" can be confirmed to originate solely from a change in Ca^{2+} by noting that the sum, $ASv_1 + Sv_2$, where $A = (S_{f2} - S_{b2})/(S_{b1} - S_{f1})$

will be constant at all Ca^{2+} concentrations *(6)*. The R_{max} and R_{min} values are essential for the calculation and are usually taken at the end of the experiment by the addition of ionomycin, or digitonin (to allow Ca^{2+} saturation) and then EGTA (to remove Ca^{2+} from the probe) (*see* **Note 2**).

3.4. Measurement Protocols

3.4.1. Fluorometry

1. Add cell suspension to quartz or UV transmissible cuvet. Keep stirred to ensure that cells remain in the illumination beam. Set temperature (37°C for mammalian inflammatory cells).
2. Set fluorometer to illuminate and emission to the appropriate wavelengths. Record single or dual wavelength data as appropriate (*see* **Table 1**).
3. Once data are constant (i.e., after warm-up time) add stimulus while recording (*see* **Fig. 1**).
4. At the end of the experiment, add ionomycin (1–4 mM) or digitonin (150 mM) to saturate the probe.
5. Once saturation has occurred, add EGTA 20 mM (*see* **Fig. 1**).
6. Note parameters listed below and calculate the cytosolic free Ca^{2+} concentration throughout the time-course using the appropriate equation given earlier and in **Fig. 1**.

3.4.2. Microfluorometery

By coupling the wavelength changer to the input port and a photomultiplier tube to the output port of a fluorescent microscope, the procedure given above can be used with individual cells. In order to reduce background signal from areas of the field not occupied by the cells (or by other cells), a pinhole in the focal plane can be useful. This can be fixed so that the cell is moved to the pinhole by the microscope stage or could be moveable. If the photomultiplier tube is replaced by a camera, then a "virtual pinhole" can be set up by binning the data from the region of the image which includes the cell of interest (*see* **Note 4**). This approach has several advantages: i) the cell is visualized and so artifacts caused by cell movement, and so on are immediately apparent, and ii) as the pinholes are electronic, several "pinholes" can be defined that read out the ratio values of more than one individual cell in the field.

It is important (in **step 6** of the earlier protocol,) that digitonin is not used for microfluorometry, as often the Ca^{2+} indicator is lost from the cell at that point (*see* **Note 3**). If this happens, then obviously the indicator is no longer within the defined (pinhole) area and the information is not meaningful. It is therefore recommended that ionomycin is used to provide the maximum and minimum signals under these conditions.

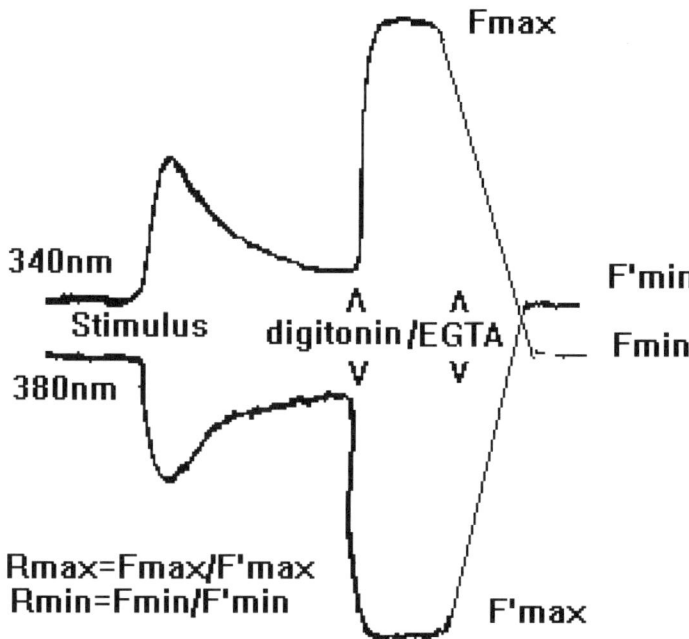

Fig. 1. A typical experiment in which cytosolic free Ca^{2+} concentration is monitored by fura2. The emission at 505 nm is recorded for excitation at 340 nm and 380 nm as indicated. A stimulus is added which produces the "Ca^{2+} signature." The addition of digitonin and then EGTA is for calibration. For a signal wavelength probe, the values of F_{max} and F_{min} are used. For a dual wavelength probes (as here) R_{max} and R_{min} are calculated as shown.

3.4.3. Flow Cytometry

Measurement of cytosolic free Ca^{2+} concentration within individual cells in a cell population is possible using flow cytometry. Time-course of Ca^{2+} changes can be achieved by addition of stimulus to the population as it passes through the machine. Caution must be exercised in the interpretation of these data as, although individual cells are being interrogated, no single cell is followed through the time-course and the same changes are merely population average changes. These often do not reflect changes at the single-cell level. For example, unless stimulus-induced Ca^{2+} spikes are synchronized within the population, these will not be observed by flow cytometry (except perhaps as an increased scatter of data points).

As with other methods, ratioing should ideally be used. Indo-1 (*see* **Table 1**) is thus the probe of choice. With a single laser line for excitation, the ratio of the two emission wavelength signals would be useful. However, the excitation wavelength of 360 nm requires a UV laser, which is not standard. As a compromise, therefore, single wavelengths indicators like fluo3 and calcium green can be used as these are more easily excited (with the 488 nm laser line).

3.5. Imaging Ca^{2+} in Individual Cells

3.5.1. Ratiometric Imaging

As well as the confidence given by the ratiometric "Ca^{2+} signature," it also permits the cytosolic free Ca^{2+} concentration within the cells to be imaged. The fluorescent intensity at any point within the 2-D microscopic image of the cell will be proportional to the amount of probe in that "line of sight." Thus, it may be brighter at the center (where the cell may be thicker) than at the edge (where the cell may be thinner). Without taking a ratio, it would not be possible to determine whether the signal at the cell edge were less because of the cell shape or because of its cytosolic free Ca^{2+} concentration. A similar argument applies to different cells with different fluorescent intensities (*see* also **Note 5**). The changing excitation wavelength is synchronized with the acquisition of images, often by a spinning filter wheel, optical chopper, or rapid-changing monochromator. These are commercially available from many sources including Spex, PTI, and Cairn Instruments. Ca^{2+} imaging is achieved by coupling the wavelength changer to the "fluorescent input" of the microscope and either a digital camera or a video camera to the "output." Digitization of the signal to provide an array of pixels each with a value that corresponds to the intensity of the fluorescence image in that region of the field is then recorded. After background subtraction, the ratio is calculated and a look-up table (LUT) used to provide color on the image corresponding to the cytosolic free Ca^{2+} concentration. With a video camera, the speed of acquisition is probably 25–30 frames/s, so that one ratio image would take about a minimum of 80 ms. Time is also taken to change wavelengths, but this is minimized by using fast filter wheels, optical choppers, or rapid changing monochromators. Often it is necessary to average a number of frames to increase the signal (with decreased time resolution) or bin pixels to increase the signal (with decreased spatial resolution, **Note 4**). The need to do either can be reduced by using intensification. In practice, useful ratio images can be acquired at rates of 1–2/s with existing equipment, but faster capture rates are possible. A problem associated with imaging is photobleaching (*see* **Note 4**) and fuller details of Ca^{2+} imaging and up-to-date technologies can be found in **ref. 2**.

3.5.2. Confocal Imaging

The single wavelength probes (e.g., fluo3 and calcium green) can only confidently be used with confocal imaging. Unlike conventional microscopy, the confocal microscope produces optical sections through the cell of a defined thickness. Therefore, the problem associated with thickness artefacts are eliminated. From the change in fluorescent intensity at a single wavelength, the free Ca^{2+} can be calculated from the law of mass action (see earlier). A particular advantage of confocal imaging in general, which can also be applied to Ca^{2+} imaging, is the ability to produce optical sections. This enables Ca^{2+} within the nucleus to be measured and slices through the cell perpendicular (xz-plane) to the normal viewing plane to be achieved. In this way, the contact between the cells and their adherent (stimulating) surfaces can be defined with precision while also measuring cytosolic free Ca^{2+} concentration *(10)*.

3.6. Rapid Ca^{2+} Measurement and Imaging

Many of the Ca^{2+} signals in inflammatory cells have time-scales that can be measured on a time-scale of seconds. However, it is now clear that these events may be composed of faster events occurring on the millisecond time-scale. There are several approaches which may be useful. A "stopped flow technique" to study the rapid kinetics of the Ca^{2+} response in populations of fura2-loaded cells has been used *(11)*. This technique depended on the rapid mixing of populations of cells with the agonist, and produced a "population averaged" Ca^{2+}rise times. Another approach is to use the confocal laser to scan a single line repeatedly (xt scanning) through individual fluo3-loaded cells. Lines can be accumulated at a rate of at least 80/s, giving a time resolution of greater than 12.5 ms with events in the cell distinguishable to about 0.1–0.2 (m resolution *(12)*.

Conventional confocal laser scanning is, however, relatively slow for whole cell imaging as a single laser beam scans sequentially left and right and up and down across the microscopic field. A faster approach is to use a rotating Nipkow disk (a series of pinpoints in the rotating disk), which scans multiple laser beams across the field at up to 360 frames/s (3 ms/frame). This promises to reveal more of the intricacies of Ca^{2+} signalling within inflammatory cells, which occur on the 10–50 ms time-scale.

3.7. Near Plasma Membrane Ca^{2+}

The addition of long hydrophobic tails to fura2 result in the production of Ca^{2+} sensing probes, which accumulate in the membranes rather than the cytosol. One such probe, FFP18 has been used to monitor near plasma membrane Ca^{2+} in neutrophils *(13,14)*. Addition of this probe to cells results in plasma membrane association of fluorescence as the C18 tail incorporates into the plasma membrane. Acetoxymethyl ester hydrolysis results in trapping of the Ca^{2+} sensing form of the indicator on the cytosolic face of the membrane as cytosolic esterases prevent "flip-flop" diffusion back to the outside. In neutrophils, which have little internal membranes, the probe remains located in the plasma membrane and reports high subplasma membrane Ca^{2+} on influx *(14)*. It is not clear whether it will be as useful in other inflammatory cell types.

3.8. Manipulating Cytosolic Free Ca^{2+}

There are a number of pharmacological agents that are useful in manipulating cytosolic free Ca^{2+} concentration listed in **Table 2**.

Cytosolic free Ca^{2+} within inflammatory cells can also be manipulated on demand by photorelease of "caged Ca^{2+}" (e.g., nitr-5), "caged Ca^{2+} chelator" (e.g., diazo-2), or caged IP_3 at defined times. These three "caged" compounds can be loaded into cells from their available acetoxymethyl-esters. However, other (nonesterified) caged compounds can also be introduced into cells by SLAM-injection *(7)*. The "caged" compound is inert until photolysis "releases the cage." In the case of "caged Ca^{2+}" and "caged Ca^{2+} chelator," the affinity of the chelator for Ca^{2+} changes dramatically on photolysis at about 360 nm. In this way, the cytosolic free Ca^{2+} concentration can be elevated or be suppressed on command *(15)*.

4. Notes

1. Remember that the de-esterification that is catalyzed enzymatically in the cell, will occur spontaneously (at a slow rate). If this occurs before presentation to the cells, the probe either will not be able to enter the cells or enter the cells in the partially de-esterified, but in the non-Ca^{2+} sensitive form. It is thus crucial to prevent hydrolysis in the stored stock solution. Hydrolysis is slowed by reduced temperature and prevented by the exclusion of water. DMSO is hydroscopic and will readily absorb water from the air. Therefore, standard laboratory-grade DMSO is not recommended. Dry DMSO can be purchased in sealed containers, preferably in smaller volumes, stored under dry gas. Another precaution that can reduce the water content of the solution is to be sure that when taking the container from the freezer (at –20°C) to let it warm up to room temperature before opening it. If this is not done, water from the air can condense on the inner surface of the container and contaminate the stock solution.
2. Obviously, extracellular Ca^{2+} must be present during the time that the Ca^{2+} chelating probe is loaded into the cells, so that it can replace Ca^{2+}, which will be bound to the probe. Otherwise, Ca^{2+} will be removed from intracellular sites. However, provided these precautions are taken, Ca^{2+} chelating probes have little obvious (adverse) effect on Ca^{2+} signaling. Alternatively, omission of extracellular Ca^{2+} during loading has been used as a deliberate strategy for "depleting cell Ca^{2+}," in order to establish a role for this ion in a particular cell activity.
3. Digitonin is often preferred when measuring cytosolic free Ca^{2+} concentration in a cell population in suspension as it ensures that all fura2 gains access to high Ca^{2+} concentration in the extracellular medium. If ionomycin is used (as it is often during Ca^{2+} imaging), it is important that sufficient ionomycin is added to produce a truly maximal fluorescence signal, as it is possible to elevate cytosolic

Table 2
Pharmacological Agents for Manipulating Ca²⁺ in Inflammatory Cells

Agent	Action and Use
Thapsigargin	Cell permeable inhibitor of store Ca^{2+}-ATPase (IC50=4–13 nM)
Thapsigargicin	Less potent and less hydrophobic analog of thapsigargin. Also disrupts lipid-protein association in biomembranes
DHQ	Releases Ca^{2+} from Ca^{2+} stores by inhibiting Ca^{2+}-ATPase activity
Cyclopiazonic Acid (CPA)	Cell permeant, reversible inhibitor of store Ca^{2+}-ATPase. Releases Ca^{2+} from the same intracellular pool as thapsigargin
BAPTA-AM and EGTA-AM	Selective intracellular Ca^{2+} chelator (Kd=110 nM) for buffering cytosolic free Ca^{2+}. Binds 1 cation per molecule
Ionomycin	A selective Ca^{2+} ionophore. Complexes with Ca^{2+} between pH7 and 9.5, Acts as efficient Ca^{2+} carrier across biological membranes
A23187	A selective (but fluorescent) Ca^{2+} ionophore.
SKF-96365 and Econazole	Inhibits receptor-mediated Ca^{2+} entry in inflammatory cells at concentrations that do not effect internal Ca^{2+} release
TMB-8	Intracellular Ca^{2+} antagonist that may block release of Ca^{2+} from intracellular stores.
U-73122	Inhibits phospholipase C (PLC) activation (IC$_{50}$=1–2 µM) and
U-73343	Analog of U-73122 thats acts as a very weak inhibitor of PLC. Suitable as negative control

free Ca^{2+} with ionophores to concentrations that are less than 1 µM. Under these latter conditions, the ionomycin signal will not correspond with R_{max} and cytosolic free Ca^{2+} concentration cannot be correctly calculated. The ratiometric dyes, unfortunately, require excitation near the UV region, which can also stimulate fluorescence from endogenous molecules in neutrophils. Consequently, the signal:noise ratio of the Ca^{2+} probe is reduced. This problem is offset by the major advantage of Ca^{2+} "signature" provided by the ratiometric dyes.

4. The information in a single pixel is limited by the noise associated with the detection system of the imager. A technique often used, called binning, is to collect the data from a pixel and its neighbors, but treat them as a single larger pixel. Binning of information on neighboring pixels will increase the signal but decrease the spatial resolution. A statistical approach can be used to determine whether small areas within the cell truly have raised Ca^{2+}. Areas of interest in the image (with n pixels) can be chosen, for comparison of their cytosolic free Ca^{2+} concentration. The areas will have statistically significant cytosolic free Ca^{2+} concentrations when

$$n = 2\left[\sigma(Z_{2\alpha} + Z_{2\beta}/\delta)\right]^2 \text{ or } \delta = \sqrt{[2/n]\left[\sigma(Z_{2\alpha} + Z_{2\beta})\right]}$$

where n is the number of pixels in each of the two areas of the image, s is the standard deviation of the distribution of Ca^{2+} values in the pixel arrays, Zx is the standard normal deviate exceeded with probability x, α is the significance level for the test, $(1-\beta)$ is the power of the test, and δ is the difference in cytosolic free Ca^{2+} concentrations *(16)*. It can be seen that the ability to detect small and localized changes in Ca^{2+} depends on both the magnitude of the Ca^{2+} change and the area it occupies. Detection of both very small and very localized Ca^{2+} changes is thus difficult and ultimately limited by the image noise, i.e., the variance (standard deviation) of individual pixels values *(17)*.

5. The major problems associated with fluorescent imaging are photobleaching and image noise. Photobleaching arises where excessive excitation results in the destruction of the fluorescent molecules and hence a reduction in the emission intensity (bleaching). Each fluorescent molecule emits about 10^4–10^5 photons/molecule before photolysis. With ratiometric methods, photobleaching is less of a problem as the ratio will remain constant during the bleaching provided that the pairs of images taken close together in time (when no significant bleaching has occurred). With nonratiometric confocal Ca^{2+} imaging, bleaching during the time of the experiment can be avoided by attenuating the laser light, and increasing the detector (photomultiplier) sensitivity so that the minimum usable emission intensity is employed.

References

1. Hallett, M. B., Hodges, R., Cadman, M., Blanchfield, H., Dewitt, S., Pettit, E. J., et al. (1999) Techniques for measuring and manipulating free Ca^{2+} in the cytosol and organelles of neutrophils. *J. Immunol. Methods* **232,** 77–88.
2. Tepikin, A. V. (2000) *Calcium Signalling: A Practical Approach.* 2nd ed. Oxford Univ. Press, Oxford, U.K., p. 230.
3. Pozzan, T., Lew, D. P., Wollheim, C.B., Tsien, R. Y., and Rink, T. J. (1983) Is cytosolic ionized calcium regulating neutrophil activation? *Science* **221,** 1413.
4. Hallett, M. B., Davies, E. V., and Pettit, E. J. (1996) Fluorescent methods for measuring and imaging the cytosolic free Ca^{2+} in neutrophils. *Methods: A Companion to Methods Enzymol.* **9,** 591–606.
5. Scanlon, M., Williams, D. A., and Fay, F. S. (1987) A Ca^{2+}-insensitive form of fura2 associated with polymorphoinuclear leukocytes-assessment and acurate Ca^{2+} measurement. *J. Biol. Chem.* **262,** 6308
6. Al-Mohanna, F. A. and Hallett, M. B. (1988) The use of fura 2 to determine the relationship between intracellular free Ca^{2+} and oxidase activation in rat neutrophils. *Cell Calcium* **8,** 17.
7. Laffafian, I. and Hallett, M. B. (1998) Lipid-assisted microinjection: introducing material into the cytosol and membranes of small cells. *Biophys. J.* **75,** 2558–2563.
8. Laffafian, I. and Hallett, M. B. (2000) Gentle micro-injection for myeloid cells using SLAM. *Blood* **95,** 3270–3271.
9. Von Tscharner, V., Deranleau, D. A., and Baggiolini, M. (1986) Calcium fluxes and calcium buffering in human neutrophils. *J. Biol. Chem.* **261,** 10,163.
10. Pettit, E. J. and Hallett, M. B. (1996) Localised and global cytosolic Ca^{2+} changes in neutrophils during engagement of CD11b/CD18 integrin visualised using confocal laser scanning reconstruction. *J. Cell Sci.* **109,** 1689–1694.

11. Sage, S. O., Pintado, E., Mahaut-Smith, M. P., et al. (1990) Rapid kinetics of agonist-evoked cytosolic free Ca^{2+} concentration in fura2-loaded human neutrophils. *Biochem. J.* **265,** 915.
12. Pettit, E. J. and Hallett, M. B. (1995) Early Ca^{2+} signalling events in neutrophils detected by rapid confocal laser scanning. *Biochem. J.* **310,** 445.
13. Davies, E. V. and Hallett, M. B. (1996) Near membrane Ca^{2+} changes resulting from store release in neutrophils: detection by FFP-18. *Cell Calcium* **19,** 355–362.
14. Davies, E. V. and Hallett, M. B. (1998) High micromolar Ca^{2+} beneath the plasma membrane in stimulated neutrophils. *Biochem. Biophys. Res. Commun.* **248,** 679–683.
15. Pettit, E. J. and Hallett, M. B. (1998) Release of "caged" cytosolic Ca^{2+} triggers rapid spreading of human neutrophils adherent via integrin engagement. *J. Cell Sci.* **111,** 2209–2215.
16. Armitage, P. and Berry, G. (1987) *Statistical Methods in Medical Research.* 2nd ed. Blackwell Scientific, Boston, MA, pp. 181–182.
17. Dewitt, S. and Hallett, M. B. (2002) Cytosolic free Ca^{2+} and calpain are required for β_2-integrin accelerated phagocytosis by human neutrophils. *J. Cell. Biol.* **159,** 181–189.

7

Detection and Visualization of Oxidase Activity in Phagocytes

Maurice B. Hallett, Caroline Cole, and Sharon Dewitt

1. Introduction

An important aspect of the function of immune phagocytes (i.e., neutrophils) is the killing of infecting microorganisms. This is achieved, after phagocytosis of the microbe, by activation of an NADPH-oxidase, which reduces oxygen to the superoxide ion in the phagosome. This has three effects. First, the superoxide that is generated is highly reactive and will react with the proteins of the ingested microbe. Second, the superoxide will dismutate to form peroxide, which is a substrate for the abundant granular protein, myeloperoxidase (*see* **Table 1**). The action of myeloperoxidase generates other reactive oxygen-containing species, including hypochlorite (*see* **Table 1**), which is also toxic for the microbe. Third, the vectorial addition of an electron to oxygen results in a decrease in H^+ ions and an elevation of intraphagosomal pH. The activity of the neutral proteases within the granules, which are initially inactive because the intragranular pH is low (about pH 4.0), is released, thus further increasing the killing environment within the phagosome. The importance of the neutrophil oxidase in combating infection is dramatically demonstrated by Chronic Granulomatous Disease (CGD), in which the oxidase fails to activate, either because of a mutation in the oxidase or because of a mutation in a signaling component *(1)*. In this congenital condition, the patient is prone to infections that are ultimately fatal. It could be argued that the "purpose" of all the other neutrophil activities (such as adherence to endothelium, extravasation, chemotaxis, and phagocytosis) is to bring the oxidase molecule to the correct place to be effective in the killing of bacteria.

From: *Methods in Molecular Biology, vol. 225: Inflammation Protocols*
Edited by: P. G. Winyard and D. A. Willoughby © Humana Press Inc., Totowa, NJ

Table 1
Myeloperoxidase Actions

Source	Enzyme	Product	Reaction
O_2	oxidase	O_2^- (superoxide)	$O_2 + e^- \rightarrow O_2^-$
O_2^-	spontaneous superoxidase dismutase	H_2O_2 (peroxide)	$O_2^- + O_2^- \rightarrow O_2 = + O_2$ (at physiol pH $O_2 = +2H^+ \leftrightarrow H_2O_2$)
H_2O_2	peroxidase	OCl^- (hypochlorite)	$H_2O_2 + Cl^- \rightarrow OCl^- + H_2O$

For molecular details of the oxidase, CGD and theoretical and chemical aspects of the oxygen-containing reactive species, see the reviews listed (*1–4*). In this chapter, assays of neutrophil oxidase activity will be presented.

2. Materials

1. Luminol is available from Sigma and other companies. A stock solution of luminol (10 m*M*) is stable at room temperature, but is best kept in the dark.
2. Cytochrome C (prepared at 15 mg/mL), superoxide dismutase (SOD; at 500 U/mL), and related enzymes are available from Sigma, Boehringer-Mannheim, and elsewhere.
3. The fluorescent probes, 2',7',-dichlorohydrofluorescein (also called 2',7',-dichlorofluorescin) and dihydrorhodamine 123, as well as a variety of variants based on "oxyBurst" are available from Molecular Probes.

3. Methods

There are i) "biochemical" assays in which the consumption of oxygen or the chemical reduction of an indicator molecule (cytochrome-*c*) can be quantified in populations of neutrophils; ii) assays which monitor (rather than measure) oxidase activity, such as the luminescent assays, some of which are catalyzed by peroxidase and so provide a less quantitative link to the oxidase itself; and iii) assays of activity within individual neutrophils.

3.1. Oxygen Consumption

The most direct measure of oxidase activity is (by definition) related to the consumption of oxygen. The concentration of oxygen in solution can be accurately measured using a polarized oxygen electrode. Commercially available electrodes are available (e.g., Rank Bros, Bottisham, UK), which are housed at the base of a chamber, can be warmed to 37°C, stirred, to prevent neutrophil sedimentation, and isolated from the atmosphere so that consumption of oxygen can be monitored (*see* **Note1**). The electrode voltage can be read as a continuous time trace either directly onto a paper chart recorder or into a computer (after A-D conversion). The precise quantitation of oxygen concentration can be made from knowledge of the initial oxygen concentration (*see* **Note 2**) and

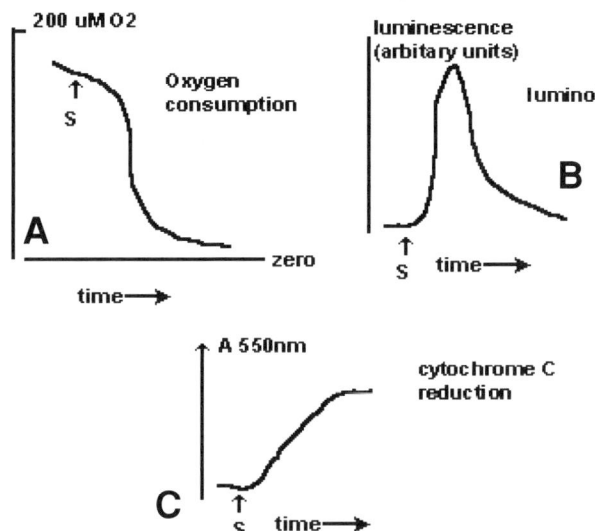

Fig. 1. Typical outputs from (**A**) oxygen consumption measurement, (**B**) luminol chemiluminescence, and (**C**) cytochrome-*c* assays for the same cellular oxidase response. Whereas in both assays (A) and (C), the product (reduced cytochrome or lack of oxygen accumulates, in (B) the product (light) does not. Assay (C), therefore, provides a direct readout of oxidase rate, whereas the rate from the other two requires the first derivative (gradient) of the reponse to be calculated.

the zero oxygen level, achieved by chemical consumption of available oxygen by the addition of excess sodium dithionite. The oxidase activity is then calculated from the rate of consumption of rate of oxygen (*see* **Fig. 1**), adjusted for the volume and cell concentration.

$$\text{Oxidase activity (moles/cell/min)} = D[O_2]t \times V_c/N_c$$

where $D[O_2]t$ is the decrease in oxygen molar concentration over t minutes; V_c is the volume of the chamber (in L), and N_c is the number of neutrophils in the chamber (i.e., cell density $\times V_c$).

It must be noted that although the oxidase produces one molecule of superoxide for every molecule of oxygen consumed (i.e., one electron transfer; *see* **Table 1**, line 1), dismutation regenerates one molecule of oxygen for every two superoxide molecules (*see* **Table 1**, line 2). This means that the overall conversion is one molecule of oxygen apparently consumed for every two electrons transferred (i.e., half the superoxide generation rate). It should also be noted that, in some cell types, the oxygen consumption rate may include mitochondria oxygen consumption. In neutrophils, this is insignificant (or totally absent), but in other cell types (such as monocytes) this may not be so. Conventionally, the experiments are performed with cyanide (1 mM) present in the medium to inhibit mitochondrial oxidase activity. The cyanide-insensitive oxygen consumption is thus taken as the phagocyte oxidase activity. However, as cyanide also inhibits peroxidase activity, it cannot be used with peroxidase-dependent assays of oxidase activity in the same way.

3.2. Cytochrome-c Reduction

Cytochrome-c is an electron acceptor that changes its absorption characteristic on reduction, and so can be used to measure electron transfer rate from the oxidase, or superoxide (2,3). An assay is described that uses inhibition by superoxide dismutase as a way of providing superoxide specificity to the assay. Ideally, a dual beam spectrophotometer with heating and stirring is required, but single-beam machines with the necessary microprocessor signal manipulation ability can also be used.

1. Cytochrome-c is prepared at 15 mg/mL; SOD at 500 U/mL; and purified cells (e.g., neutrophils at 10^6/mL).
2. Two spectrophotometer cuvets (1 mL volume) are prepared each with 700 μL HEPES buffered Krebs medium (*see* **Chapter 5**), 100 μL of cell suspension, and 100 μL of cytochrome-c solution.
3. To the reference cuvet is added 100 μL SOD solution and to the sample cuvet Krebs medium (100 μL). These are placed in the spectrophotometer and allowed to temperature equilibrate.
4. The absorbance difference between the reference and sample at 550 nm is recorded continually against time.
5. Stimuli are added to both cuvets at a defined time (*see* **Note 4**) and the rate of increase in absorbance recorded (*see* **Fig. 1**).
6. The extinction coefficient for cytochrome c reduction at 550 nm is 2.1×10^4 M^{-1} cm^{-1}, and the rate of superoxide production (S) can be calculated as (for a 1-cm pathlength)

$$S \text{ (moles/min/}10^6\text{cells)} = 10^6 \times (DAt/2.1 \times 10^4) \times V/C$$

DAt = change in absorbance over t min; V = volume of reactants in L; C = cell number in cuvet, which here is 10^5.

3.3. Luminescent Assays

There are several lumigenic probes for oxidase activity in neutrophils. These include luminol, lucigenin (5), and coelenterazine (6). The assays require a luminometer, which can either be a simple home-built device as there are no complex optics required (merely a housing and a photomultiplier tube with power supply and read out), or can be purchased commercially (e.g., Berthold, LKB, and so on) and can include multitube access for multiple time-courses.

Lucigenin and coelenterazine is used to monitor superoxide, whereas luminol requires peroxidase activity for light generation. All protocols are essentially similar.

3.3.1. Luminol Protocol

1. Neutrophils are isolated and counted and suspended in HEPES-buffered Krebs medium (*see* **Chapter 5**) at about 10^6–10^7/mL and kept on ice until required (*see* **Note 3**)
2. A stock solution of luminol (10 mM) is stable at room temperature, but is best kept in the dark.
3. HEPES-buffered Krebs medium (0.9 mL) is added to the reaction tube together with 100 µL of neutrophil suspension and 1 µL of luminol (final concentration 10 µM and 10^6 cells).
4. The reaction tube is placed into luminometer to warm to 37°C. (Also, some plasticware has phosphorescence, so a period of "dark adaptation" is useful to reduce background signal.)
5. The luminescent signal is recorded for at least 30 s before the addition of stimulus (e.g., f-met-leu-phe (0.1–1 µM) plus cytochalasin B (5 µg/mL), phorbol myristate acetate (100 nM), and so on (*see* **Note 4**).
6. The luminescent record gives the instantaneous rate of oxidase activity, rather than the cumulative effect as with oxygen consumption (*see* **Fig. 1**).

3.4. Flow Cytometry Based Assay

The use of fluorescence rather than absorbance gives an improved sensitivity that enables oxidant events to be measurable in individual neutrophils. The methods rely on the conversion of non-(or weakly) fluorescent molecules such as 2'7'dichloro**hydro**fluores**cein** (also called 2'7'dichlorofluores**cin**) or dihydrorhodamine 123 to their highly fluorescent analogues (2'7'dichloro-fluores**cein** and rhodamine 123, respectively) by oxidation. It is likely that many of the products of the neutrophil oxidase system (including those generated by myeloperoxidase) play a part in the oxidation and so this approach is not useful for dissecting which oxygen-containing molecular species are involved in a particular response. However, the "switching-on" of the fluorescence depends initially on the activation of the oxidase and is thus very useful for establishing timing *(7)*. The probes are available as their membrane permeant diacetate esters and are loaded in the cells as with the ester Ca^{2+} indicators (*see* **Chapter 6**). Standard flow cytometry at the fluorescein or rhodamine excitation wavelength is then used to follow population trends in oxidase activity following stimulation of the population.

A modification of this technique is to couple the oxidant indicator to a particle or immune complex for phagocytosis (*see* **Chapter 5**). Molecular Probes has a series of reagents (called OxyBurst reagents) that are useful for this. "Fc OxyBurst" is an immune complex with the probe already covalently attached. With this approach, the stimulus and the probe are one, and oxidase activity within the phagosome only is monitored.

3.5. Microscopic Assays

In order to follow oxidase activation within an individual neutrophil behavior, microscopic techniques that monitor neutrophil oxidase activity are useful.

3.5.1. NBT Reduction

Nitroblue tetrazolium is reduced to an insoluble dye by the active oxidase. Thus, in the presence of the stain, neutrophils with active oxidase are stained black. Although this technique is useful for quantifying the number of cells that are active, it cannot be quantified or give an indication of the time-course of the response.

3.5.2. Fluorescent Microscopy

The fluorescent approaches described earlier for flow cytometry are also applicable to fluorescent microscopy. Amine-reactive OxyBurst derivatives can be covalently linked to zymosan or other particles. These can be visualized both outside and within the cell, and the oxidase status of each cell or phagosome within the cell monitored. When coupled with single-cell techniques for inducing phagocytosis (*see* **Chapter 5**), the timing of oxidase activation within individual phagosomes is possible *(7)*.

3.5.3. Luminescence

Although chemiluminescence is less "user-friendly" than fluorescence, it is possible with supersensitive photon counting cameras (e.g., Hamamatsu, Photek, and so on) to detect the spatial distribution of photon emission microscopically from luminol *(8)*. This can be superimposed on the image of the cell to discover the timing and number of neutrophils responding.

4. Notes

1. The design of the oxygen chamber is important so that additions can be made to the cells without oxygen also being introduced. The design by Rank Brother (Bottisham, UK) has a lid with a small diameter bore hole in place. This permits the lid to be lowered onto the face of the cell suspension within the chamber, as the hole acts as an escape for air above the liquid. The same hole can be used for the addition of stimuli using a small volume (1–10 µL) syringe.
2. The concentration of oxygen in solution depends on the atmospheric pressure (which does not usually vary by much, but for accuracy can be found on a daily

basis), and the solubility of oxygen (which depends on temperature and ionic strength and protein concentration). The relationship is given by Henry's Law, i.e., $[O_2] = \alpha\ P/22.4$, where P is the partial pressure (in atmospheres) and α is the Bunsen solubility coefficient. The solubility coefficient depends on temperature and composition of the medium and can be found from tables in **ref. 9**. For HEPES-buffered Krebs medium, the Bunsen solubility coefficient is approx 0.023 and the oxygen concentration can be taken as approx 203 μM. Remember that for gases, the solubility decreases as the temperature increases (i.e., bubbles appear as water is warmed). It is, therefore, important that all reagents are equilibrated to the same temperature before experimenting.
3. Whole blood can also be used after dilution to prevent excessive absorption of light by hemoglobin, but can be more difficult to standardize, as a result of variation in neutrophil/monocyte number, lipid, serum, and so on.
4. When adding stimuli, it is important that there is not excessive dilution of the reaction mixture. Although this can be taken into account, it is often easier to add the stimulus in a small volume. For example, f-met-leu-phe or PMA are stimuli that can be dissolved in DMSO at 1000X greater concentration than required (f-met-leu-phe is easily soluble at 1 mM). One microliter of this stock can then be added to the reaction mixture (1 mL) without increasing the reaction volume significantly. Also the solvent (DMSO) is maintained at a nontoxic level (0.1%).

References

1. Segal, A. W. (1996) The NADPH oxidase and chronic granulomatous disease. *Mol. Med. Today* **2,** 129–135.
2. Segal, A. W. and Abo, A. (1993) The biochemical basis of the NADPH oxidase of phagocytes. *T.I.B.S.* **18,** 43–47.
3. Packer, L., Ed. (1984) Oxygen radical in biological systems. *Methods in Enzymol.* **105**.
4. Greenwald, R., Ed. (1985) *CRC Handbook for Oxygen Radical Research.* CRC, Boca Raton, FL.
5. Dahlgren, C. and Karlsson, A. (1999) Respiratory burst in human neutrophils. *J. Immunol. Methods* **232,** 3–14.
6. Lucas, M. and Solano, F. (1992) Coelentrazine is a superoxide anion sensitive chemiluminescent probe- its usefulness in the assay of respiratory burst in neutrophils. *Anal. Biochem.* **206,** 273.
7. Dewitt, S. and Laffafian, I., and Hallett, M. B. (2003) Phagosomal oxidative activity during integrin (CR3)-mediated phagocytosis by neutrophils. *J. Cell. Sci.,* in press.
8. Sukazi, E., Kobayashi, H., Kodama, Y., Masujima, T., and Terakawa, S. (1997) Video-rate dynamics of exocytotic events associated with phagocytosis in neutrophils. *Cell Motil. Cytoskeleton.* **38,** 215–228.
9. Altman, P. L. and Dittmer, D. S., Eds. (1974) *Biology Data Handbook.* vol III, FASEB, p. 1571.

8

Measurement of Complement Activation

Tom Eirik Mollnes

1. Introduction

Complement is a humoral defense system that protects the host from microorganisms by inducing an inflammatory reaction at the site of invasion. However, complement activation is not limited to microbial protection, but is generally activated in any tissue damage irrespective of the stimulus that initiated the reaction. Thus, complement is a double-edged sword which, when activated improperly, may contribute to inflammation and tissue damage. Weisman et al. demonstrated in 1990 that specific complement inhibition markedly reduced tissue damage in experimental myocardial infarction (*1*), a number of animal and clinical studies have documented that activation of complement contributes to the ischemia/reperfusion injury in general, and to the pathophysiology of various autoimmune diseases, trauma, systemic inflammatory response syndrome, septicemia, and transplant rejection (for review, *see* **refs.** *2–5*).

Traditional complement tests are based on functional haemolytic activity (CH50) or immunochemical quantification of single components. These tests are valuable for detection of complement deficiencies. However, in order to measure activation of complement, specific activation products need to be quantified. Various indirect methodological approaches have been used to detect complement activation products. These have now largely been replaced by sensitive and specific enzyme immunoassays (EIA) based on monoclonal antibodies (MAb) directed against neoepitopes, i.e., antigenic determinants exposed in the activation products but hidden in the native components (*6*). When an antineoepitope specific MAb is used as capture antibody in EIA, only the actual activation product will bind. After washing, there are no native components left in the well that can compete with the activation product, and a second antibody that is not necessarily neoepitope-specific can then be used for detection. By this approach, the amount of an activation product can be quantified directly in a plasma sample without any pretreatment.

When complement is activated, a number of neoepitopes are exposed in the different activation products. Fig. 1 schematically illustrates activation of the complement system where known neoepitopes exposed in activation products defined by specific MAbs are illustrated with asterisks. Commercial kits are available for quantification of activation products both from the classical, alternative, and terminal pathways. However, these are generally expensive and not always of sufficient quality. Thus, an alternative for those experienced with both complement research and EIAs, is to design their own assays based on commercially available antibodies or antibodies obtained from colleagues. The assay described in this chapter is based on the MAb aE11 *(7)*, specific for a neoepitope in the human terminal SC5b-9 complement complex (TCC) (**Fig. 2**). TCC is the final complement activation product, indicating that the terminal pathway has been activated to its end. It is less prone to in vitro activation than the other activation products and is a reliable indicator of complement activation. Assays for other activation products are, however, useful to define the initial activation pathway(s) involved. These assays are designed principally in the same way as the TCC assay, using appropriate antibodies for the respective products. Most of the MAbs available are directed against human proteins, but some crossreact with other species, whereas others are specially designed for experimental animal models *(8)*.

In vivo complement activation can be measured in plasma or other body fluids. Because complement activation readily occurs in vitro, a prerequisite for reliable results reflecting the in vivo situation is that the samples are obtained, prepared, and stored according to strict guidelines as described in **Subheadings 2.1.** and **3.1.**. Similarly, if in vitro studies are performed to evaluate the effect of various complement activators or inhibitors, it is important that the same guidelines are followed after the incubation period is finished in order to avoid further and undesired activation.

2. Materials

1. Test samples are collected in tubes containing ethylenediamine tetraacetic acid (EDTA) giving a final concentration of 10–20 mM EDTA in the sample (*see* **Note 1**).
2. 96-well microtiter plates (e.g., Nunc-ImmunoPlate MaxiSorp).
3. Coating buffer: Phosphate-buffered saline (PBS), pH 7.4 (*see* **Note 2**).
4. Capture antibody: Neoepitope specific MAb to an activation product, e.g., mouse MAb aE11 to a neoepitope of human TCC.

Complement Activation

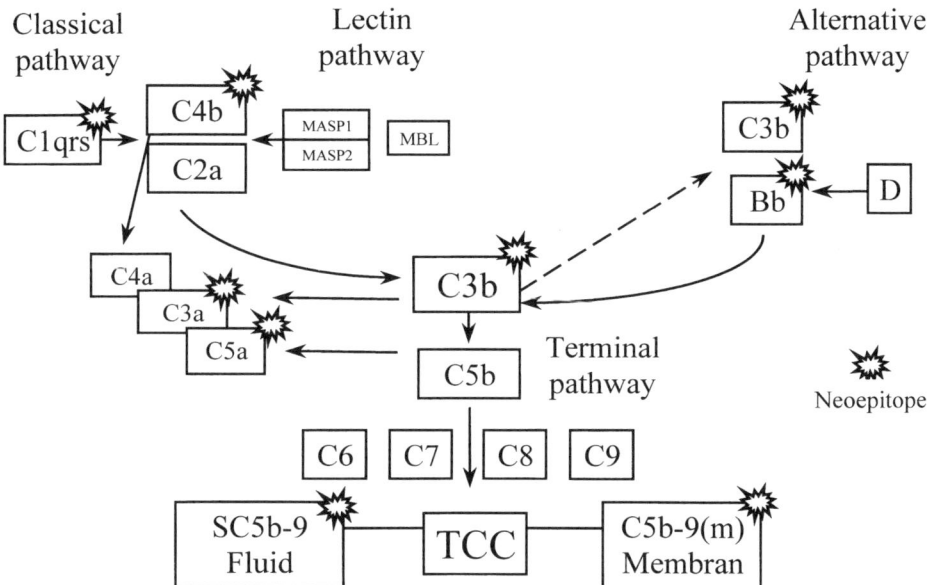

Fig. 1. Schematic illustration of the activation products generated when complement is activated. There are three initial activation pathways: the classical pathway which is activated through C1q by immune complexes, CRP, and other substances, the lectin pathway that is activated through binding of mannose binding lectin (MBL) to, e.g., bacterial surfaces, and the alternative pathway that is activated by foreign surfaces through factor D cleaving B when B is bound to C3b. Asterisks indicate exposure of neoepitopes that have been defined by specific monoclonal antibodies. Using these antibodies as capture antibodies in enzyme immunoassays, classical pathways activation can be detected by complexes between C1r/C1s and C1-inhibitor, classical and lectin pathway activation can be detected by C4b/C4c, alternative pathway can be detected by Bb, all initial pathways are covered by activation of C3 as detected by C3a, C3b/C3c or C3d, and terminal pathway activation is detected by C5a or the terminal C5b-9 complex (TCC). The latter exists in two forms: the membrane bound C5b-9(m) (membrane attack complex) and the soluble SC5b-9, both exposing the same neoepitope. The illustration is simplified and does not cover all complement activation products.

5. Washing buffer: PBS containing 0.1 % Tween-20.
6. Antigen buffer: PBS containing 0.2% Tween-20 and 10 mM EDTA (final conc).
7. Plasma or other samples to be tested (*see* **Note 3**).
8. Internal reference(s) with known concentration.
9. Standard.
10. A serum pool from healthy blood donors ($n>3$).
11. Zymosan.

12. Antibody buffer: PBS containing 0.2% Tween-20.
13. Antibody, preferably biotinylated (*see* **Notes 4** and **5**); e.g., MAb antihuman C6 for detection of TCC.
14. Peroxidase conjugated avidin and antibody buffer.
15. H_2O_2.
16. ABTS (2,2 azino-di(3-ethyl)-benzthiazoline sulfonate).
17. Substrate buffer: 0.15 M sodium acetate buffer, pH 4.0.

3. Methods
3.1. Test Samples

1. Draw blood directly into the Vacutainer tube containing EDTA (10–20 mM final conc.)
2. Turn tube gently 4–5 times to ensure mixing of EDTA.
3. Place tube immediately (or max after 30 min) on ice or in refrigerator.
4. Centrifuge for 15 min at 1500g (cool centrifugation).
5. Remove plasma carefully (avoid cellular elements), transfer it into Cryotubes and store immediately at –70°C (*see* **Note 6**).

3.2. Enzyme Immunoassay

1. Dilute capture antibody, e.g., MAb aE11 for TCC detection, in coating buffer to a final immunoglobulin concentration of 1 µg/mL (*see* **Note 7**). Add 50 µL antibody solution to each well (*see* **Note 8**). Incubate at +4°C for at least 16 h (can usually be stored for a few weeks).
2. Wash the plates at room temperature three times in washing buffer (*see* **Subheading 2.5.**). Volume: 200–300 µL per well.
3. Standard, reference sample(s), and test samples are diluted in antigen buffer. Keep buffer and samples cool (on crushed ice). Titrate the standard twofold in six to eight steps (*see* **Note 9**). Add all standard and samples in triplicate, 50 µL to each well. Incubate at +4°C for 1 h. Wash as described in **Subheading 3.2.2**.
4. To prepare the standard (*see* **Note 10**), add 10 mg zymosan per mL serum to a serum pool that has been prewarmed to +37°C (the recommended amount of zymosan is in substantial excess and will give a reproducible degree of activation). Incubate at +37°C for 1 h with continuous mixing. Centrifuge at 10,000g for 45 min. Remove supernatant carefully to avoid contamination with zymosan particles and store in small aliquots at –70°C.
5. Dilute detection antibody, e.g., biotinylated anti-C6 MAb for TCC detection, in antibody buffer (*see* **Note 11**). Add 50 µL antibody solution to each well. Incubate at +37°C for 45 min. Wash as described in **Subheading 3.2.2**.
6. Dilute peroxidase-conjugated avidin in antibody buffer and add 50 µL to each well. Incubate at +37°C for 45 min. Wash as described in **Subheading 3.2.2**.
7. Substrate is prepared by adding ABTS (final conc. 0.3 mM) and H_2O_2 (final conc. 2.4×10^{-3}%) to substrate buffer immediately prior to use. Add substrate rapidly, 100 µL to each well, and incubate at room temperature until the upper standard

Complement Activation

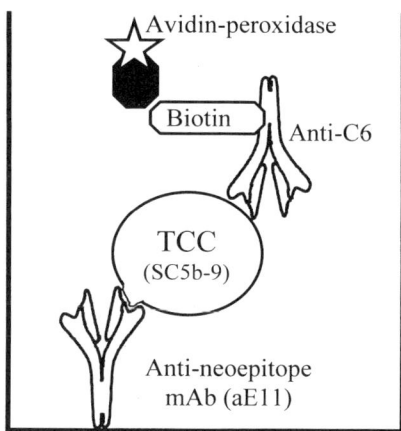

Fig. 2. Schematic illustration of an EiA based on a MAb reacting with a neoepitope exposed in a complement activation product; in this case, the terminal SC5b-9 complex (TCC). MAb aE11 reacts with a neoepitipe exposed in C9 during assembly of the complex. The detection antibody is directed against another part of the molecule, in this case by a biotinylated MAb recognizing C6. A complex of avidin and peroxidase is added. Avidin has high affinity to biotin and peroxidase is the active enzyme reacting with the final color-developing substrate solution.

reaches an optical density of approx 1.0 (usually 20–30 min) (see **Note 12**).

8. Read in a spectrophotometer for 96-well microtiter plates at 410 nm using 490 as reference filter (see **Note 13**). Calculation can be made automatically by the reader or by an external computer. Reference values should be within defined limits to accept the setup. Indicate final values corrected for dilution; i.e. corresponding to the amount in undiluted plasma (see **Note 14**).

4. Notes

1. EDTA is used to block calcium and magnesium and thereby inhibit all initial pathways of complement. Citrate is insufficient for this purpose and heparin cannot be used. EDTA may, however, be replaced by nafomastate mesilate (FUT-175).
2. Some capture MAbs work better if diluted in 0.05 M sodium carbonate buffer, pH 9.6.
3. Serum cannot be used for evaluation of in vivo complement activation because in vitro activation readily occurs if the guidelines for sample collection are not followed (carefully study **Subheading 3.1.**).
4. If the antibody is not biotinylated, this can easily be done as follows: 1) Dialyze the antibody (1 mg/mL) against 0.1 M NaHCO$_3$, pH 8.0, overnight at +4°C. 2) Add 200 µL of biotin-N-hydroxysuccinimide ester dissolved in dimethyl sulfoxide (2 mg/mL) to 1 mL of IgG (1 mg/mL) and incubate at room temperature

for 2–4 h. 3) Dialyze against PBS, pH 7.4, overnight at +4°C and store in aliquots at –70°C.
5. Biotinylated antibodies generally work very well in these types of assays and are recommended. Alternative principles for detection of activation products are directly enzyme-labeled antibody, antibody from another species followed by an enzyme-labeled antispecies antibody, or an MAb of another subclass than the capture antibody followed by an antisubclass specific enzyme-labeled antibody.
6. Ensure that the sample is kept cool during the whole process from sampling to freezing. Furthermore, the time from sampling to freezing should optimally not exceed 4 h.
7. Final antibody concentration should be titrated in the range of 0.1–10 µg/mL for each new batch of antibody to obtain optimal conditions. Culture supernatant or ascitic fluid may be used as alternative to purified immunoglobulin.
8. It is recommend that the edge wells of the plates are not used since they will often give false high values. Fill edge rows with buffer throughout the whole procedure until the last step where substrate is added to the whole plate.
9. If the standard is made according to the guidelines in **Subheading 3.2.**, it can be repeatedly diluted twofold from approx 1/200.
10. The standard described for the present TCC assay (**Subheading 3.2.**) is based on zymosan, which activates the alternative pathway. If activation products of the classical pathway are to be detected, heat aggregated IgG (HAIGG) can be used, which will give similar amounts of C3 activation products and TCC as zymosan. HAIGG standard is made as follows: 1) Make a 10 mg/mL solution of human IgG in PBS. 2) Incubate in glass tubes in a water bath at +63°C for 15 min. 3) Cool immediately on crushed ice. The HAIGG preparation can be stored at –20°C. 4) Add 1 mg of HAIGG per mL serum to a serum pool which has been prewarmed to +37°C. 5) Incubate at +37°C for 30 min with continuous mixing. 6) Centrifuge at 6000g for 30 min. 7) Remove supernatant and store in small aliquots at –70°C.
11. Optimal dilution of the reagent should be made for each new batch.
12. Stopping solution is usually not required if the reagents have been titrated optimally and the colour formation is rather slow. If stopping solution is required, 50–100 µL of 1% sodium dodecyl-sulfate in water or 12.5% H_2SO_4 can be used.
13. If all wells are blank and no color formation occurs, two pitfalls should be considered: Tween-20 in the coating buffer will prevent the capture antibody from binding to the plastic and NaN_3 (sodium azide) in the conjugate or substrate buffer will block the activity of peroxidase.
14. International standards for complement activation products are as yet not available, except for those included in the commercial kits. A definite advantage in using activated serum as standard is its stability and its suitability for use in many of the actual assays. Such a standard can be defined to contain a certain amount of arbitrary units (AU) per mL of all activation products present in the standard, e.g., 1000 AU/mL of TCC as recommended for the present standard.

References

1. Weisman, H. F., Bartow, T., Leppo, M. K., Marsh, H. C., Jr., Carson, G. R., Concino, M. F., et al. (1990) Soluble human complement receptor type 1: in vivo inhibitor of complement suppressing post-ischemic myocardial inflammation and necrosis. *Science* **249**, 146–151.
2. Asghar, S. S. and Pasch, M. C. (2000) Therapeutic inhibition of the complement system. *Front Biosci.* **5**, E63–E82.
3. Sahu, A. and Lambris, J. D. (2000) Complement inhibitors: a resurgent concept in anti-inflammatory therapeutics. *Immunopharmacology* **49**, 133–148.
4. Makrides, S. C. (1998) Therapeutic inhibition of the complement system. *Pharmacol. Rev.* **50**, 59–87.
5. Kirschfink, M. (1997) Controlling the complement system in inflammation. *Immunopharmacology* **38**, 51–62.
6. Mollnes, T. E. and Harboe, M. (1993) Neoepitope expression during complement activation - a model for detecting antigenic changes in proteins and activation of cascades. *Immunologist* **1**, 43–49.
7. Mollnes, T. E., Lea, T., Harboe, M., and Tschopp, J. (1985) Monoclonal antibodies recognizing a neoantigen of poly(C9) detect the human terminal complement complex in tissue and plasma. *Scand. J. Immunol.* **22**, 183–195.
8. Link, C., Hawlisch, H., Vilsendorf, A. M. Z., Gyleruz, S., Nagel, E., and Köhl, J. (1999) Selection of phage-displayed anti-guinea pig C5 or C5a antibodies and their application in xenotransplantation. *Mol. Immunol.* **36**, 1235–1247.

9

Measurement of Matrix Metalloproteinase Activities in the Medium of Cultured Synoviocytes Using Zymography

Linda Troeberg and Hideaki Nagase

1. Introduction

Human synovial cells in culture, particularly those obtained from patients with rheumatoid arthritis, secrete a number of matrix metalloproteinases (MMPs) into the culture medium. Enzymes secreted include collagenases (MMP-1, MMP-13), gelatinases (MMP-2 and MMP-9), and stromelysin 1 (MMP-3). These enzymes are usually secreted as inactive zymogens, which can be activated in vitro by treating with proteinases or mercurial compounds such as 4-aminophenyl mercuric acetate (APMA) *(1)*. The activity of these enzymes, both in their zymogen and mature form, can be analyzed by zymography. This electrophoretic technique, described as early as 1966 *(2)*, allows visualization of the number and approximate size of proteinases in complex biological samples *(3)*. A protein substrate, often gelatin, is copolymerized with the polyacrylamide gel, and samples are electrophoresed in sodium dodecyl sulfate (SDS). Following electrophoresis, the resolved proteinases are renatured by exchange of the SDS for a nonionic detergent, such as Triton X-100. The gel is then incubated in a buffer suitable for proteinase activity, enabling the renatured proteinases to hydrolyze the copolymerized protein substrate in a zone around their electrophorezed position. Once stained, these zones of digestion are clearly visible as light areas against the darkly stained protein background. This simple technique is highly sensitive, particularly for gelatinases A and B (MMP-2 and MMP-9), picogram quantities of which can be detected *(4)*. Some applications and limitations of the technique are described.

2. Materials
2.1. Equipment and Supplies

1. Minigel electrophoresis system, for example, BioRad Mini-PROTEAN 3 apparatus (gel dimensions 8.5 × 6.5 × 0.75 cm).
2. Power supply (200 V, 500 mA).
3. 37°C incubator.

2.2. Reagents

Reagents should be of electrophoresis or ultrapure grade. *See* **Note 1** for alternative buffer systems.

1. 30% (w/v) acrylamide, 0.8% (w/v) *N,N'*-methylene-*bis*-acrylamide stock solution (*see* **Note 2**).
2. TEMED (*N,N, N',N'*-tetramethyl ethylene diamine).
3. 10% (w/v) ammonium persulfate in H_2O (store at 4°C, stable for 2 wk).
4. Molecular mass standards, for example BioRad low range SDS-PAGE standards.

2.3. Stock Solutions

1. 4X Lower gel buffer: 110 mM amediol, 47 mM HCl, 0.02% NaN_3 (store at 4°C, stable for at least 1 mo).
2. 4X Upper gel buffer: 84 mM amediol, 62 mM HCl, 0.02% NaN_3 (store at 4°C, stable for a least 1 mo).
3. Sucrose solution: 50% (w/v) sucrose, 0.03% (v/v) toluene, 0.02% NaN_3 (store at 4°C, stable for a least 1 mo).
4. 10X Protein substrate solution: *see* **Note 3** for alternative substrates and *see* **Note 4** for instructions on dissolving gelatin (8 mg/mL in lower gel buffer) or casein (20 mg/mL in 0.1 M NaOH) (both stored at –20°C, stable for at least 1 mo).
5. 4X Upper reservoir buffer: 41 mM amediol, 40 mM glycine, 0.4% (w/v) SDS (store at 4°C, stable for a least 1 mo).
6. 4X Lower reservoir buffer: 62.5 mM amediol, 50 mM HCl (store at 4°C, stable for at least 1 mo).
7. 2X Sample loading buffer: 2% (w/v) SDS, 0.1% (w/v) bromophenol blue, 40% (v/v) glycerol (store at 4°C, stable for at least 1 mo).
8. Staining solution: 0.125% (w/v) coomassie blue R-250, 62.5% (v/v) methanol, 25% (v/v) acetic acid (store at room temperature, stable).
9. Destaining solution: 30% (v/v) methanol, 1% (v/v) formic acid (store at room temperature, stable).
10. Zymogram developing buffer: 50 mM Tris-HCl, pH 7.5, 200 mM NaCl, 5 mM $CaCl_2$, 0.02% NaN_3 (store at 4°C, stable for a least 1 mo).
11. Zymogram renaturing buffer: 2.5% (w/v) Triton X-100 in zymogram developing buffer (store at 4°C, stable for at least 1 mo).

Table 1
Composition of Zymogram Lower Gels

Reagent	Volume required per gel			
	6% gel	7.5% gel	10% gel	12% gel
Acrylamide:*bis* acrylamide solution	0.8 mL	1.0 mL	1.32 mL	1.61 mL
Lower gel buffer	1.0 mL	1.0 mL	1.0 mL	1.0 mL
Protein solution	0.4 mL	0.4 mL	0.4 mL	0.4 mL
50% sucrose	0.86 mL	0.86 mL	0.86 mL	0.86 mL
H_2O	0.94 mL	0.74 mL	0.42 mL	0.13 mL
Ammonium persulfate	14 µL	14 µL	14 µL	14 µL
TEMED	1.5 µL	1.5 µL	1.5 µL	1.5 µL

3. Methods

The buffer system used for gel electrophoresis is based on the method of Bury *(5)*.

3.1. Preparation of Gels and Electrophoresis

1. Clean the glass electrophoresis plates with water and then wipe with ethanol. Assemble the gel casting apparatus according to the manufacturer's instructions.
2. Choose what percentage acrylamide gel to cast depending on the molecular mass of the proteinase activity to be visualized. Higher molecular mass activities resolve better on lower percentage gels, whereas lower molecular mass activities resolve better on higher percentage gels. For MMPs, we usually run 10% gels, which resolve well between 14 and 100 kDa. **Table 1** shows the composition of 6%, 7.5%, 10%, and 12% acrylamide gels.
3. Mix the components of the lower gel according to Table 1 and swirl to ensure thorough mixing. Once the ammonium persulfate and TEMED have been added, the gel will start to polymerize, so prepare the mixture immediately before use. Pour the mixture into the casting stand to about 4/5 of the height of the gel. Carefully overlay the gel with a layer of H_2O to exclude atmospheric oxygen, which interferes with polymerization. Leave to polymerize for about 45 min. When polymerization is complete, a clear line will be visible at the interface between the gel and the overlay. *See* **Note 5** for polymerization troubleshooting. Decant the water overlay and blot any remaining water with a wick of filter paper from the side of the glass plates.

Table 2
Composition of Zymogram Upper Gels

Reagent	Volume required per gel
Acrylamide:*bis* acrylamide solution	142 µL
Upper gel buffer	285 µL
50% sucrose	285 µL
H$_2$O	428 µL
Ammonium persulfate	14 µL
TEMED	— µL

4. Mix the components of the upper gel according to **Table 2** and after brief swirling, pour into the casting stand immediately. Insert the well comb, taking care not to trap bubbles under the comb. The upper gel polymerizes much faster than the lower gel (approx 5–10 min), so work as swiftly as possible. Leave to polymerize for about 15–20 min.
5. Prepare samples by mixing 5–20 µL of sample with an equal volume of sample loading buffer. Note that this buffer contains no reducing agents or EDTA, as these reagents would inactivate MMPs. Do not boil the sample, as this will also inactivate MMPs.
6. Assemble the gel in the electrophoresis apparatus according to the manufacturer's instructions. Dilute the upper and lower reservoir buffers and add to the respective chambers. The lower reservoir buffer can be reused several times. Load samples into the wells and electrophorese at 150 V until the bromophenol blue tracker dye reaches the bottom of the gel (about 45 min for a 10% gel).

3.2. Developing and Staining

1. After electrophoresis, disassemble gel apparatus and place gels in a plastic or glass container in zymogram renaturing buffer (approx 20 mL). Wash for 1 h, replacing the solution four times during this period (approx 4×15 min). Incubate one gel per container so that all areas of each gel are thoroughly washed. Place the gels on a rotary shaker, if available.
2. Rinse gels briefly in zymogram developing buffer, and then incubate in about 30 mL of this buffer at 37°C for 4 h or overnight. If incubating overnight at 37°C, ensure that the container is airtight to prevent evaporation. *See* **Note 6** for guidelines of incubation times.
3. Decant the zymogram developing buffer and add Coomassie blue stain solution. Stain for 30 min to 1 h, then destain thoroughly using multiple changes of destaining solution until the clear bands of MMP activity are visible against the dark blue background. The gel can be stored in destaining solution. For long-term storage, gels can be scanned or dried using a commercial gel drier.

3.3. Examples and Interpretation of Results

3.3.1. Molecular Species and M_r

Figure 1 shows Coomassie blue-stained gelatin (**A** and **B**) and casein (**C** and **D**) zymograms of recombinant MMPs. The gelatin and casein backgrounds stain dark blue, whereas the regions of MMP activity show up as lightly stained or clear zones. Gels A and C were incubated at 37°C for 4 h, whereas B and D were incubated for 16 h. Comparing the area of digestion after 4 and 16 h gives an indication of the substrate preference of the various MMPs. For example, although proMMP-2/MMP-2 are clearly visible after 4-h incubation (A, lanes 3–6), MMP-1 is only clearly visible after 16-h incubation (A, lanes 1 and 2 compared with B, lanes 1 and 2). This indicates that gelatin is a better substrate for MMP-2 than for MMP-1. Note also that much less MMP-2 (100 pg) than MMP-1 (500 ng) or MMP-3 (100 ng) is required to produce a similar zone of digestion. Comparing A and B with C and D, it is clear that gelatin is better than casein for detection of all three tested MMPs, with clearer zones of digestion evident. The main advantage of casein gels is that MMP-2 does not digest this substrate under the conditions used (D, lanes 3–6), enabling discrimination between this enzyme and other MMPs that may be present in the sample, for example MMP-1, (**D**, lanes 1 and 7), and MMP-3 (C, lanes 1 and 7). As discussed in Note 6, detection of MMP-1 and MMP-3 is more difficult on zymograms incubated for 16 h (**D**) than on those incubated for 4 h (**C**). This may be caused by diffusion of casein from the gel, producing a paler background with poorer contrast.

Zymography permits the detection of proteinases present within a sample by visualization of a zone of substrate digestion. This includes MMP zymogens and inhibitor-bound MMPs which are not active in the culture medium. This characteristic of zymography can be useful and has enabled the study of proMMP-2 activation by zymography *(6)*, but researchers must take care when predicting in vivo enzyme activity from zymogram data. MMPs are usually released from cells as inactive zymogens, which undergo processing of their propeptide to generate the lower molecular mass, fully active form. The zymogen is maintained by interaction of a cysteine residue in the propeptide and the catalytic zinc in the active site *(1)*. Treatment of zymogens with SDS disrupts this interaction, allowing autocatalytic activation of the zymogen when the gel is renatured and developed. Activity is thus seen at the molecular mass of the zymogen (e.g., **B**, bands **a, c, e**). This zymogram-dependent activation should not be confused with in vitro activation by proteinases or APMA, which is carried out prior to electrophoresis. For example, proMMP-1 (*see* **Fig. 1B**, band **a**, 55 kDa) is converted to active MMP-1 (43 kDa, band **b**) by treatment with

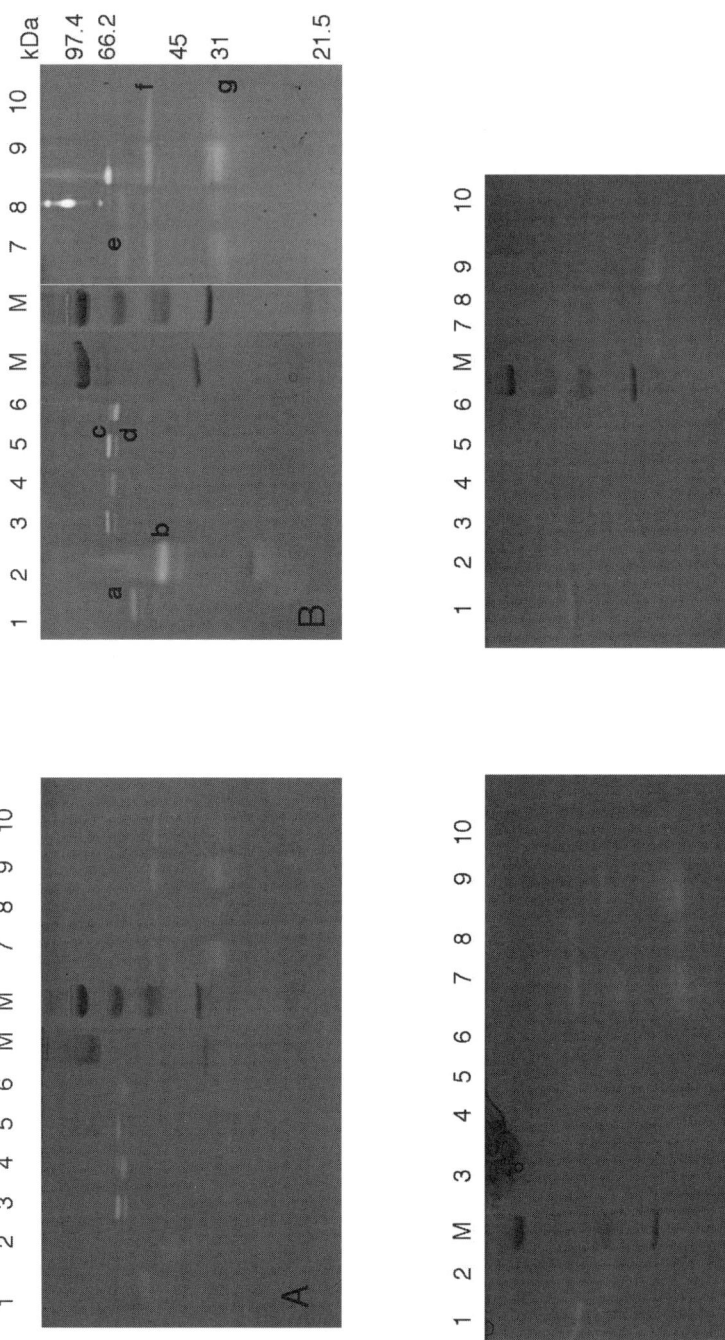

Fig. 1. Gelatin and casein zymograms of recombinant MMPs. (A) Gelatin zymogram (10% acrylamide, 4-h incubation at 37°C) showing migration of recombinant proMMP-1 (500 ng, lane 1), APMA-activated recombinant MMP-1 (500 ng, lane 2), proMMP-2/MMP-2 purified from the medium of human cervical fibroblasts (300 pg in lane 3, 100 pg in lane 5), APMA-activated proMMP-2/MMP-2 (300 pg in lane 4, 100 pg in lane 6), recombinant proMMP-3 (500 ng in lane 7 and 100 ng in lane 8) and APMA- activated recombinant MMP-3 (500 ng in lane 9 and 100 ng in lane 10). APMA treated samples were prepared by incubation with 1.5 mM

(*continued*)

APMA prior to electrophoresis. Furthermore, MMPs are often present in biological samples complexed with their natural inhibitors, the tissue inhibitors of metalloproteinases (TIMPs). These complexes dissociate upon treatment with SDS and as both enzyme and inhibitor remain immobilized at their electrophorezed positions during renaturation and development, they are not able to reassociate, enabling visualization of previously TIMP-bound MMPs *(6)*.

Whereas the position of the bands relative to the molecular mass markers can be used as a guide to their molecular mass, the incorporation of a protein substrate into the gel retards the migration of proteins through the gel in nonlinear manner, so that accurate assessment of molecular mass is difficult on a zymogram *(7)*. Standard MMPs, commercially available from numerous sources, can be run alongside the samples for comparison, as shown in **Fig. 2**. Alignment of one's band of interest with a standard MMP, although suggestive, cannot be taken as proof of identity. At best, zymogram analysis allows identification of, for example, a "72-kDa gelatinase." Because proMMP-2 has a molecular mass of 72 kDa, it would be tempting to identify a band of this apparent M_r as proMMP-2, but active MMP-9 has a similar molecular mass of 68 kDa *(8)* and these molecular masses cannot be reliably discriminated, especially given the reduction in molecular mass brought about by the protein substrate *(7)*. Further characterization, such as immunoprecipitation of the activity by a specific antibody, is required for unequivocal identification.

Proteinase inhibitors can be added to the renaturing and developing buffers to establish the class of proteinase responsible for the activity seen. For example, metalloproteinases are inhibited by EDTA (10 mM), cysteine proteinases by E-64 [L-trans-epoxysuccinyl-leucylamido(4-guanidino)butane 10 µM], serine proteinases by PMSF (phenyl methyl sulfonyl fluoride, 1 mM) and aspartic proteinases by pepstatin A (10 µM).

Fig. 1. *(continued)* APMA for 1 h at 37°C. BioRad low range molecular mass markers (M) are phosphorylase b (97.4 kDa), bovine serum albumin (66.2 kDa), ovalbumin (45 kDa) and carbonic anhydrase (30 kDa). (**B**) Gelatin zymogram (10% acrylamide, 16-h incubation at 37°C) showing the same sample as in **A**. Band **a** indicates proMMP-1 (55 kDa), which is converted by APMA-treatment to mature MMP-1 (**b**, 43 kDa). ProMMP-2 (**c**, 72 kDa) is converted to mature MMP-2 (**d**, 68 kDa) by APMA treatment (compare lanes 3 and 5, and 4 and 6). Recombinant proMMP-3 (**e**, 57 kDa) is converted by treatment with APMA to mature MMP-3 (**f**, 45 kDa) and the catalytic domain of MMP-3 (**g**, 28 kDa). Note that this recombinant proMMP-3 sample (lanes 7 and 8) contains some activated MMP-3 and MMP-3 catalytic domain. Zones of digestion are paler than in **A**, possibly because casein has diffused out of the gel during the increased incubation time. (**C**) Casein zymogram (10% acrylamide, 4-h incubation) showing the same samples as in **A**. (**D**) Casein zymogram (10% acrylamide, 16-h incubation) showing the same samples as in **A**. Zones of digestion are paler that in **C**, possibly because casein has diffused out of the gel during the increased incubation time.

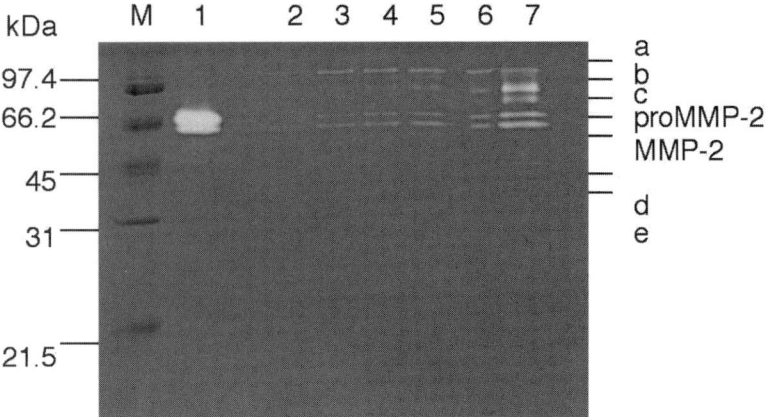

Fig. 2. Gelatin zymograms analyzing MMP production by cultured synovial membranes. Hyman synovial tissue, taken from various tendon locations, was cultured in vitro for 48 h according to standard protocols. Culture supernatants were collected and diluted 10-fold before analysis by gelatin zymography (10% acrylamide, 16-h incubation). Lane 1 shows recombinant proMMP-2/MMP-2 control (240 pg). Lanes 2–7 show increasing amounts of the one in ten dilution of culture supernatant. Lane 2, 2 μL; lane 3, 4 μL; lane 4, 6 μL; lane 5, 8 μL; lane 6, 10 μL; lane 7, 12 μL. The identity of bands **a** and **e** is unknown. Based on their size, bands **b** and **c** are likely to be proMMP-9 and MMP-9, respectively, whereas **d** is likely to be the 45-kDa MMP-2 catalytic domain, lacking the C-terminal hemopexin domain. Further diagnostic analysis (e.g., immunoprecipitation) is, however, required to confirm this preliminary identification.

3.3.2. Quantitation

Within a certain range, the area of substrate digestion is proportional to the amount of enzyme present. Using a known concentration of enzyme, one can construct a standard curve (such as in **Fig. 3**) and estimate the concentration of samples run alongside. Such studies require careful optimization and a prior knowledge of the identity of the proteinase analyzed. As little as 1–10 pg of MMP-2 (see **Fig. 3** and **ref. 9**) and 32 pg MMP-9 *(4)* can be detected on gelatin zymograms, whereas Gogly et al. *(10)* report detecting as low as 0.1 pg of MMP-1 on collagen zymograms.

4. Notes

1. Although we routinely use the buffer system described by Bury *(5)*, many other SDS-PAGE systems have been successfully used by others *(11)*.
2. Unpolymerized acrylamide is mutagenic, carcinogenic, and neurotoxin. It can be absorbed into the body by inhalation, through the skin and by ingestion. Consult the laboratory safety procedures before use and always wear gloves when han-

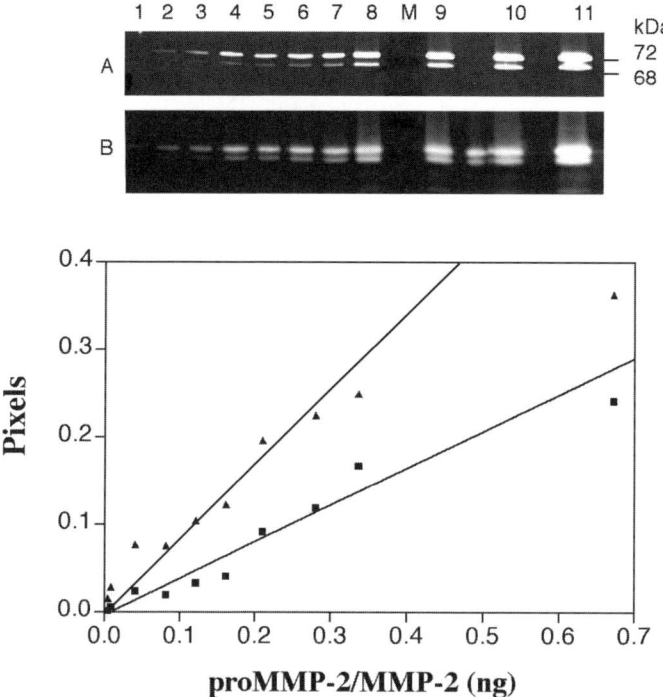

Fig. 3. Quantitation of proMMP-2/MMP-2 activity on gelatin zymograms. Various concentrations of recombinant proMMP-2/MMP-2 were analyzed on a 10% acrylamide gel incubated at 37°C for either 4 h (**A**) or 16 h (**B**). Molecular mass markers (**M**) are as in Fig. 1. Lane 1, 2 pg: lane 2, 4 pg; land 3, 8 pg; lane 4, 40 pg; lane 5, 80 pg; lane 6, 120 pg; lane 7, 160 pg; lane 8, 210 pg; lane 9, 280 pg; lane 10, 340 pg, and lane 11, 670 pg. Areas of digestion were quantified using a BioRad GS-710 Calibrated Imaging Densitometer and Quantity One (Version 4.2.1) software. The scanned image was inverted and the background subtracted, giving dark bands on a pale background. The pixels in the 72- and 68-kDa bands were quantified and plotted against the concentrations of pro-MMP-2/MMP-2 as determined by absorbance at 280 nm (extinction coefficient = 122 800 M^{-1} cm^{-1}). The relationship between pixels and enzyme concentration is linear up to approx 0.2 arbitrary pixel units in this example. The bands visible between lanes 9 and 10 in B originate from overflow of neighbouring lanes. This is a common problem with high concentrations of gelatinases and is best avoided by leaving lanes empty between samples, as shown here.

dling. To minimize risk of inhalation of the powder, it is safer to buy a premade solution of acrylamide and N,N'-methylene-*bis*-acrylamide. Do not dispose of unpolymerized acrylamide solutions in the sewer system—rather add ammonium persulfate and TEMED to polymerize, and then discard according to local regulations.

3. Other proteins that are digested by the MMPs of interest and remain soluble in the buffer system required for electrophoresis can be used instead of gelatin. Gelatin is the most widely used substrate *(6,12)*, as it is readily available, economical, and serves as a substrate for several MMPs. The sensitivity, however, varies depending on the MMP to be detected, and gelatin zymograms are far more sensitive for gelatinases (MMP-2 and MMP-9) than for collagenases or stromelysins (*see* **Fig. 1**). Here, we also give examples of casein zymograms, but other proteins such as collagen *(10)*, fibronectin *(13)*, and fibrinogen *(13)* have also been used. As an alternative to Coomassie staining of an immobilized protein substrate in the gel, a fluorescent protein or peptide can be incorporated and visualized using a UV transilluminator *(14,15)*. This method has the advantage that the gel can be visualized in the developing buffer, without prior fixation or staining. This permits the researcher to visualize the development of product over time and eliminates the uncertainty inherent in estimation of a suitable development time.
4. To ensure a uniformly stained gel background, the protein substrate must be fully dissolved before incorporation into the gel. Gelatin is soluble in lower gel buffer and casein is soluble in 0.1 M NaOH. Both solutions require heating to 37°C with occasional vortexing until no undissolved material is visible.
5. Crosslinking of acrylamide monomers by N, N'-methylene-*bis*-acrylamide is initiated by ammonium persulfate and accelerated by TEMED. Aging of the ammonium persulfate solution is the most common cause of failure to polymerize and we do not recommend storing the solution at 4°C for longer than 2 wk.
6. Many factors must be taken into consideration when deciding on an appropriate incubation time and it is often useful to test various incubation times to determine which one gives a reasonable zone of digestion with good background contrast. The incubation time required to produce suitable bands depends both on the concentration of MMPs present in the sample, and the rate with which they hydrolyze the protein substrate used. To analyze high concentrations of MMP, a 4-h incubation is often sufficient and we routinely incubate gelatin zymograms for 4 h when analyzing gelatinases. Longer incubation times will produce larger zones of digestion, which is desirable for low concentrations of enzyme, but inappropriate with high concentrations of a strong gelatinase (e.g., MMP-2), where overnight digestion can produce a smear of digestion behind the band, making it difficult to discriminate between adjacent zones. Increased incubation times are also sometimes accompanied by paler background staining, which adversely affects contrast. This may be caused by the fact that protein substrate is not completely immobilized in the gel and is able to slowly diffuse from the gel into the solution.

Acknowledgment

This work was supported by a Wellcome Trust Grant 057508. The authors thank Abhilash Jain for providing human synovium-conditioned medium.

References

1. Nagase, H. (1997) Activation mechanisms of matrix metalloproteinases. *Biol. Chem.* **378**, 151–160.
2. Barrett, A. J. (1966) Chondromucoprotein-degrading enzymes. *Nature* **211**, 1188–1190.
3. Heussen, C. and Dowdle, E. B. (1980) Electrophoretic analysis of plasminogen activators in polyacrylamide gels containing sodium dodecyl sulfate and co-polymerized substrates. *Anal. Biochem.* **102**, 192–202.
4. Leber, T. M. and Balkwill, F. R. (1997) Zymography: a single step staining method for quantitation of proteolytic activity on substrate gels. *Anal. Biochem.* **249**, 24–28.
5. Bury, A. F. (1981) Analysis of protein and peptide mixtures. Evaluation of three sodium dodecyl sulfate-polyacrylamide gel electrophoresis buffer systems. *J. Chromatogr.* **213**, 491–500.
6. Itoh, Y., Ito, A., Iwata, K., Tanzawa, K., Mori, Y., and Nagase, H. (1998) Plasma membrane-bound tissue inhibitor of metalloproteinases (TIMP)-2 specifically inhibits matrix metalloproteinase 2 (gelatinase A) activated on the cell surface. *J. Biol. Chem.* **273**, 24,360–24,367.
7. Hummel, K. M., Penheiter, A. R., Gathman, A. C., and Lilly, W. W. (1996) Anomalous estimation of protease molecular weights using gelatin-containing SDS-PAGE. *Anal. Biochem.* **233**, 140–142.
8. Ogata, Y., Itoh, Y., and Nagase, H. (1995) Steps involved in activation of pro-matrix metalloproteinase 9 (progelatinase B)-tissue inhibitor of metalloproteinases-1 complex by 4-aminophenylmercuric acetate and proteinases. *J. Biol. Chem.* **270**, 18,506–18,511.
9. Kleiner, D. E. and Stetler-Stevenson, W. G. (1994) Quantitative zymography: detection of picogram quantities of gelatinases. *Anal. Biochem.* **218**, 325–329.
10. Gogly, B., Groult, N., Hornebeck, W., Godeau, G., and Pellat, B. (1998) Collagen zymography as a sensitive and specific technique for the determination of subpicogram levels of interstitial collagenase. *Anal. Biochem.* **255**, 211–216.
11. Hawkes, S. P., Hongxia, L., and Taniguchi, G. T. (2001) Zymography and reverse zymography for detecting MMPs and TIMPs, in *Matrix Metalloproteinase Protocols* (Clark, I. M., ed.), Humana Press, Totowa, NJ, pp. 399–410.
12. Jain, A., Nanchahal, J., Troeberg, L., Green, P., and Brennan, F. (2001). Production of cytokines, vascular endothelial growth factor, matrix metalloproteinases, and tissue inhibitor of metalloproteinases 1 by tenosynovium demonstrates its potential for tendon destruction in rheumatoid arthritis. *Arthritis Rheum.* **44**, 1754–1760.
13. Feitosa, L., Gremski, W., Veiga, S. S., Elias, M. C., Graner, E., Mangili, O. C., et al. (1998) Detection and characterization of metalloproteinases with gelatinolytic fibronectinolytic and fibrinogenolytic activities in brown spider (*Loxosceles intermedia*) venom. *Toxicon* **36**, 1039–1051.
14. Quesada, A. R., Barbacid, M. M., Mira, E., Fernandez-Resa, P., Marquez, G., and Aracil, M. (1997) Evaluation of fluorometric and zymographic methods as activity assays for stromelysins and gelatinases. *Clin. Exp. Metastasis* **15**, 26–32.
15. Yasothornsrikul, S. and Hook, V. Y. (2000). Detection of proteolytic activity by fluorescent zymogram in-gel assays. *Biotechniques* **28**, 1166–1168.

10

Measurement of Aggrecanase-Generated Interglobular Domain Catabolites in the Medium and Extracts of Cartilage Explants Using Western Blot Analysis

Clare E. Hughes, Christopher B. Little, and Bruce Caterson

1. Introduction

Cartilage explant cultures and chondrocyte cultures have been routinely used to study the degradative mechanisms involved in joint destruction that lead to disease states such as osteoarthritis and rheumatoid arthritis. Stimulation of these culture systems with catabolic cytokines or chemical agents such as retinoic acid leads to an increase in the release of catabolites and enzymes into the culture medium. Detection of these catabolites using neoepitope antibodies can be used as indicators for the activity of degradative enzymes responsible for the breakdown of the tissue. Catabolites released include aggrecan interglobular domain (IGD) fragments, whereas enzymes include the aggrecanases (ADAMTS-4, TS-5, and-TS-1) as well as a number of matrix metalloproteinases. Monoclonal antibodies have been developed that specifically recognize the new N- and C-terminal amino acid sequences generated by aggrecanase cleavage of the IGD in aggrecan between ^{373}E-^{374}A (human sequence enumeration). These mouse monoclonal antibodies have been named BC-3 and BC-13 *(1,2)*. BC-3 recognizes the new N-terminal sequence ARGSVIL... and BC-13 recognizes the new C-terminal ...NITEGE in the IGD of aggrecan. These same amino acid sequences are not recognized in the intact molecule. Furthermore, the specific N- or C-terminal amino acid is essential for epitope recognition by these antibodies. Catabolites are separated by sodium dodecyl sulfate-polyacrylamide gel electrophoresis (SDS-PAGE) and transferred to a nitrocellulose membrane, which are then immuno-blotted with either the N- or C-terminal neoepitope antibodies.

From: *Methods in Molecular Biology, vol. 225: Inflammation Protocols*
Edited by: P. G. Winyard and D. A. Willoughby © Humana Press Inc., Totowa, NJ

A standard curve of immunostaining intensity vs dilution of a known amount of aggrecanase-generated IGD fragment for antibody BC-3 allows semiquantitative analysis of unknown samples. An example of such semiquantitative analysis could be used for assessing dose-dependent inhibition of aggrecanase activity by a panel of inhibitors.

2. Materials

2.1. Equipment and Supplies

1. Mini gel electrophoresis system, for example, Xcell Surelock Mini-Cell apparatus (suppliers Invitrogen).
2. Power supply (e.g., BioRad PowerPac 200, 200V, 2.0A).
3. Novex Tris-Glycine Gels 1.5 mm/10 well 4–12% or 10% (Invitrogen, Catalog number EC6038 and EC6078, respectively).
4. BioRad Mini Trans-Blot Transfer Cell.
5. Nitrocellulose membrane (for example, Schleicher&Schuell Protran Nitrocellulose transfer membrane 0.2 µm).
6. Filter paper (Whatman 3mm Chromatography paper).
7. Microtiter plate reader (for example, Labsystems Multiskan MS).
8. Flatbed scanner (for example, AGFA ARCUS II).

2.2. Reagents

All reagents should be of electrophoresis grade or equivalent.

1. Gel running buffer: 25 mM Tris-HCl, pH 8.1–8.4 (*see* **Note 1**), 192 mM glycine, 0.1% (w/v) SDS (store at 4°C stable for 3–6 mo).
2. Transfer buffer: 25 mM Tris-HCl, pH 8.1–8.4 (*see* **Note 1**), 192 mM glycine, 20%(v/v) methanol (store at 4°C. Can be reused up to five times).
3. Sample buffer: 0.125 M Tris-HCl, pH 6.8 with 4% (w/v) SDS, 20% (v/v) glycerol, 0.01% (w/v) bromophenol blue (store at room temperature).
4. AP Buffer: 100 mM Tris-HCl, pH 9.8, 100 mM NaCl, 5 mM MgCl$_2$.
5. Substrate solution: 10 mL AP buffer + 66 µL NBT + 33 µL BCIP. The BCIP/NBT Promega Color development Substrate (5-bromo-4-chloro-3-indolyl-phosphate/Nitro blue tetrazolium) is supplied by Promega.
6. Wash buffer: 50 mM Tris-HCl, pH 7.4, 200 mM NaCl, 0.02% (w/v) NaN$_3$.
7. Blocking solution: 5% (w/v) bovine serum albumin (BSA) fraction V supplied by Sigma A-9647) in wash buffer.
8. Antibody solution: 1% (w/v) BSA in wash buffer.
9. Deglycosylation buffer (1X): 100 mM Tris-acetate, pH 6.5. 10X = 1 M Trizma pH to 6.5 using acetic acid (*see* **Note 2**).
10. Chondroitin sulfate (CS) stock solution: 0.5 mg chondroitin sulfate C (sodium salt from shark cartilage, Sigma C-4384) in 1 mL MilliQ water (or equivalent). Store at –20°C.
11. Dimethylmethylene blue (DMMB; Serva catalog number 20335) solution: dissolve 32 mg 1,9,-dimethylmethylene blue in 20 ml ethanol overnight with orbital

rotation at room temperature. In a 2 L cylinder add 1.5 L of MilliQ water (or equivalent grade); 59 mL 1 M NaOH, 7 mL of 98% Formic acid. Add the dissolved DMMB to this solution and make to 2 L with MilliQ water. Stir for 2 h (*see* **Note 3**). Store the solution in a light proof bottle (Stable for up to 12 mo).

3. Methods

3.1. Preparation of Standard Curve Samples

1. Dissolve a suitable preparation of cartilage aggrecan in 100 mM Trizma pH 7.5, 50 mM NaCl, 1 mM CaCl$_2$, such that the final concentration is 1 mg/mL glycosaminoglycan (GAG) as determined using the DMMB assay (see later). Incubate 50 µL with 0.5 µg recombinant ADAMTS-4 (obtained from Genetics Institute, Boston, MA) for 14–16 h at 37°C.
2. Add 5 µL of 10X deglycosylation buffer to the 50 µL digest. Then add chondroitinase ABC (for example, Sigma protease free preparation; 0.01 U/10 µg GAG), keratanase (Seikagaku; 0.01 U/10 µg GAG) and keratanase II (Seikagaku; 0.0001 U/10 µgGAG) and digest for 2 h at 37°C (*see* **Note 4**). Dialyze the sample against MilliQ water (or equivalent grade) and lyophilize to dryness using a Speed Vac (*see* **Note 5**).
3. The resulting sample can then be reconstituted in sample buffer (at 1 µg/µL GAG equivalent) containing 10% (v/v) mercaptoethanol and a twofold serial dilution of this digest (equivalent to 20, 10, 5, 2.5, 1.25, 0.625, 0.3135 µg GAG) can then be separated on a 4–12% SDS-polyacrylamide gel as described later.

3.2. Preparation of Unknown Samples

1. Generate aggrecanase cleaved aggrecan IGD neoepitopes by treatment of cartilage explant cultures with catabolic inducing agents such as IL-1, retinoic acid, or TNF-α *(2)*. Media samples containing aggrecanase-generated aggrecan catabolites are processed directly. However, cartilage plugs should be extracted using 4 M guanidinium chloride using previously described methods and dialyzed against MilliQ water *(2)*.
2. Determine the glycosaminoglycan concentration of the samples using the DMMB assay as follows:
   a) Prepare chondroitin sulfate standards (0, 10, 20, 30, 40 µg/mL) from the CS stock solution (0.5 mg/mL).
   b) Prepare appropriate dilutions of media and cartilage extract samples from explant cultures. For example 20 mg wet weight of young bovine or porcine articular cartilage cultured in 1 mL serum free medium for 4 d would release 5 µg GAG/mg under control conditions; 25 µg GAG/mg in the presence of 10^{-6} M retinoic acid and 40 µg GAG/mg in the presence of 10 ng/mL IL-1. Thus, these samples would require dilutions of approx 1:4; 1:20; and 1:40, to be within the linear range of the standard curve (*see* **Note 6**).
   c) Add 40 µL of each standard (0, 10, 20, 30, 40 µg/mL in triplicate) into the wells of a 96-well microtiter plate and 40 µL of appropriately diluted sample into separate wells on the same plate (in duplicate).

d) Add 200 µL/well of DMMB solution and measure immediately at 525 nm using a microplate reader (e.g., Labsystems Multiskan, MS). Program the plate reader according to the manufacturer's instructions to calculate a linear standard curve and the concentrations of the unknown samples.
3. Take 10 µg GAG from each unknown media sample or the extract from an equal wet weight of tissue (*see* **Note 7**), add an appropriate volume of 10X deglycosylation buffer and make up to 500–1000µL with 1X deglycosylation buffer. Add chondroitinase ABC, keratanase, and keratanase II, as described earlier and digest for at least 2 h at 37°C. Samples can then be dialyzed (using 12–14,000 cut-off dialysis tubing) against MilliQ grade water and lyophilized to dryness using a Speed Vac.
4. The media samples can then be reconstituted at 1 µg/µL GAG equivalent in sample buffer containing 10%(v/v) mercaptoethanol. The cartilage extracts can be reconstituted in an equal volume of sample buffer (containing 10% [v/v] mercaptoethanol /wet weight of tissue). Boil the samples for 5 min.
5. Samples are then ready for separation on 4–12% gradient gels for catabolites detected using the mouse monoclonal antibody BC-3 or on 10% slab gels for catabolites detected using the mouse monoclonal antibody BC-13 as described later. *See* **Subheading 1.** for a discussion of these two monoclonal antibodies.

3.3. Gel Electrophoresis of Aggrecan IGD Catabolites

1. Precast gels should be assembled into the gel electrophoresis apparatus according to the manufacturer's protocol. Pour gel running buffer into the upper and lower buffer chambers.
2. Load prestained molecular mass standards (for example, Precision Protein Standards™ supplied by BioRad, molecular weight range 10–250 kDa) and aggrecan standards into the wells of one gel and unknown samples into the wells of a second gel. Electrophorese at 150 V until the bromophenol blue tracker dye reaches the bottom of the gel (about 90 min).
3. Just prior to the gels finishing, soak the nitrocellulose membrane and four sheets of filter paper/gel in transfer buffer.
4. Remove the gels from the cassettes according to the manufacturer's instructions and place in the transfer cassettes according to the manufacturer's protocol (BioRad system). Fill the transfer tank with the transfer buffer and transfer for 1 h at 100 V (*see* **Note 8**).

3.4. Western Blotting

All blotting steps are performed at room temperature with agitation on a platform rocker. Membranes are placed in flat-bottomed 15 × 18 cm trays (2/ tray). 10 mL of solution is sufficient for all incubation steps. 30–40 mL is used for all washing steps.

1. After transfer, remove the nitrocellulose membranes and block for a minimum of 1 h in Blocking solution.

2. Briefly rinse the membranes twice in wash buffer and incubate in primary antibody (BC-3 1:100 hybridoma supernatant or BC-13 1:100 hybridoma supernatant) diluted in antibody solution for 1 h or overnight (*see* **Note 9** and **10**).
3. Rinse the membrane briefly three times in wash buffer and then apply secondary antibody [Promega alkaline phosphatase-conjugated anti-mouse IgG (H & L)] diluted in antibody buffer (1:7500) and incubate for 1 h.
4. Rinse the membranes 3 × 10 min in wash buffer and then add substrate solution and allow color to develop typically for 10–30 min.
5. Stop color development with three washes in MilliQ water and dry membranes on filter paper.

3.5. Examples and Interpretation of Results

3.5.1. Standard Curve of N-Terminal IGD Catabolites

Fig. 1A shows a Western blot of ADAMTS-4 generated aggrecan IGD fragments detected using antibody BC-3 (recognizing the neoepitope sequence ARGSVIL...). Lanes 1–8 represent a serial dilution of the digested aggrecan (20 µg–0.15625 µg aggrecan as determined using the DMMB assay prior to deglycosylation). Digestion of aggrecan with ADAMTS-4 produces approx eight molecular weight species of IGD catabolites from 250 kDa to 45 kDa. The most prominent two species generated having molecular weights of 148 kDa and 70 kDa. All of the bands have the same N-terminus ARGS... as defined by their reactivity with BC-3. The heterogeneity results from variable C-terminal truncations. A heterogeneous population of aggrecan metabolites accumulate within the cartilage with age *(3)* and are present in the aggrecan preparation that was digested with ADAMTS-4. Subsequent IGD cleavage of this heterogeneous aggrecan population by ADAMTS-4 releases BC-3 positive catabolites. The smallest BC-3 positive catabolite resulting solely from ADAMTS-4 cleavage of full-length aggrecan (E^{374}-E^{1480}, bovine sequence enumeration) is approx 250 kDa *(4)*. The proteinases responsible for the *in situ* generation of C-terminally truncated aggrecan that are subsequently cleaved within their IGD by ADAM-TS4, so generating BC-3 positive fragments below 250 kDa, are unknown. In order to obtain semiquantitative data, the density of any chosen molecular weight catabolite can be calculated using commercially available programs, for example, NIH image analysis software (available from http://rsb.info.nih.gov/nih-image/). Density of bands may be measured as peak density *(5)* or integrated pixel density *(6,7)*. These values can then be plotted against the concentration of GAG loaded per lane and a line of regression generated. An example of such a plot is shown in **Fig. 1B** where the density of the 148 kDa catabolite was calculated and plotted versus GAG concentration/lane. A straight-line plot was obtained giving a linear regression value of 9.7. Similar analysis of the 70 kDa band showed that the density plateaux at the highest

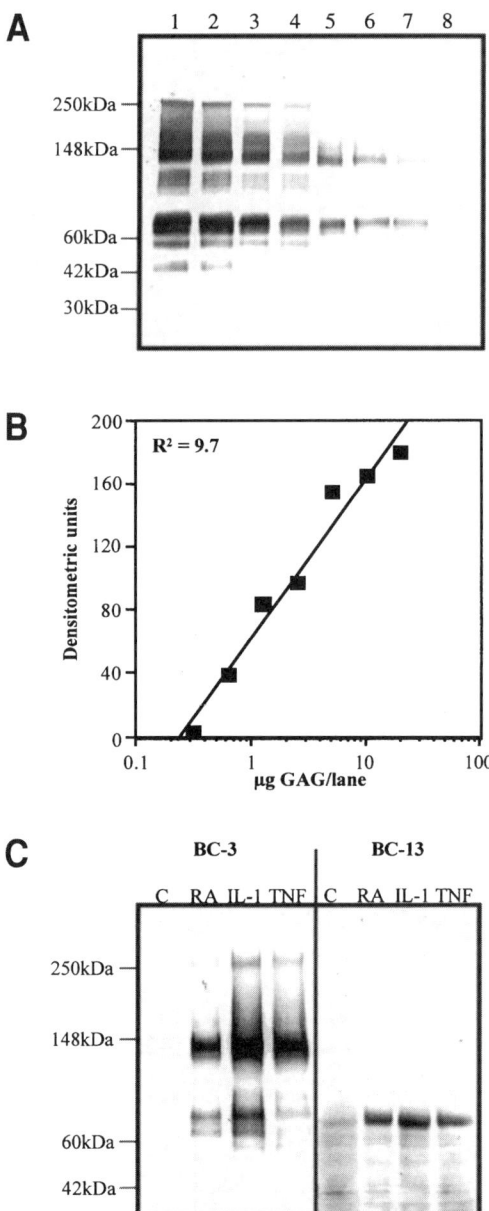

Fig. 1. Western blot analysis of aggrecanase generated aggrecan IGD metabolites. **(A)** BC-3 Western blot (4–12% Tris-HCl/glycine gel) of recombinant ADAMTS-4 digested bovine aggrecan. Twofold serial dilutions of aggrecan were loaded in lanes 1–8 (20, 10, 5, 2.5, 1.25, 0.625, 0.3125, 0.15625 μg GAG/lane, respectively). Migration position of pre-stained molecular markers are shown on the left. **(B)** Semi-log plot

3.5.2. Analysis of N- and C-Terminal IGD Catabolites Generated in Explant Cultures

Figure 1C shows Western blot analysis of IGD catabolites from the media (BC-3) and cartilage extracts (BC-13) treated without (C) or with either retinoic acid (RA), IL-1, or TNF. Analysis using monoclonal antibody BC-3 gave no staining in the control cultures. However, in the presence of catabolic stimuli BC-3-positive metabolites were detected. The range of molecular weights reflects those generated by the digest of aggrecan with ADAMTS-4 (*see* **Fig. 1A**). The BC-3 gels were loaded on an equal GAG basis and therefore increased band staining is indicative of a greater proportion of any given fragment. Hence, one would interpret IL-1 and TNF to be more potent catabolic agents than RA based upon the increased intensity of the 148 kDa band. This interpretation only applies for the experimental conditions used as biological variations could occur due to species or age of animals.

BC-13 detects the C-terminal neoepitope ...NITEGE remaining on G1 after cleavage by aggrecanases. These gels were loaded using the extract from an equal wet weight of tissue (1 mg/lane). A standard curve such as that generated for BC-3 in Fig. 1A could be generated from the ADAMTS-4 digest using BC-13. The BC-13 Western blot in Fig. 1C demonstrates that significantly more aggrecanase generated G1 metabolites are present in articular cartilage after catabolic stimulation. The coordinate increase of BC-13 and BC-3 positive metabolites demonstrate that primary cleavage of the aggrecan IGD by aggrecanases is occurring in situ in these explant cultures. Increased release of BC-3 positive catabolites may in some cases not be reflected by increased BC-13 positive catabolites in the cartilage extracts. This could be because of the fact that the BC-13 positive G1 metabolites can be released from the tissue *(8)* and/or further cleaved by other proteinases such as matrix metalloproteinases *(2)*.

Fig. 1. *(continued)* of the densitometric analysis of the 148 kDa band from (**A**). (**C**) Western blot analysis (4–12% Tris-HCl/glycine gel) of aggrecanase generated aggrecan IGD metabolites from explant cultures of porcine articular cartilage. Explants were cultures for 4 d in serum-free medium in the absence (C) or presence of 10^{-6} M retinoic acid (RA), 10 ng/mL IL-1, or 100 ng/mL TNF. For BC-3 blot of media samples, 10 µg GAG equivalent was deglycosylated and separated as described **Subheading 3**. For the BC-13 blot of cartilage extracts, 1 mg wet weight equivalents were deglycosylated and separated as described in **Subheading 3**.

**Table 1
Neoepitope Antibodies Recognizing Aggrecan Cleaved in the IGD by Aggrecanases**

Ab Name	Ab Type	Epitope	Reference
BC-3	Mouse monoclonal	ARGSVIL.	*(1)*
T767	Rabbit polyclonal	ARGSVIL..	*(9)*
R663*	Rabbit polyclonal	ARGVI...	*(10)*
Anti-ARG	Rabbit polyclonal	ARGSVIL..	*(11)*
71	Rabbit monoclonal	ARGSV...	*(12)*
BC-13	Mouse monoclonal	..NITEGE	*(2)*
Anti-NITEGE	Rabbit polyclonal	..NITEGE	*(13)*
AGG-C	Rabbit polyclonal	..NITEGE	*(14)*
I19C	Rabbit polyclonal	..NITEGE	*(15)*
Anti-ITEGE	Rabbit polyclonal	..NITEGE	*(16)*
RAM 3.2	Rabbit polyclonal	..NITEGE	*(17)*

*This antibody is reported to also recognize EARGSVIL.

3.5.3. Neoepitope Antibodies

Neoepitope antibodies recognizing aggrecan cleaved in the IGD by aggrecanases have been made by a number of laboratories (*see* **Table 1**).

It is important to consider species related sequence differences. For example the aggrecanase generated IGD neoepitope in mouse aggrecan is ALGSVIL.... and this sequence is not recognized by BC-3.

4. Notes

1. The pH of the gel running buffer and transfer buffer will be between pH 8.1 and 8.4. It should not be necessary to adjust the pH value.
2. Chondroitinase ABC requires the presence of acetate for maximum activity.
3. Check the absorbance of the DMMB solution against MilliQ water as a blank at 525 nm and 592 nm. Absorbance readings should be approximately 0.3 and 1.4, respectively.
4. The keratanase and keratanase II are essential for BC-3 epitope exposure.
5. This sample could be run on 4–12% gradient SDS-PAGE gels by direct addition of an equal volume of 2X sample buffer, rather than the described dialysis and drying steps. However, the larger volumes necessary for analysis of cultures media samples and cartilage extracts usually necessitates dialysis.
6. The DMMB assay has a short dynamic range and samples must be within the linear range of the standard curve.
7. To standardize the loading of samples on to the gels, different methods need to be employed for media and extracts, based on the particular aggrecan catabolites present in these two samples. In culture media, predominantly GAG-bearing catabolites are released, and thus in order to compare the relative abundance of

the different N-terminal neoepitope-bearing catabolites, these samples are loaded on an equal GAG basis. Control cultures release significantly less GAG compared with catabolically stimulated cultures, thus loading on an equal GAG basis removes the potential bias of analyzing significantly less aggrecan fragments in control lanes. In contrast, the G1-bearing aggrecan molecules retained within the cartilage matrix would be a mixture of intact monomers containing the GAG-attachment domains, and the free G1 domains that result from cleavage within the IGD. In control cultures, the cartilage extract contains a significantly higher GAG content than cartilage from catabolically stimulated cultures, therefore, these samples are loaded on the basis of an equivalent wet weight of tissue. For extracts, we routinely analyze 1 mg wet weight equivalents.
8. It is important to have the transfer buffer at 4°C as the ice block alone is not sufficient to cool the unit. We recommend use of the BioRad Mini Trans-Blot Transfer Cell system, as in our experience it has given the most consistent transfer results.
9. If comparisons between samples are made then incubation times should remain constant.
10. For experimental samples it is advisable to run "a no primary antibody control." Western blotting is performed exactly as described except that the primary antibody incubation step is excluded. Any band evident on the no primary antibody control indicates nonspecific binding of secondary antibody. This is particularly a problem with cartilage extracts from human tissue that may contain immunoglobulin. This problem is minimized by use of the Promega secondary antibody listed in the reagents section.

Acknowledgment

This work was supported by the Arthritis Research Campaign, UK and Wellcome Trust. Dr. Clare Hughes is an ARC Research Fellow.

References

1. Hughes, C. E., Caterson, B., Fosang, A. J., Roughley, P. J., and Mort, J. S. (1995) Monoclonal antibodies that specifically recognize neoepitope sequences generated by 'aggrecanase' and matrix metalloproteinase cleavage of aggrecan: application to catabolism in situ and in vitro. *Biochem. J.* **305,** 799–804.
2. Little, C. B., Flannery, C., Hughes, C. E., Mort, J. S., Roughley, P. J., Dent, C., and Caterson, B. (1999) Aggrecanase versus matrix metalloproteinases in the interglobular domain catabolism of articular cartilage aggrecan in vitro. *Biochem. J.* **344,** 61–68.
3. Vilim, V. and Fosang, A. J. (1994) Proteoglycans isolated from dissociative extracts of differently aged human articular cartilage: characterisation of naturally occurring hyaluronan-binding fragments of aggrecan. *Biochem. J.* **304,** 887–894.
4. Tortorella, M. D., Pratta, M. A., Liu, R., Austin, J., Ross, O. H., Abbaszade, I., et al. (2000) Sites of cleavage by recombinant human aggrecanase-1 (ADAMTS-4). *J. Biol. Chem.* **275,** 18,566–18,573.

5. Hughes, C. E., Little, C. B., Büttner, F. H., Bartnik, E., and Caterson, B. (1998) Differential expression of aggrecanase and matrix metalloproteinase activity in chondrocytes isolated from bovine and porcine articular cartilage. *J. Biol. Chem.* **273,** 30,576–30,582.
6. Sandy, J., Gamett, D., Thompson, V., and Verscharen, C. (1998) Chondrocyte-mediated catabolism of aggrecan: aggrecanase-dependent cleavage induced by interleukin-1 or retinoic acid can be inhibited by glucosamine. *Biochem. J.* **335,** 59–66.
7. Kashiwagi, M., Tortorella, M., Nagase, H., and Brew, K. (2001) TIMP-3 is a potent inhibitor of ADAMTS-4 (Aggrecanase 1) and ADAMTS-5 (Aggrecanase2). *J. Biol. Chem.* **276,** 12,501–12,504.
8. Sztrolovics, R., White, R., Poole, A., Mort, J., and Roughley, P. (1999). Resistance of small leucine-rich repeat proteoglycans to proteolytic degradation during interleukin-1-stimulated cartilage catabolism. *Biochem. J.* **339,** 571–577.
9. Billington, C., Clark, I., and Cawston, T. (1998) An aggrecan-degrading activity associated with chondrocyte membranes. *Biochem. J.* **336,** 207–212.
10. Vankemmelbeke, M., Ilic, M., Handley, C., Knight, C., and Buttle, D. (1999) Coincubation of bovine synovial or capsular tissue with cartilage generates a soluble "Aggrecanase" activity. *Biochem. Biophys. Res. Commun.* **255,** 686–691.
11. Sandy, J. D. and Verscharen, C. (2001) Analysis of aggrecan in human knee cartilage and synovial fluid indicates that aggrecanase (ADAMTS) activity is responsible for the catabolic turnover and loss of whole aggrecan whereas other protease activity is required for C-terminal processing in vivo. *Biochem J.* **358,** 615–626.
12. Cai, L., Yin, J., Starovasnik, M., Hogue, D., Hillan, K., Mort, J., and Filvaroff, E. (2001). Pathways by which interleukin 17 induces articular cartilage breakdown in vitro and in vivo. *Cytokine.* **16,** 10–21.
13. Lark, M. W., Gordy, J. T., Weidner, J. R., Ayala, J., Kimura, J. H., Williams, H. R., et al. (1995) Cell-mediated catabolism of aggrecan. Evidence that cleavage at the "aggrecanase" site (Glu 373-Ala 374) is a primary event in proteolysis of the interglobular domain. *J. Biol. Chem.* **270,** 2550–2556.
14. Sztrolovics, R., Alini, M., Roughley, P. J., and Mort, J. S. (1997) Aggrecan degradation in human intervertebral disc and articular cartilage. *Biochem. J.* **326,** 235–241.
15. Sugimoto, K., Takahashi, M., Yamamoto, Y., Shimada, K., and Tanzawa, K. (1999). Identification of aggrecanase activity in medium of cartilage culture. *J. Biochem.* **126,** 449–455.
16. Mercuri, F. A., Doege, K. J., Arner, E. C., Pratta, M. A., Last, K., and Fosang, A. J. (1999) Recombinant human aggrecan G1-G2 exhibits native binding properties and substrate specificity for matrix metalloproteinases and aggrecanase. *J. Biol. Chem.* **274,** 32,387–32,395.
17. Bayliss, M., Hutton, S., Hayward, J., and Maciewicz, R. (2001) Distribution of aggrecanase (ADAMts 4/5) cleavage products in normal and osteoarthritic human articular cartilage: the influence of age, topography and zone of tissue. *Osteoarthritis Cartilage* **9,** 553–560.

11

In Vitro Model of Human Articular Cartilage Degradation

William D. Shingleton

1. Introduction

Rheumatoid arthritis is characterized by inflamed joints with proliferating synovium and erosion of cartilage and bone. Eventually, loss of articular cartilage leads to a necessity for joint replacement surgery. Elucidation of the mechanisms of cartilage degradation are key to understanding the pathogenesis of rheumatoid arthritis.

Hyaline cartilage is a fiber-reinforced gel produced and maintained by surprisingly few chondrocytes. Articular cartilage consists of 70–80% water, which is held in the structure by negatively charged proteoglycans. The water creates a swelling force that is resisted by a scaffold of type II collagen fibers. Proteoglycans are held within this scaffold. However, water can move from a loaded region to an unloaded region and return when the compressive force is removed. This gives cartilage its unique load bearing properties (for review, *see 1*).

Proteoglycan is rapidly lost during cartilage degradation but can be readily replaced by the chondrocytes if conditions allow *(2)*. Loss of proteoglycan always occurs before collagen degradation can be observed *(3)* and once the collagen is lost it cannot be replaced. Therefore, cartilage collagen degradation represents the irreversible step in cartilage degradation *(4)*.

The study of human articular cartilage degradation in vitro can been hampered by availability of tissue; maximal use of what cartilage is available is, therefore, advantageous. Often, the most reliable source is from joint replacement surgery. This tissue is macroscopically variable. To maintain consistency, it is important to dissect only macroscopically normal tissue (*see* **Note 1**). Normal articular cartilage can be obtained from postmortem specimens. This tissue is preferable as it has not been subjected to degradative stimuli, but can be difficult to obtain. Cartilage collagen degradation in human articular cartilage is difficult to study because not all specimens respond. In our hands, only 50% of the specimens studied released collagen fragments and the maximal release observed was 25% of the total collagen contained in the tissue.

If human cartilage is not available, articular cartilage from porcine (pigs trotters) or bovine metacarpal or metatarsal-phalangeal joints could be used. These can be obtained from local abattoirs (*see* **Note 2**). Cartilage from these animals will be normal, but young. This should be considered when interpreting results.

A cytokine stimulus is necessary to induce the chondrocyte to degrade its extracellular matrix in a reasonable time frame. From animal models using bovine nasal and bovine or porcine articular cartilage, proinflammatory cytokines such as interleukin 1 (IL-1) or tumor necrosis factor-α (TNF-α) will induce cartilage degradation. These cytokines work in human tissue but to a lesser degree. Indeed these agents, although always inducing the degradation of proteoglycan, do not always induce collagen degradation in animal tissue. A combination of IL-1α and oncostatin M (OSM) *(5,6)* will always induce cartilage collagen degradation in animal cartilage and is the most successful combination to induce some collagen release in human articular cartilage.

As a measure of proteoglycan degradation, the release of glycosaminoglycan (GAG) is determined by a modification of the 1,9-dimethylmethylene blue (DMB) dye binding assay *(7)*. As a measure of collagen degradation, the levels of hydroxyproline (OHPro) are determined *(8)*. The quantity of GAG and collagen remaining in the cartilage is also determined and the results are expressed as the percentage of the total present in the sample at the start of culture (*see* **Note 3**).

2. Materials
2.1. Cartilage Dissection
1. Sterile scalpel handles and blades, rats tooth forceps.
2. Square Petri dishes (Sterilin, Stone, UK).
3. Dulbecco's phosphate buffered saline (PBS; Life Technologies, Paisley, UK) supplemented with penicillin (100 U/mL; Life Technologies), streptomycin (100 µg/mL; Life Technologies), gentamycin (50 µg/mL; Sigma, Poole, UK), and nystatin (40 U/mL; Life Technologies).

2.2. Cartilage Culture
1. Tissue culture plates (24 well; Corning/Costar, High Wycombe, UK).
2. Dulbecco's modified Eagle's medium (DMEM) containing 25 mM HEPES (Life Technologies) supplemented with glutamine (2 mM; Life Technologies) penicillin (100 U/mL; Life Technologies), streptomycin (100 µg/mL; Life Technolo-

gies), gentamycin (50 µg/mL; Sigma, Poole, UK), and nystatin (40 U/mL; Life Technologies).
3. Interleukin 1α (1 ng/mL; R&D Systems, Abingdon, UK).
4. Oncostatin M (10 ng/mL; R&D Systems).
5. Phosphate buffer: 0.1 M NaH$_2$PO$_4$ (0.1 M, 137 mL) plus 0.1 M Na$_2$HPO$_4$ (63 mL) check pH is 6.5.
6. Papain (BDH, Poole, UK): 25 mg/mL in phosphate buffer.
7. Cystine HCl (Sigma): 50 mM in phosphate buffer.
8. Ethylenediamine tetraacetic acid (EDTA) (Sigma): 51 mM in phosphate buffer.

2.3. Proteoglycan Degradation

1. 1,9-dimethylmethylene blue (DMB; BDH).
2. DMB buffer: 40 mM glycine, 41 mM NaCl, 9.5 M HCl, make up to 1 L with distilled water, pH to 3.0). Add 16 mg DMB and check the absorbance at 515 nm is 0.31. Store at room temperature in a brown bottle.
3. Flat bottom microtiter plates (Sterilin).
4. PBS to dilute samples.
5. Chondroitin sulfate (bovine trachea, Sigma; 1 mg/mL stock in phosphate buffer). This may be stored in aliquots at –20°C.

2.4. Collagen Degradation

1. Concentrated hydrochloric acid (HCl 12 N, BDH).
2. Hot block at 105°C.
3. Acid resistant vacuum dryer (Savant Speed-Vac, Life Sciences International, Basingstoke, UK).
4. Chloramine T (BDH): 7% w/v in water, diluted 1:5 in acetate-citrate buffer. Made up immediately before use.
5. Acetate-citrate buffer: 57 g sodium acetate, 37.5 g trisodium citrate, 5.5 g citric acid, 358 mL propan-2-ol per L of distilled water.
6. p-Dimethyaminobenzaldehyde (DAB; Sigma) 20 g dissolved in 30 mL 60% perchloric acid (BDH). Diluted 1:3 in propan-2-ol immediately before use.
7. Hydroxyproline (OHPro; Sigma. 1 mg/mL stock dissolved in water). This may be stored in aliquots at –20°C.
8. Plastic plate sealers (ICN Biomedicals, Basingstoke, UK).

2.5. Cytotoxicity Assay

1. Any commercially available kit, e.g., Cytotox 96 (Promega, Southampton, UK).

3. Methods
3.1. Cartilage Dissection (see Note 1)

1. Place the tissue in a Petri dish lid, and hold firmly with the forceps. Cut full depth cartilage from the subchondral bone. Place the cartilage slices in the Petri dish base and cover with a small amount of PBS.

2. Cut the cartilage slices into small pieces approx 2 mm^2 (*see* **Note 4**).
3. Wash the pieces 3× with PBS (*see* **Note 5**).

3.2. Cartilage Culture

1. Place three pieces of cartilage into each well of a 24-well plate.
2. Add 1 mL DMEM to the wells and incubate overnight to allow the cartilage to equilibrate (*see* **Note 6**).
3. Remove and discard the culture medium and replace with fresh DMEM with and without test reagents, four wells per treatment.
4. Harvest the medium at appropriate time-points (*see* **Note 7**) and replace with fresh medium ± cytokines. Terminate the experiment at day 14. Store media supernatants at −20°C until assayed.
5. Transfer the remaining cartilage pieces to screw capped tubes for papain digestion and immediately add 350 µL phosphate buffer.
6. Add 100 µL papain, 50 µL cystine HCl, and 50 µL EDTA solution (*see* **Note 8**) and incubate overnight at 65°C. Remove from incubator and add 450 µL phosphate buffer. Store at 4°C until assay and at −20°C thereafter.

3.3. Proteoglycan Degradation Assay

1. Prepare a standard curve from 0 to 40 µg/mL in 5 µg intervals. Dilute the 1 mg/mL stock in phosphate buffer.
2. Dilute media and papain digest samples in phosphate buffer (*see* **Note 9**). Add 40 µL of sample and standards to duplicate wells of a microtitre plate.
3. Add 250 µL of DMB solution to each well and read the absorbance at 530 nm immediately (*see* **Note 10**).
4. Determine the concentration of GAG (µg/mL) in the unknowns from the standard curve, correcting for any dilution used.
5. To calculate GAG release from the explant culture, determine the total amount in each well by addition of the GAG released at each time point to that in the papain digest. Express GAG release under the various culture conditions as a percentage of the total GAG:

$$\% \text{ GAG Release} = [\text{GAG in medium} / \text{total GAG}] \times 100$$

Four wells are used for each condition. Therefore the results can be expressed as a mean ± standard deviation. Different treatments can be compared to each other or control by using an unpaired, two tailed Students T test. An example of results obtained is given in **Fig. 1**.

3.4. Collagen Degradation Assay

1. Add 200 µL of medium or digest sample to a screw-capped tube, add an equal volume of conc. HCl, secure the lid, and hydrolyze overnight at 105°C (*see* **Note 11**).
2. Allow the samples to cool and pulse centrifuge the tubes.
3. Neutralize the samples by drying in the Speed-Vac. Once dry, add 200 µL water.

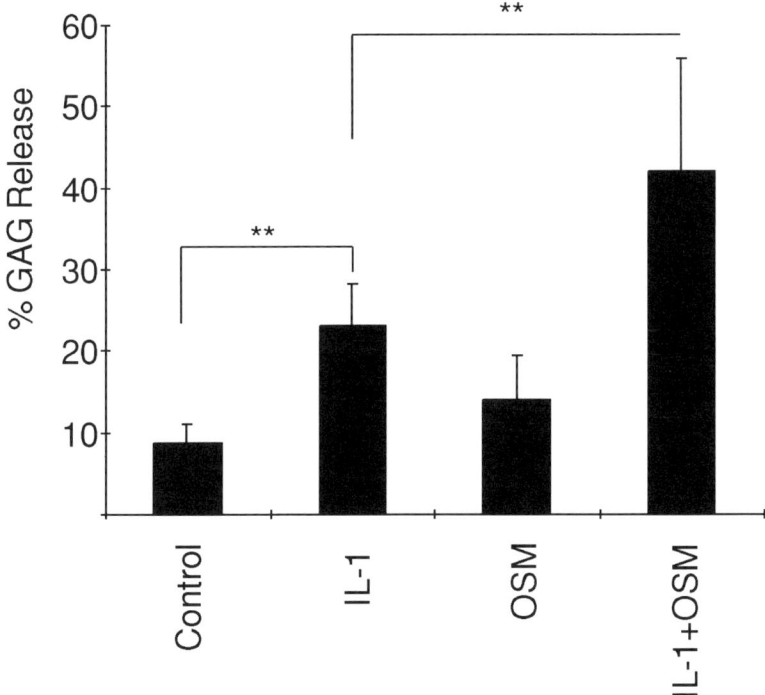

Fig. 1. Percentage release of GAG from human articular cartilage cultured in the presence of IL-1α (1 ng/mL), OSM (10 ng/mL), or IL-1α+OSM (1+10 ng/mL). Medium was harvested at d 7 following stimulation and assayed for GAG as described in **Subheading 3.3.** Data expressed as mean ±2 standard deviation. Statistical significance was tested using the Students T test (** = $p < 0.01$).

4. Prepare a standard curve from 0 to 30 μg/mL in 5 μg intervals by diluting the stock OHPro in water.
5. Add 40 μL of hydrolyzed sample and standards in duplicate to a microtitre plate. Dilute the samples in water if required (*see* **Note 12**).
6. Add 25 μL chloramine T solution to each well using a multichannel pipet. Note the start time. Wait 4 min since time zero and add 150 μL of DAB solution in the same sequence.
7. Gently wipe the top of the plate and seal with a sticky plastic plate sealer and incubate at 65°C for 35 min.
8. Allow plates to cool for a few minutes and read at 560 nm.
9. Determine the concentration of OHPro (μg/mL) in the unknowns from the standard curve, correcting for any dilution used.
10. To calculate OHPro release from the explant culture, determine the total amount in each well by addition of the OHPro released at each time point to that in the

papain digest. Express OHPro release under the various culture conditions as a percentage of the total OHPro (*see* **Note 13**):

% OHPro Release = [OHPro in medium / total OHPro] × 100

Results can be presented as described in **Subheading 3.3.5**.

4. Notes

1. Normal articular cartilage has a shiny off-white appearance. In older patients, the cartilage will be yellowish in color. The surface should be smooth and even in texture. Avoid areas that are roughened, scored, or worn away. If the appearance looks normal, but the cartilage seems swollen or thicker than normal, this may indicate that the collagen scaffold has begun to degrade and the cartilage volume has increased because of the swelling pressure created by the water and proteoglycan components of the tissue. This partially degraded tissue may also appear less shiny. This can be tested by pushing a scalpel blade vertically into the cartilage until it meets the subchondral bone. If the depth of cartilage is more than 2–3 mm the cartilage is best avoided or the fact at least noted. A cartilage that looks macroscopically normal is no guarantee that the tissue is normal if it has been dissected from a diseased joint.
2. Ensure you ask only for joints from legs that have been cut above the joint, to avoid the opening of the joint capsule. Trotters will come cleaned, as they would be destined for human consumption, bovine material will not. I recommend thorough cleaning away from the culture cabinet, followed by skinning of the limb. Great care is required when skinning to avoid puncturing the joint capsule. Once in the tissue culture cabinet, open the joint and proceed in a similar manner to that described earlier.
3. Results are expressed as percentage of total, to reduce the variability between replicates. It is very difficult to cut even-sized pieces of cartilage form the articular cartilage. There is no reason not to express your results as µg/mL if you prefer, but it must be remembered that hydroxyproline accounts for only 13% of the amino acid content of collagen.
4. You may prefer to score the cartilage while on the bone before slicing it off. However, it can be difficult to control the size of the cartilage chips.
5. Transfer the cartilage pieces to a 30-mL universal tube, fill with PBS supplemented antibiotics and allow to sit for 5 min. Repeat this twice. Contamination can be a problem with primary culture, this step both dilutes and kills any contamination that may be present. If possible the tissue should also be collected from theatre in a sterile container (Nalgene, 500 mL autoclaveable wide necked jar) containing approx 100 mL PBS supplemented with antibiotics. This keeps the tissue viable for up to 24 h as well as helping to reduce contamination.
6. The aim of this protocol is to create a model of cartilage breakdown; therefore, the presence of serum is avoided as it contains chondroprotective agents such as insulin-like growth factor-1 *(9,10)*. The absence of serum was also shown not to affect the viability of the tissue and cartilage in serum free culture for 8–9 d can respond to serum and other growth factors *(11)*.

7. To monitor GAG release, it may be necessary to harvest the medium at day 3 as well. For collagen degradation, it is unlikely that any hydroxyproline will be detected at day 7. However, some may have been released by day 10. There is no need to culture beyond day 14. If the tissue has not responded by day 14 of continuous stimulation it is not going to.
8. Mix 10 mL papain, 5 mL cysteine HCl, and 5 mL EDTA solution together. The papain suspension dissolves, and 200 μL of the combined solution can be added to each tube.
9. To estimate the dilution factor required prior to assay, dilute one sample from each of the four replicates 1:10, 1:20, 1:50, and 1:100 (or as required), incubate with DMB dye along with the zero and 40 μg/mL standards. Determine by eye which dilution will fall within the standard curve and apply to the sample and remaining replicates in the assay.
10. Plates should be read as soon as possible following addition of DMB and excessive mixing avoided. GAG/DMB complexes aggregate with time and will precipitate leading to a decrease in absorbance.
11. Hydroxyproline is an amino acid specific to collagens, which have to be hydrolyzed to constituent amino acids to allow assay of OHPro.
12. In general media samples will be on scale neat and digests on scale at 1:10.
13. To determine the total amount of OHPro released throughout the culture period, add the values obtained at each time-point before dividing by the total. Express results as cumulative release.

Acknowledgment

The author would like to thank the patients and orthopedic surgeons of the Freeman Hospital, Newcastle upon Tyne, and the Queen Elizabeth Hospital, Gateshead for provision of tissue at joint replacement. WDS was supported by a grant from GlaxoSmithKline.

References

1. Muir, H. (1995) The chondrocyte, architect of cartilage - Biomechanics, structure, function and molecular biology of cartilage matrix macromolecules. *BioEssays* **17,** 1039–1048.
2. Page-Thomas, D. P., King, B., Stephens, T., and Dingle, J. T. (1991) In vivo studies of cartilage regeneration after damage induced by catabolin/interleukin-1. *Ann. Rheum. Dis.* **50,** 75–80.
3. Billinghurst, R. C., Wu, W., Ionescu, M., Reiner, A., Dahlberg, L., Chen, J., et al. (2000) Comparison of the degradation of type II collagen and proteoglycan in nasal and articular cartilages induced by interleukin-1 and the selective inhibition of type II collagen cleavage by collagenase. *Arthritis Rheum.* **43,** 664–672.
4. Jubb, R. W. and Fell, H. B. (1980) The breakdown of collagen by chondrocytes. *J. Pathol.* **130,** 159–162.
5. Cawston, T. E., Ellis, A. J., Humm, G., Lean, E., Ward, D., and Curry, V. (1995) Interleukin-1 and Oncostatin M in combination promote the release of collagen

fragments from bovine nasal cartilage in culture. *Biochem. Biophys. Res. Commun.* **215,** 377–385.
6. Cawston, T. E., Curry, V. A., Summers, C. A., Clark, I. M., Riley, G. P., Life, P. F., et al. (1998) The role of OSM in animal and human cartilage collagen turnover and its localisation within the rheumatoid joint. *Arthritis Rheum.* **41,** 1760–1771.
7. Farndale, R. W., Buttle, D. J., and Barrett, A. J. (1986) Improved quantitation and discrimination of sulphated glycosaminoglycans by use of dimethylmethylene blue. *Biochim. Biophys. Acta* **883,** 173–177.
8. Bergman, I. and Loxley, R. (1963) Two improved and simplified methods for the spectrophotometric determination of hydroxyproline. *Anal. Chem.* **35,** 1961–1965.
9. Luyten, F. P., Hascall, V. C., Nissley, S. P., Morales, T. I., and Reddi, A. H. (1988) Insulin-like growth factors maintain steady-state metabolism of proteoglycans in bovine articular cartilage explants. *Arch. Biochem. Biophys.* **267,** 416–425.
10. Tyler, J. A. (1989) Insulin-like growth factor 1 can decrease degradation and promote synthesis of proteoglycan in cartilage exposed to cytokines. *Biochem. J.* **260,** 543–548.
11. Hascall, V. C., Handley, C. J., McQuillan, D. J., Hascall, G. K., Robinson, H. C., and Lowther, D. A. (1983) The effect of serum on biosynthesis of proteoglycans by bovine articular cartilage in culture. *Arch. Biochem. Biophys.* **224,** 206–223.

II

IN VIVO MODELS OF INFLAMMATION

12

In Vivo Models of Inflammation

Introduction to Part 2

Derek A. Willoughby

1. Introduction

This section is dedicated to in vivo models of inflammation, a necessary procedure for the discovery of appropriate usage of new therapeutic agents despite its problems (*see* essay later in this book by Professor David Blake). It is surprising that despite the increasing numbers of new antiinflammatory agents, of which none are perfect, there are certain models that are being used today under similar conditions to those described some decades ago. Such a model system is the acute inflammation in the mouse ear, which has recently been extensively reviewed by Professor Miklós Gábor, who has also contributed to this section of the book.

A further method widely favored by the pharmaceutical industry is the carrageenan-induced rat paw edema used in both rat and mouse. Dr. Chris Morris has described these methods. Indeed, it was using the carrageenan rat paw model that Charley Winter of Merck, Sharpe & Dohme demonstrated the antiinflammatory activity of indomethacin. This procedure is still a primary screen for new cyclooxygenase-2 (COX-2) inhibitors, as described in Part 3 of this book, in the chapter by Dr. Chi-Chung Chan. Certain groups use the rat pleural model of inflammation. In this, the carrageenan is not injected into the rat paw, but into the pleural cavity. The inflammation follows a similar time-course, the difference being that whereas the paw-edema model permits an easy measurement of paw swelling, the closed pleural cavity permits harvesting of the entire exudate, allowing quantification of the fluid phase and enumeration of the different cell types that have migrated. These inflammatory exudates and cells may be examined for expression of certain genes associated with the inflammatory response. The mediators may be analyzed over a complete time-course. This has led to the concept of a sequential release of mediators.

The use of the pleural cavity for the study of such mechanisms is described by Dr. Adrian Moore for nonimmune and different immune types of inflammation. It is obvious that if a compound is suspected of inhibiting a certain mediator or gene expression in inflammation, then it must be tested in the model when that system is active. However, it is commonplace to examine agents which are, e.g., alleged COX-2 inhibitors at one standard time-point in the paw edema model. Yet, if at that time-point there is no participation of the COX-2 enzyme and its products, this is obviously a time-wasting exercise. We have found over the years that different strains of rats have differing mediator time-course responses. Similarly different types of carrageenan will cause a differing time release of certain cytokines. Changing of the housing conditions of the test animals may also lead to a differing time-course of the release of mediators. Very importantly with an irritant like carrageenan, which exerts a proinflammatory effect by activation of the alternate pathway of the complement system, if there is an infection within the housing, those animals will have activated their complement cascade and will subsequently not give an inflammatory response to carrageenan, because of a depleted complement system.

These are obviously only a few of the factors that may result in differing responses from laboratory to laboratory. Yet all too often, groups measure anti-inflammatory activity to carrageenan paw edema at one time-point. It is tiresome, indeed time consuming, but each group should carry out detailed time-courses in which many of the proinflammatory factors are measured under their own local conditions. For such measurements, we suggest the use of a closed body cavity, say pleural cavity, or even an artificial closed cavity such as the air pouch, described by Drs. Paul Colville-Nash and Toby Lawrence. The labor of determining precise temporal and spatial distribution of proinflammatory factors is invaluable.

2. Cell Patterns in Inflammatory Exudates

It was recognized for many years that the pattern of cell migration during the acute inflammatory response was initially migration of polymorphonuclear leucocytes (PMNs), followed by macrophages or mononuclear cells (MNs). There were various hypotheses for the changing cell population in acute inflammatory exudates. In relation to joint inflammation, it was not known which cell was the precursor to the macrophage. It was widely assumed to be derived from the fibroblast of the tissues, suggesting it had not migrated. Subsequently, it was found that the inflammatory MN was derived from the circulating blood monocyte which, following migration into the extravascular space, divided, and resulted in macrophage cells. Today we are aware that not only are there specific factors attracting cell types to the site of inflammation (chemokines), but that the all important factors appear to be adhesion molecules for different leukocyte subsets, thus causing a specific type of cell to adhere to the vascular endothelium prior to migration.

The methods used to study some of these factors are described by Professor Mauro Perretti and Dr. Stephen Getting. This area is fascinating not only because of the underlying mechanisms for sustaining specific cell type migration, but also because of the actual dominance of different cell types during the evolution of the inflammatory response. Thus, the first cell type to migrate to provide an innate immune response is the PMN. This will actively phagocytose foreign material and these cells dominate the site of inflammation. However, shortly thereafter in nonspecific acute responses, the next cell to dominate in the exudates is the MN. This often is a dramatic switch in cell type. Now it has clearly been shown that a major contributing factor to this apparent removal of PMNs and replacement by MNs is not only a change in chemokines and adhesion molecules, but apoptosis of the PMNs. Once these cells are dead, they are rapidly removed by the MNs that act a) as a second line of defense and b) as workers cleaning the site of damaged tissue fragments, dead PMNs, to allow normal healing or resolution to proceed. Some of the methods applied to the study of wound healing are described in the following chapter by Dr. Annette Tomlinson and Professor Mark Ferguson.

The studies involving cell migration and cellular behavior are very interesting. It is important to stress to colleagues who may be brilliant genetic scientists or biochemists, but have little understanding of the basic inflammatory response, certain points. The most important of these is an appreciation that analysis of inflamed tissue removed at differing time points after its initiation corresponds to the examination of what is essentially a totally different tissue in terms of its cellular composition. Thus, at the outset, analysis of a pleural exudate would reveal certain factors–it must be appreciated that at that time point, these factors are associated with a tissue composed of PMNs. An exudate examined later will be composed of MNs, so that strictly one is not, on a cellular composition basis, examining like with like.

Further, factors that are potential traps involving cells in the inflammatory response are, in particular, the behavior of cells following different stimuli. If certain irritants are injected into the intradermal of subcutaneous tissues, they will provoke an ongoing inflammatory response known as a granuloma. This is the tissue that is formed in rheumatoid arthritis, and results in pannus formation that both invades and destroys cartilage, as described by Professor Sharon Wahl et al. and also by Drs. Paul Colville-Nash and Toby Lawrence. Histological examination following the injection of different irritants into the skin using a simple hematoxylin and eosin (H & E) staining could show similar onset of granulomas. However, more detailed examination of these sites will reveal that "irritant (a)" is initiating granuloma by constant monocyte migration and transformation of these cells into macrophages. "Irritant (b)" is initiating its granuloma by massive local proliferation of macrophages. "Irritant (c)" has produced a massive number of long-lived macrophages with no further contribution from migrating cells or local proliferation. "Irritant (d)" produces an ongoing onset to granuloma formation by a mixture of all three mechanisms, namely proliferation, migration, and long-lived cells. To study the effects of potential therapeutic agents on these types of experimental granulomata, obviously is fraught with hazard without a complete understanding of the cellular kinetics of the chronic tissue. Thus, if the experimental model is not dependent on migration, blocking adhesion receptor sites is not going to be effective. If the model is dependent on proliferation, it will require an antiproliferative mechanism.

As we move on to the study of chronic tissue, which has an innate ability to erode cartilage within joints, there are other factors important for its growth and development, namely angiogenesis or neovascularization. For any tissue that is rapidly growing, it needs nutrients that are supplied by the accompanying growth of new blood vessels. The blockade of their development impairs tissue growth. Drs. Chandon Alam and Mike Seed have described methods used to study angiogenesis. Angiogenesis represents another potential therapeutic target in that its suppression will block this aggressive tissue's progressive development.

It does seem that long-term treatment with such agents would be much safer with some type of targeting to the site of inflammation. Indeed, as we develop a greater understanding of the inflammatory process, one is drawn to the conclusion that many of the factors involved in inflammation may also have key physiological roles, thus requiring direct targeting to the site of the inflammatory response. It was of course the concept that COX-2 was expressed only at the site of inflammation that was so exciting, providing the possibility to have nonsteroidal antiinflammatory drugs (NSAIDs) with no gastrointestinal side effects. Indeed, the prediction of reduced gastrointestinal side effects thus far appears to be correct. Time will permit the full evaluation of these agents. Yet is inhibition of the inflammatory response (as expressed in the in vivo models) about to be described? The effect that we are searching for in RA and OA, are agents that treat the underlying pathology of the disease, not the symptoms alone, e.g., swelling, pain, heat, improve but cartilage degradation progresses or is even accelerated. Thus symptomatic treatment with NSAIDs improves the quality of life of the patient, yet, in fact, their inactivity on real pathological change may ultimately have an untoward long-term effect.

Many examples of chronic inflammation have a basic driving immune basis. Mention has been made of the pleural cavity as a model of both antibody and cell-mediated inflammation. A further area that is very important in terms of immune mechanisms is the process of graft rejection. Methods for studying this are well described by Dr. Isabelle Binet and Professor Kathryn Wood. With the ever-increasing numbers of grafts, there is a constant search for new immunosuppressant agents using the methods described by these authors.

Professor Brendan Whittle et al. describe a model of colitis, which may be used as a form of inflammatory bowel disease. These basic methods for studying the action of novel antiinflammatory bowel disease agents also suggest the need for studying side effects of existing antiinflammatory agents. Professor Whittle is an expert in this area of gastroirritancy.

The important topic of reperfusion injury and screening for effective therapeutic agents is covered by Professor C. Thiemermann et al. in two chapters where they describe in detail methods for drug discovery in antiischaemic cardiac reperfusion and kidney reperfusion. These are very important therapeutic areas and many groups are showing increasing interest.

In conclusion, it is hoped that the next section of this book will prove invaluable to those working in the in vivo area of inflammation. The editors recognize that there could have been many more such chapters.

13

Carrageenan-Induced Paw Edema in the Rat and Mouse

Christopher J. Morris

1. Introduction

Carrageenin, from the Irish word "carraigin" meaning Irish moss, refers not only to a species of red alga *Chondrus crispus* found along rocky areas of the Atlantic coast of the British Isles, Europe, and North America, but also refers to its mucopolysaccharide extract, discovered by the British pharmacist Stanford in 1862. The name was later changed to carrageenan so as to comply with the "-an" suffix for polysaccharides. Structurally, the carrageenans are a complex group of polysaccharides made up of repeating galactose-related monomers and are of three main types; lambda, kappa, and iota (*see* **Chapter 33, Note 1**). Each has their own gel characteristics which are all thermally reversible. The lambda form does not gel strongly at room temperature and is injectable to induce an inflammatory response. Inflammation induced by carrageenan, originally described by Winter *(1)*, is acute, nonimmune, well-researched, and highly reproducible. Cardinal signs of inflammation—edema, hyperalgesia, and erythema—develop immediately following subcutaneous injection, resulting from action of proinflammatory agents—bradykinin, histamine, tachykinins, complement and reactive oxygen, and nitrogen species. Such agents can be generated *in situ* at the site of insult or by infiltrating cells. Neutrophils readily migrate to sites of inflammation and can generate proinflammatory reactive oxygen and other species. The inflammatory response is usually quantified by increase in paw size (edema) which is maximal around 5 h postcarrageenan injection (*see* **Fig. 1**) and is modulated by inhibitors of specific molecules within the inflammatory cascade. The nonsteroidal antiinflammatory drug (NSAID) indomethacin is a clinically useful example (*see* **Fig. 1**). The model, therefore, has had, and will continue to have, a vital role in novel drug development.

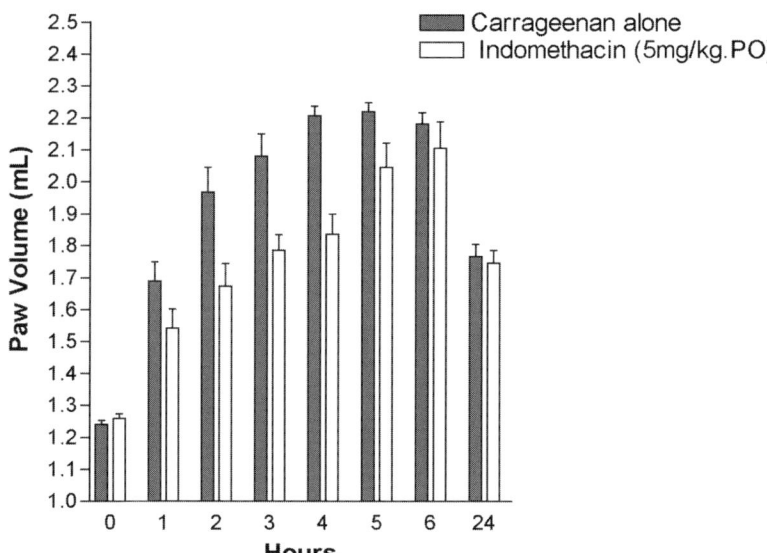

Fig. 1. Inflammatory response post-carrageenan injection.

2. Materials

1. Animals

Species:	Rat	Mouse
Strain:	Wistar, Albino	Swiss
Sex:	Male	Male
Weight:	165–220 g	25–35 g

   Healthy animals were kept in approved plastic cages, with metal mesh lids and bottoms, at a temperature of $20 \pm 2°C$ and were exposed to a 12-h light dark cycle. Food and water was supplied *ad libitum* throughout the duration of the study.
2. Carrageenan (lambda form, FMC Marine Colloids Division, NJ, or type IV, Sigma-Aldrich, Poole, UK) was prepared as a 1% W/V solution in 0.9% saline, no more than 24 h before use. Carrageenan powder becomes extremely sticky on contact with water and may form lumps that are difficult to dissolve. Complete solution of solid material is vital to prevent blockage of the hypodermic needle bore and potential injury to the investigator by pressurized ejection of the needle from the syringe or breakage of the syringe barrel in the hand (*see* **Note 1**).
3. 25-gauge hypodermic needles five-eighths-in long. Becton Dickinson, Oxford, UK. www.bd.com
4. 1-mL disposable plastic syringes. Becton Dickinson, Oxford, UK. www.bd.com
5. 100-µL gastight syringe. Hamilton Co., 1700 series, Cat. No. 81001 www.hamiltomcompany.com
6. Plethysmometer, Cat. No. 7150 www.ugobasile.com
7. Digital calipers with computer link. Digimatic 500, www.mitutoyo.com

3. Methods

3.1. Induction of Inflammation

1. Animals are weighed, randomized into groups ($n=6$), and kept for 1 wk to acclimatize to the laboratory conditions. This helps to keep stress levels low, which is important for the development of a good inflammatory response.
2. All animals were marked on the tail with an indelible pen for identification.
3. If required, test compounds are administered to animals at an appropriate timepoint before carrageenan injection. The timing will depend on the pharmacological profile of the compound or may be determined by time-course studies. Effects of unknown compounds are usually compared to reference compounds whose pharmacology and action in this model are known. NSAIDs [such as indomethacin (5 mg/kg per-orally)] are good examples (*see* **Subheading 3.5.**).
   This model is unsuitable for comparative studies where individual drugs cause a significant fall in blood pressure. This compromises the oedematous response.
4. Volume of preinjection paw/paws measured immediately prior to carrageenan injection. (For more details, *see* **Subheading 3.2.**).
5. 100 µL (rat) or 25 µL (mouse) of a 1% solution of lambda carrageenan in 0.9% saline is injected subcutaneously into the plantar region of the left hind paw. Injections are performed in lightly anesthetized (ketamine hydrochloride, 20 mg/kg, intraperitoneal) animals using a five-eighths-in, 25-gauge needle inserted into the pad region of the glabrous skin on the underside of the paw. The injection site lies close to the center of the plantar region, an important point in relation to the mouse which does not have a well-defined pad region on the underside of the hindpaw (*see* **Note 2**).
6. Carrageenan injected and control paw volumes are measured hourly as required from 1–6 h and again at 24 h (For more details, *see* **Subheading 3.2.**)
7. Animals are killed after the final assessment and paws removed by cutting at the tibio-tarsal level. Paws may then be used for a wide variety of assays linked to the inflammatory response, though detailed protocols are beyond the scope of this chapter. Paw tissue may be examined immunohistochemically or by *in situ* hybridization for cellular localization and quantification of specific proteins, i.e., growth factors, cytokines, tachykinins, or homogenized and extracted for the measurement of, for example, prostaglandin E2 and elastase activity *(2)* and cyclooxygenases *(3)*. Edema fluid may also be removed by centrifugation of whole paws and direct measurement of specific molecules made *(4)*.

3.2. Quantification of Paw Swelling

In the case of the rat paw, there are three commonly used methods, the one selected being dependent on equipment available and personal preference. Results from the various methods correlate well *(5)*.

1. The most basic method (which is not suitable for mice), requiring minimal equipment but much practice, is measurement of paw circumference (PC) by a length of cotton thread looped round the paw at the metatarsal level and gently tightened.

The loop is then carefully opened out and its length measured to the nearest millimetre with a ruler. Accurate measurement is dependent on near immobility of the paw and to this end rats are placed in a plastic cylinder (20 × 6 cm), and the tail and paws left free. The preinjection PC of the left hind paw is measured followed by hourly measurements of the same paw as detailed in **Subheading 3.1.6**.
2. Edema may also be assessed by measurement of paw thickness in the dorsal-plantar axis at the metatarsal level by caliper. The point of measurement should be premarked on the top of the foot with an indelible pen for reference at subsequent measurements. If modern electronic digital calipers are used, multiple measurements may be made at a given time-point and the results fed directly into a computer. An index of paw thickness is calculated as mean difference of paw thickness (Δ paw thickness/thickness of the contralateral paw).
3. The most convenient, rapid, and accurate assessment technique and the one most applicable to the mouse paw is plethysmometry. A plethysmometer directly measures changes in paw volume by water displacement and consists of two vertical water-filled interconnecting perspex tubes (*see* **Fig. 2A,B**). The larger one (A -18-mm diameter) is used to measure fluid displaced by the paw, a volume change that is precisely mirrored in the smaller tube containing a transducer. The transducer is linked to a decoder capable of digitally displaying volumes and/or feeding data directly to a computer.

The paw is immersed in vessel A until a fixed and visible anatomical point on the ankle and the chamber water meniscus coincide. At this point, several recordings are made. The most visible point at the ankle is the lateral malleolus and a line should be marked on the skin just above this protrusion with an indelible pen to allow easy and accurate repeated measurement. Accuracy is also helped by keeping the foot steady during the measurement process.

The volume of both the contralateral and injected paws can be measured at each time-point and a volume increase calculated by subtraction. A far simpler and equally effective protocol is to measure the left paw volume for each animal prior to carrageenan injection and then at hourly intervals (*see* **Note 3**).

3.3. Results and Statistics

Values are expressed as mean ± standard error of the mean (SEM). Data were analyzed by analysis of variance (ANOVA) followed by *post hoc* analysis with a one-tailed Dunnett's *t*-test for multiple comparisons. Comparisons are made with preinjection values or with the contralateral paw as appropriate to the protocol adopted.

3.4. Applications

Inhibition of carrageenan-induced inflammation has been shown to be highly predictive of antiinflammatory drug activity in human inflammatory disease and doses of NSAIDs in this model correlate well with effective dose in patients *(6)*. Using antagonists of various mediators of inflammation, Di Rosa et al. *(7)* showed that the inflammatory response to carrageenan consisted of three

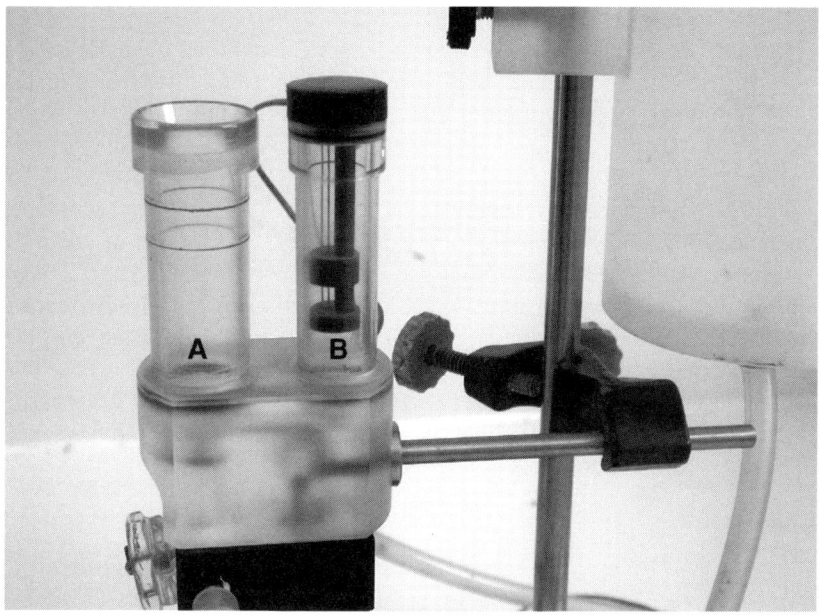

Fig. 2. A water displacement plethysmometer.

phases. The primary phase mediated by both histamine and 5-hydroxytryptamine, is followed by a secondary kinin-mediated phase notably the endogenous nonapeptide bradykinin produced by kallikrein. Novel histamine H_3-receptor agonists *(8)* bradykinin agonists *(9)* and bradykinin receptor antagonists *(10)* have been assessed in this model. The final phase is attributed to local production of prostaglandins (PG), especially those of the E series. The precursor of both PGs and thromboxanes is PGH_2, derived from arachodonic acid by the action of cyclooxygenase (COX) enzymes. Inhibition of these enzymes is the basis of action of the NSAIDs of major clinical importance in the treatment of pain and inflammation *(11)*. Carrageenan paw edema has, therefore, been a vital tool in the development of NSAIDs and recently developed novel COX inhibitors. A role for neutrophil derived reactive oxygen species, nitric oxide, and peroxynitrite in carrageenan-induced inflammation has also been identified and a number of specific inhibitors have been identified *(2,12)* which have potential clinical use.

Recently, the paw edema model has become popular as a model of localized inflammatory pain. Several behavioural and electrophysiological studies have shown that, after injection of carrageenan, initial edema development is followed by a period of allodynia, which peaks around 4 h after inoculation and lasts 24–96 h *(13)*.

The literature on pharmacology and specific modulation is extensive.

4. Notes

1. The lumpy carrageenan problem may largely be avoided by adding the powder to saline at 4°C and immediately stirring rapidly to facilitate even distribution. Any remaining lumps are very difficult to dissolve and should be dispersed by homogenisation. Warming to 50°C with stirring speeds up the solubilization process.
2. At injection, the needle should be directed along the center line of the paw for a distance of 6 mm in the direction of the toes and at an angle of about 5° to the plantar surface. The needle point should be bevel downward and a new needle should be used for each injection. Slow injection of the viscous carrageenan, followed by brief gentle massage of the plantar region with a finger, gives good distribution in the tissue.
3. Some authors measure the baseline foot volume immediately after carrageenan injection to negate the effect of the injected fluid volume. Experiments in this laboratory show that this is not necessary.

References

1. Winter, C. A., Risley, E. A ., and Nuss, G. W. (1962) Carrageenan-induced edema in hind paw of the rat as an assay for anti-inflammatory drugs. *Proc. Soc. Exp. Biol.* **111,** 544–547.
2. Rioja, I., Ubeda, A., Terencio, M., Guillen, I., Riguera, R., Quintela, J. M., et al. (2000) An inflammatory ditriazine inhibiting leukocyte functions and expression of inducible nitric oxide synthase and cyclo-oxygenase-2. *Eur. J. Pharmacol.* **397,** 207–217.
3. Nantel, F., Denis, D., Gordon, R., Northey, A., Cirino, M., Metters, K. M., et al. (1999). Distribution and regulation of cyclooxygenase-2 in carrageenan-induced inflammation. *Br. J. Pharmacol.* **128,** 853–859.
4. Smith, C. J., Zhang, Y., Koboldt, C. M., Muhammad, J., Zweifel, B. S., Shaffer, A., et al. (1998) Pharmacological analysis of cyclo-oxygenase 1 in inflammation. *Proc. Natl. Acad. Sci. USA* **95,** 13,313–13,318.
5. Eschalier, A., Kayser, V., and Guilbaud, G. (1989). Influence of a specific 5-HT3 antagonist on carrageenan-induced hyperalgesia in rats. *Pain* **36,** 249–255.
6. Otterness, I. G., Wiseman, E. H., and Gans, D. (1979). A comparison of the carrageenan edema test and the ultraviolet light-induced erythema test as predictors of the clinical dose in rheumatoid arthritis. *Agents Actions* **9,** 177–183
7. Di Rosa, M., Giroud, J. P., and Willoughby, D. A. (1971). Studies of the mediators of the acute inflammatory response induced in rats in different sites by carrageenan and turpentine. *J. Pathol.* **104,** 15–29.
8. Rouleau, A., Stark, H., Schunack, W., and Schwartz, J-C. (2000). Anti-inflammatory and anti-nociceptive properties of BP 2-94, a histamine H3-receptor agonist prodrug. *J. Pharmacol Expt. Ther.* **295,** 219–225.
9. Wirth, K., Hock F. J., Albus, U., Linz, W., Alpermann, H. G., Anagnostopoulos, H., et al. (1991). Hoe 140 a new potent and long-acting bradykinin antagonist. *Br. J. Pharmacol.* **102,** 774–777.

10. Asano, M., Hatori, C., Inamura, N., Sawai, H., Hirosumi, J., Fujiwara, T., et al. (1997). Effects of a nonpeptide bradykinin B2 receptor antagonist FR167344, on different in-vivo animal models of inflammation. *Br. J. Pharmacol.* **122,** 1436–1440.
11. Vane, J.R. and Botting, R. M. (1995). New insights into the mode of action of anti-inflammatory drugs. *Inflamm. Res.* **44,** 1–10.
12. Jadot.G., Michelson, A.M., and Puget K. (1986) Anti-inflammatory activity of superoxide-dismutases: inhibition of carrageenan induced edema in rats. *Free. Rad. Res. Commun.* **1,** 395–403.
13. Fletcher, D., Kayser, V., and Gilbaud, G. (1996). Influence of timing on the analgesic effect of bipuvicaine and epinephrine infiltration in carrageenan injected rats. *Anaesthesiology* **84,** 1020–1026.

14

Pleural Models of Inflammation

Immune and Nonimmune

Adrian R. Moore

1. Introduction

The inflammatory response is complex. It involves selective and temporal migration of specific cell types to the affected site, fluid exudation, and usually (given time) some form of resolution. These events are orchestrated by a plethora of mediators that act sequentially to give rise to the ever-changing pattern of pathology. Many of these mediators are now identified and we are beginning to understand at a molecular level the intracellular signal transduction pathways activated when cells are exposed to these mediators.

The immune system of mammals is broadly similar across species. Inflammatory mediators in rodents usually have counterparts of high homology in humans. Inflammatory models in rodents are, therefore, invaluable in investigating inflammatory mechanisms and for testing novel antiinflammatory therapies that may be applicable to humans. Nevertheless, care should always be exercised when extrapolating from animal models to humans and certain mediators will vary enormously in their significance across species.

Rodent models of inflammation need to be robust and refined so as to allow inflammatory exudates to be harvested at various time-points for cytological, biochemical, and molecular biological analysis. In this regard, cavity models of inflammation offer distinct advantages over the ever-popular paw edema *(1)* and cutaneous models *(2)*. Inflammatory exudates can be harvested relatively simply from the peritoneum *(3)*, pleural cavity *(4)*, and air pouch (formed on the dorsum of an animal by the simple subcutaneous injection of air) *(5)* . Inflammatory irritants can be directly injected into a cavity to produce a "nonimmune" inflammatory response. Alternatively, a variety of active immune hypersensitivity reactions can be induced by the injection of antigen into previously sensitized animals. Such reactions may be further dissected by injection of antigens into "naïve" animals that have received sensitized T cells or serum by adoptive transfer from sensitized animals. These are passive models in that the challenged animal has not been sensitized. The Arthus reaction can be induced passively by injection of antibody systemically and antigen locally. This mimics the situation in sensitized animals but it is more common (given the cost of antibodies) to reverse the routes of administration of antigen and antibody to give a reverse passive Arthus reaction.

The choice of which cavity model of inflammation is suitable for a given study depends in part on the species used and the question to be addressed. Pleurisy is technically difficult in the mouse (although not impossible). Murine peritonitis is, therefore, a popular model. In rats, where pleurisy is straightforward, accurate quantification of exudates volume is easier than in peritonitis where visceral organs interfere with exudate collection. Air pouches offer their own distinct advantages and are discussed in detail elsewhere in this book.

Only a few pleural models will be described here in detail, but once the technique is mastered, the reader will quickly become aware of its versatility and how to manipulate the model to their own ends. However, this versatility has given rise to a multitude of published models, the results from which can be difficult to compare. Even "standard" models such as carrageenan pleurisy can vary according to the type of carrageenan used, its batch, amount injected, strain of animal, and so on. The reader is advised to use the literature as a guide but not to select specific time-points for study without first establishing a full time-course in their own laboratory.

2. Materials

All reagents may be purchased from Sigma Chemical Co. (Poole, Dorset, UK) unless otherwise stated.

3. Methods
3.1. General Method for Pleurisy Induction

1. Male Wistar rats (B&K Universal Ltd, Aldborough, Hull, UK) from about 180–220 g are ideal subjects. In any individual experiment, the weight range should be no more than about 20 g.
2. Rats are anesthetised with a suitable gaseous anesthetic such as halothane or isofluorane.
3. The animal is laid on its right flank and the skin over the thorax moisted with 70% ethanol.
4. A small cut is made to expose the intercostal muscles.
5. A 21-gauge needle that has been reduced in length to about 6 mm (bend and

break the needle at the appropriate point) is used to inject the irritant into the pleural cavity at the level of the fifth to sixth intercostals space (*see* **Note 1**).
6. The wound is closed with a wound-closure clip or with tissue glue and the animal allowed to recover from the anesthetic.
7. At time intervals appropriate to the experiment, animals are killed by overexposure to anesthetic.
8. The musculature of the thorax and upper abdomen is exposed and the muscle incised to reveal the xiphisternum. This should be gripped firmly with forceps and the diaphragm perforated just below the cartilage. Two cuts either side of the sternum enable a flap to be reflected to reveal the thoracic cavity.
9. 1 mL of phosphate-buffered saline (PBS) containing an anticoagulant such as heparin at 10 U/mL is introduced to the cavity.
10. Using a plastic Pasteur pipet, the exudates can be recovered into suitable tubes (*see* **Notes 2–6**).
11. The volume of recovered exudates can be determined either by collection into graduated tubes or by collecting into weight matched tubes and noting the change in weight.
12. Cells may be counted by hand using a hemocytometer or more conveniently using a Coulter counter.
13. The recovered exudate volume multiplied by the cell count/mL gives the total cells.
14. The true exudate volume can be calculated from the recovered exudate volume by subtraction of the 1 mL lavage volume.
15. Differential cell counts can be performed on smears or cytospin preparations (*see* **Note 7**).

3.2. Carrageenan Pleurisy (6) (see Notes 8–11)

1. Lambda carrageenan is prepared as a 1% solution in sterile saline.
2. 0.15 mL is injected intrapleurally.
3. The inflammatory response peaks at about 24 h.

3.3. Pleurisy Induced by Crystals (see Note 12)

A number of arthritic conditions result in crystal deposition. These include gout (urate crystals), pseudogout (calcium pyrophosphate), and osteoarthritis (hydroxyapatite). The inflammatory potential of these crystals can be readily assessed by injection in to the pleural cavity.

1. Monosodium urate crystals are prepared by boiling an equal mix of 0.03 M uric acid and 0.03 M sodium hydroxide. After filtering through a 3-µm Acropor membrane filter (AN-3000, Gelman, Ann Arbor, MI), sodium chloride is added to a concentration of 0.1 M to accelerate and improve the quality of the crystals (7).
2. Calcium pyrophosphate dihydrate crystals are prepared by mixing a calcium nitrate solution (0.1 M final concentration) with acidified sodium pyrophosphate (0.025 M final concentration in $Na_2P_2O_7$ and 0.03 M HNO_3). Crystals form after about 1 d at 60°C.

3. Any pyrogenic contaminants can be inactivated by heating the crystals to 180°C for 3 h.
4. Crystals for injection should have an average length of about 10 µm. Morphology can be checked by scanning electron microscopy and the purity checked by X-ray diffraction.
5. Prepare a 1% suspension in sterile saline for intrapleural injection (*see* **Note 13**). Sonicate to prevent clumping and mix continuously to avoid sedimentation.
6. Inject 1 mL into the pleural space.
7. Crystal inflammation tends to be maximal at 6–12 h.

3.4. Methylated Bovine Serm Albumin (mBSA) Pleurisy (10) (see Notes 14 and 15)

1. mBSA is prepared in sterile saline at 10 mg/mL (*see* **Note 16**). This is mixed to an emulsion with an equal volume of incomplete Freund's adjuvant (IFA).
2. Rats are anesthetised with a gaseous anaesthetic and the base of the tail is shaved.
3. Rats are injected intradermally with 0.1 mL of the mBSA/IFA emulsion at the base of the tail (*see* **Note 17**).
4. After 12 d, rats are injected intrapleurally with 0.1 mL of mBSA prepared in sterile saline at 10 mg/mL.
5. The inflammatory response peaks between 24 and 48 h.

3.5. Reverse Passive Arthus (RPA) Reaction (11) (see Notes 18–20)

1. Rats are anesthetised with a suitable gaseous anaesthetic.
2. BSA is prepared at 5 mg/mL in sterile saline. A volume of 0.2 mL is injected intravenously.
3. After 20 min, rats are again anesthetised and injected intrapleurally with 0.2 mL polyclonal rabbit anti-BSA antibody at 1 mg/mL in sterile saline.
4. The inflammatory response peaks at about 6 h.

4. Notes

1. The blunted needle aforementioned creates a resistance when pushing through into the pleural space. A distinct "pop" is felt as the needle passes through allowing the experimenter to know that the needle is correctly placed. The rounded tip also minimises the chances of injecting directly into the lungs.
2. Blood contaminated exudates should be rejected.
3. For biochemical analysis exudates should be collected onto ice and centrifugation used to prepare cell free exudate and cell pellets.
4. It may be necessary to include a standard protease inhibitory cocktail in the lavage solution to protect polypeptide mediators, enzymes, and other proteins from degradation. Cell pellets treated in this way are suitable for Western blotting.
5. *Ex vivo* production of inflammatory mediators into exudates may be minimized by incorporating appropriate inhibitors in the lavage solution. For example,

indomethacin is often included in the lavage when exudates are to be assayed for cyclooxygenase products.
6. Exudate cells may be removed for cell culture ex vivo. In which case, cell culture medium may be more appropriate than PBS for lavage.
7. In addition to routine cytological analysis, cell preparations may be used for immunocytochemistry, enzyme cytochemistry or *in situ* hybridization.
8. Carrageenan is a natural extract from seaweed and will be subject to batch variation.
9. Carrageenan exists in many forms, lambda carrageenan is described as nongelling.
10. Carrageenan provokes a complement dependent inflammation.
11. Considerable literature exists on the action of drugs on carrageenan induced inflammation although the majority of this is using the paw edema model.
12. Calcium pyrophosphate dihydrate crystals produce a complement independent inflammatory response *(9)*.
13. Crystals are usually injected as a weight/volume suspension. Care should be taken in comparing responses to different crystals because in addition to their chemical composition, numbers of crystals and their size will affect the magnitude of the response.
14. mBSA has direct irritant properties. In nonsensitized animals this response has resolved by 24 h. In sensitized animals, the continuing inflammation at 24 h is representative of a delayed type hypersensitivity reaction.
15. If studies are being conducted with immunomodulators, dosing over the period of sensitization or over the challenge period may provide useful information as to mode of action.
16. mBSA is not readily soluble, but will form an opalescent solution.
17. A good intradermal injection will appear white and is clearly visible under the epidermis.
18. RPA is quicker and more convenient than active sensitization protocols provided the investigator is not concerned with antigen uptake and presentation.
19. A variety of protein antigens and antibodies can be used in this procedure. Immunoglobulins and antiimmunoglobulin antisera are popular and readily available commercially. If a monoclonal antibody is contemplated, ensure it is of a complement fixing isotype.
20. Amounts of antigen and antibody administered should be taken as a guide and some preliminary dose ranging studies are recommended.

References

1. Winter, C. A., Risley, E. A., and Nuss, G. W. (1963) Anti-inflammatory and antipyretic activities of indomethacin 1-(p chlorobenzoyl)-5-methoxy-2-methyl-indole-3-acetic acid. 369–376.
2. Eipert, E. F. and Miller, H. C. (1975) Contact sensitivity in mice measured with thymidine labeled lymphocytes. *Immunol. Commun.* **4,** 361–372.

3. Murch, A. R. and Papadimitriou, J. M. (1981) The kinetics of murine peritoneal macrophage replication. *J. Pathol.* **133,** 177–183.
4. Spector, W. G. and Willoughby, D. A. (1957) Histamine and 5 hydroxytryptamine in experimental pleurisy. 57–65.
5. Selye, H. (1953) On the mechanism through which hydrocortisone affects the resistance of tissue to injury.1207–1213.
6. Di Rosa, M. Giroud, J.-P., and Willoughby, D. A. (1971) Studies on the mediators of the acute inflammatory response induced in rats in different sites by carrageenan and turpentine. *J. Pathol.* **104,** 15–29.
7. Roberge, C. J., de Medicis, R., Dayer, J.-M., Rola-Pleszczynski, M., Naccache, P. H. and Poubelle, P. E. (1994) Crystal induced neutrophil activation. V. Differential production of biologically active IL-1 and IL-1 receptor antagonist. *J. Immunol.* **152,** 5485–5494.
8. Denko, C. W. and Whitehouse, M. W. (1976) Experimental inflammation induced by naturally occurring microcrystalline calcium salts. *J. Rheumatol.* **3,** 54–62.
9. Willoughby, D. A., Dunn, C. J., Yamamoto, S., Capasso, F., Deporter, D. A., and Giroud, J. P. (1975) Calcium pyrophosphate-induced pleurisy in rats: a new model of acute inflammation. *Agents Actions* **43,** 221–224.
10. Willis, D., Moore, A. R., and Willoughby, D. A. (2000) Heme oxygenase isoform expression in cellular and antibody-mediated models of acute inflammation in the rat. *J. Pathol.* **190,** 627–634.
11. Yamamoto, S., Dunn, C. J., Deporter, D. A., Capasso, F., Willoughby, D. A., and Huskisson, E. C. (1975) A model for the quantitative study of Arthus (immunologic) hypersensitivity in rats. *Agents Actions* **5,** 374–377.

15

Models of Acute Inflammation in the Ear

Miklós Gábor

1. Introduction

Methods were earlier described *(1)* for the determination of proinflammatory mediators and biochemical markers, models of acute inflammation and pain (use of implanted sponges to study the acute inflammatory response, pleurisy and pouch models, and so on), models of nonarthritic inflammatory disorders and tissue injury (cutaneous models, eye models, models of acute pulmonary inflammation, animal models of inflammatory bowel disease, and so on), and animal models of arthritis (rat adjuvant arthritis, chronic remittent erosive arthritis, monoarticular antigen-induced arthritis, and cartilage proteoglycan-induced arthritis).

Additional inflammation models were recently published *(2)*: comparison of adjuvant and streptococcal cell wall-induced arthritis in the rat, murine collagen-induced arthritis, angiogenesis, allergen-induced airway inflammation and airway hyperreactivity in mice, skin inflammation, and so on.

As concerns pharmacological applications, ear edema induced by different irritants provides a range of skin inflammation models suitable for the evaluation of both topically and systemically administered synthetic agents, substances of plant origin, plant extracts, marine products, and so on *(3)*.

The topical route of administration of different drugs (e.g., corticosteroids) is preferred in eczema, atopic and seborrheic dermatitis, psoriasis, and other conditions.

Many models of inflammation have been developed; those that involve the skin offer particular advantages: 1) The ear model is a quick and simple method; 2) it requires small quantities of substances; 3) it provides well-reproducible results; and 4) it is accompanied by low possibilities of error and gives rapid results.

For studies of the antiinflammatory effects of different agents, we earlier also developed combined models *(4–6)*. Simultaneously with the induction of carrageenan or zymosan paw edema in rats, an acetone solution of croton oil was applied to the ear of the same animals.

Our methods have various advantages: 1) the rapid performance of screening tests; 2) time saving; 3) the more economic use of the experimental animals; and 4) the simplicity of the technique. Details of these models will be reviewed in this chapter.

2. Materials *(see* Note 1)

1. Croton oil (Sigma Chemical Co.). Light-sensitive. Solutions in acetone are made fresh as required. Toxic on inhalation, in contact with the skin, and if swallowed. Irritating to the eyes and respiratory system. Possible risk of irreversible effects. Possible carcinogen. Stored at room temperature.
2. 12-0-Tetradecanoylphorbol 13-acetate (TPA) (Sigma Chemical Co., St. Louis, MO). Approximately 99% (TLC). Keep under argon. Sensitive to humidity. Stock solutions can be stored at $-20°C$ for several months. TPA is a potent inflammatory agent and known tumor promoter. Use appropriate safety procedures. Stored at $-18°C$.
3. Cantharidin (Sigma Chemical Co.). Light-sensitive. Humidity-sensitive. Cantharidin is an epidermal irritant and produces vesicles and bullae on human skin. Stored at room temperature.
4. Mustard oil (Merck KGaA, Darmstadt, Germany). Allyl isothiocyanate. Flammable, toxic. It produces a prompt skin irritation. Longer contact may result in vesication. As vapor, as oil or in solution, it causes strong irritation of the conjunctival, nasal, and bronchial mucosae. Store at $+2°C$ to $+8°C$.
5. Arachidonic acid (Sigma Chemical Co.). Purity approx 99% (capillary GC), from porcine liver. Solutions are kept under nitrogen. Stored below $0°C$.
6. Dithranol (anthralin). (Hermal, Kurt Herrmann, Hamburg, Germany). Light-sensitive. Dithranol is a powerful irritant and should be kept away from the eyes and tender parts of the skin. Severe dermatitis may occur with a solution of 2%. Solutions should be prepared fresh daily. Stored in airtight containers in a refrigerator at $4°C$.
7. Ethyl phenylpropiolate (Sigma-Aldrich Chemical Co., Sheboygan, WI). Purity 98%. May be harmful on inhalation, ingestion, or skin absorption. May cause skin and eye irritation. Stored in airtight containers in a refrigerator at $4°C$.
8. Mezerein (Sigma Chemical Co.). From the plant of *Daphne mezerium*. A second-stage tumor promoter and inflammatory agent. Stored at $-0°C$.
9. Zymosan from *Saccharomyces cerevisiae* (Sigma Chemical Co.). The suspension is made fresh as required. Stored at $+2°C$ to $+8°C$.
10. Capsaicin (Fluka S.A., Buchs, Switzerland). Natural; ~65% (HPLC). Sensitive to air. Toxic if swallowed. Irritating to eyes and skin. Stored at $4°C$.
11. Carrageenan (Sodium carrageenan; Viscarin, Marine Colloids Inc., Springfield, NJ). Stored at room temperature.

12. Acetone: spectrophotometric grade.
13. 90% ethanol. Store at –20°C.
14. Oditest (The Dyer Co., Lancaster, PA): special micrometer.
15. Plethysmometer UB/7140 for measuring swelling of the rat paw (edema) (Hugo Sachs Electronic, March-Hugstetten, Germany).

3. Methods *(see* Notes 2 and 3*)*
3.1. Croton Oil-Induced Ear Inflammation
3.1.1. Mouse Ear Inflammation

1. Use male mice weighing 28–32 g each *(see* **Note 4**).
2. Dissolve croton oil in acetone (35 µg/10 µL) and apply topically, dropwise, from a Hamilton syringe within 30 s to the inner surface of the right ear of the mice.
3. Apply the same volume of acetone (10 µL) to the other ear.
4. Use warm air from an electric hair dryer for a few seconds to evaporate the solvent.
5. After 4 h, sacrifice the animals with an overdose of diethyl ether and cut off the ears.
6. Cut out a disk from the middle part of each ear, using a punch 6 mm in diameter.
7. Weigh these disks on a torsion balance. Express the extent of the edema as the difference in weight of the disks from the inflamed and the control ear *(6,7)*.

3.1.2. Rat Ear Inflammation

1. Use male rats weighing 60–100 g each *(see* **Note 4**).
2. Dissolve the test compound in acetone containing croton oil (5% v/v, 40 µL) and apply simultaneously to the inner surface of each of the ears.
3. Treat the control groups of animals with croton oil only or with vehicle (40 µL acetone).
4. 6 h later, sacrifice the animals and remove the ears.
5. Punch out standard sized disks (5 mm in diameter) and weigh the disks.
6. Calculate the mean weight of the ear disks and, hence, the percentage decrease in ear weight from that of the croton oil controls *(8)*.

3.2. 12-0-TPA-Induced Ear Inflammation

1. Use female mice 5–8 wk old.
2. Dissolve TPA in acetone (125 µg/mL, i.e., 2.5 µg/20 µL) and deliver 10 µL to each of the inner and outer surfaces of the right ear of the mice by means of an automatic microliter pipet.
3. Apply Oditest dial calipers to the tip of the ear for ear-thickness determinations *(see* **Note 3**).
4. After 4 h, sacrifice the animals by cervical dislocation, remove the ears immediately with sharp scissors, and cut out plugs 8 mm in diameter from the tip with a biopsy punch.
5. Weigh the plugs immediately to the nearest 0.1 mg.
6. The extent of the inflammation induced by TPA is assessed in terms of the increase in weight of the right ear punch biopsy over that of the left ear *(9,10)*.

3.3. Cantharidin-Induced Ear Inflammation

3.3.1. Mouse Ear Inflammation

1. Use male mice weighing 20–30 g.
2. Apply a solution of cantharidin (25 µg/10 µL) in acetone with an automatic pipet to the inner surface of one ear. Leave the other ear untreated.
3. After 6 h, sacrifice the mice, and amputate and weigh the ears.
4. The difference in weight between the inflamed and noninflamed ears is taken as a measure of the response *(11)*.

3.3.2. Rat Ear Inflammation

1. Use 21- to 22-d-old male rats weighing 50–60 g.
2. Anesthetize the animals (0.12 ml Chloropent ip; the rats remain anesthetized for approx 3 h).
3. Apply cantharidin (400 µg/ear) solution topically to the outer surface of one ear via a hypodermic syringe with a 22-gauge needle. Employ a standardized vehicle, consisting of a mixture of 1 part ethanol, 1.5 parts collodion (USP), 2 parts acetone, and 3 parts anhydrous diethyl ether by volume.
4. Sacrifice the animals 72 h after topical application of the cantharidin solution.
5. Cut out disks with a # 3 cork borer (9/32" diameter) and weigh each tissue sample to the nearest 0.1 mg.
6. Express the extent of the edema as the difference in weight of the disks from the inflamed ear and the vehicle-treated control ear *(12)*.

3.4. Mustard Oil Inflammation in Mouse Ear Skin

1. Use 6-wk-old male mice weighing 30–35 g.
2. Anesthetize the animals with pentobarbital sodium (50 mg/kg, ip).
3. Dilute allyl isothyocyanate with mineral oil to concentrations of 0.5–20% (v/v). Apply 20 µL of solution topically to both surfaces of one ear of each mouse (application of mineral oil has no effect on ear thickness).
4. Use 5% mustard oil to study the inflammatory response of the irritant.
5. Examine the edema response 30 min after the application of mustard oil by measuring the increase in thickness at the edge of the ear before and at various times after the development of inflammation, using dial calipers (*see* **Note 5**).
6. The extent of edema is expressed as the increase in ear thickness *(13)*.

3.5. Ethyl Phenylpropiolate-Induced Ear Inflammation

1. Use male rats weighing 90–100 g.
2. Dissolve ethyl phenylpropiolate (EPP) in acetone (50 mg EPP/mL) and apply topically to both ears in a volume of 20 µL/ear side.
3. Measure the ear thickness before induction and after 2 h with a special micrometer (Oditest) (*see* **Note 5**).
4. Express the extent of the edema as the individual gain in ear thickness *(14)*.

3.6. Dithranol-Induced Mouse Ear Inflammation

1. Use male mice weighing 28–32 g each.
2. Dissolve dithranol (30 µg/10 µL) in acetone and apply topically, dropwise, from a Hamilton syringe within 30 s to the inner surface of the right ear.
3. Apply a similar volume of acetone (10 µL) to the other ear.
4. Use an electric hair dryer for a few seconds to evaporate the solvent.
5. After 24 h, kill the animals with an overdose of diethyl ether and cut off the ears.
6. Cut out disks from the middle part of each ear, using a sharp punch 6 mm in diameter.
7. Weigh these disks on a torsion balance. Express the extent of the edema as the difference in weight of the disks from the inflamed and the control ear *(6,15)*.

3.7. Arachidonic Acid-Induced Ear Inflammation

1. Use male mice, weighing 28–32 g each.
2. Dissolve arachidonic acid in acetone (2 mg/10 µL) and apply topically, dropwise, from a Hamilton syringe within 30 s to the inner surface of the right ear of the mice.
3. Apply the same volume of acetone (10 µL) to the other ear.
4. Use an electric hair dryer for a few seconds to evaporate the solvent.
5. After 1 h, sacrifice the animals with an overdose of diethyl ether and cut off the ears.
6. Cut out a disk from the middle part of each ear, using a sharp punch 6 mm in diameter.
7. Weigh these disks on a torsion balance. Express the extent of the edema as the difference in weight of the disks from the inflamed and the control ear *(16)*. (For the original methods, *see* **ref. 17**.)

3.8. Capsaicin-Induced Mouse Ear Inflammation

1. Use male mice weighing 28–32 g each.
2. Dissolve capsaicin in 90% alcohol (40 µg/10 µL) and apply topically, dropwise, from a Hamilton syringe within 30 s to the inner surface of the right ear of the mice.
3. Apply the similar volume of alcohol (10 µL) to the inner surface of the other ear.
4. Use warm air from an electric hair dryer for a few seconds to evaporate the solvent.
5. After 60 min, sacrifice the animals with an overdose of diethyl ether and cut off the ears.
6. Cut out a disk from the middle part of each ear, using a sharp punch 6 mm in diameter.
7. Weigh these disks on a torsion balance. Express the difference in weight of the disks from the inflamed and the control ear *(18)*.

3.9. Zymosan-Induced Mouse Ear Inflammation

1. Use female mice weighing 20–25 g.
2. Apply 1% zymosan as a sterile saline suspension. Administer 20 µL of zymosan

intradermally with a Hamilton microsyringe with a 27-gauge needle into one of the ears, about 5 mm from the edge of the lobe. Controls receive vehicle.
3. Sacrifice the animals 4 h after the intradermal application of 1% zymosan.
4. Cut off both earlobes and weigh the ears.
5. Calculate the extent of the edema by subtracting the wet weight of the untreated ear from that of the treated one of the same animal *(19)*.

3.10. Carrageenan-Induced Mouse Ear Inflammation

1. Use male mice, 6–7 wk old.
2. Inject the mice intradermally in the external ear with 25 µL of 1%-carrageenan via a microsyringe with a 27-gauge needle.
3. Kill the animals with an anesthetic overdose.
4. Cut out the injection sites with an 8-mm gasket punch for weight measurement, 4 h after the intradermal injection.
5. Express the extent of the edema by weighing the punched-out ear tissue in the treated and in the control group *(20)*.

3.11. Mezerein-Induced Ear Inflammation

1. Use male mice weighing 25–30 g.
2. Dissolve mezerein in acetone (6.5 µg/20 µL) and apply 10 µL of the solution topically to both surfaces of the right ear of the mice.
3. Apply the same volume of acetone (10 µL) to both surfaces of the left ear.
4. Measure the thickness of the ears using dial calipers prior to the experiment and 4 h after the induction of inflammation. Apply the calipers near the tip of the ear, just distal to the cartilaginous ridges and record the thickness.
5. Express the extent of the edema as the increase in ear thickness caused by the inflammatory challenge *(21)*.

3.12. Combined Methods

3.12.1. Simultaneously Induced Zymosan Paw Edema and Croton Oil Ear Edema in Rats

1. Use male rats weighing 130–135 g.
2. Apply 0.1 mL of a 1% suspension of zymosan by subplantar injection in the right hind paw of the rat.
3. Apply the same volume (0.1 mL) of physiological saline to the other hind paw of the rat.
4. Determine the extent of the edema in conscious animals 30 min after subplantar injection with the mercury displacement method or with a plethysmometer.
5. Apply an acetone solution of croton oil (100 µg/10 µL) dropwise, within 30 s, with a Hamilton syringe to the inner surface of the right ear of the same animals simultaneously with the induction of zymosan paw edema.
6. Apply an identical volume of acetone (10 µL) to the inner surface of the other ear.
7. Evaporate the solvent by means of a current of warm air.

8. After 4 h, sacrifice the animals under diethyl ether anesthesia and cut off their ears.
9. Cut out disks 6 mm in diameter with a sharp punch from comparable areas of the ears and weigh the wet disks with mg accuracy on a torsion balance.
10. Express the extent of the edema in terms of the difference in weight of the inflamed ear and the control ear *(22)*.

3.12.2. Simultaneously Induced Carrageenan Paw Edema and Croton Oil Ear Edema in Rats

1. Use male rats weighing 130–135 g.
2. Administer 0.1 mL of a 0.5% suspension of carrageenan via subplantar injection into the right hind paw of rats. (The suspension contains 500 µg carrageenan in a volume of 0.1 mL). Apply the same volume (0.1 mL) of physiological saline to the other hind paw.
3. Determine the extent of the edema in conscious animals, 4 h after the subplantar injection, with a plethysmometer.
4. Dissolve croton oil in acetone (100 µg/10 µL) and apply the solution dropwise within 30 s with a Hamilton syringe to the inner surface of the right ear of the same animals simultaneously with the induction of carrageenan paw edema.
5. Apply the same volume of acetone (10 µL) to the inner surface of the other ear.
6. Evaporate the solvent by means of a current of warm air.
7. After 4 h, kill the animals under diethyl ether anesthesia and cut off their ears.
8. Cut out disks 6 mm in diameter with a sharp punch from comparable areas (middle part) of the ears and weigh the wet disks with mg accuracy on a torsion balance.
9. Express the extent of the edema in terms of the difference in weight of the inflamed and the control ear *(23)*.

4. Notes

1. Croton oil is a relatively crude mixture of many constituents and varies in its irritant properties from batch to batch and with aging.
   12-0-Tetradecanoylphorbol 13-acetate is a potent inflammatory agent and a known tumor promoter.
   Before the application of dithranol, it is advisable to purify the substance by recrystallizing it from a mixture of acetic acid and water (90:10). For elicitation of dithranol dermatitis, a fresh solution of the irritant must be prepared just prior to its application.
   Arachidonic acid solutions should be prepared fresh daily.
   Acetone should be of spectrophotometric grade and from a freshly opened bottle. Generally 10 µL of solution is applied to each of the inner and outer surfaces of the ear. This volume covers the ear adequately without excessive drainage or dripping.
2. There are considerable differences in skin irritation between mouse strains. As an example, C 57 BL/6 mice are most sensitive and SENCAR mice most resis-

tant to dithranol (anthralin)-induced skin (ear) irritation *(22)*.

It is, therefore, advisable to carry out preliminary experiments to establish the effective dose of the applied skin irritant for the mouse strain used in the laboratory. In the combined methods, it is suitable to use rats of the Wistar strain.

3. In view of diurnal variations, the examinations are carried out at the same time of day, in the morning. It is important to reestablish the dose-response to inflammatory agents regularly in order to maintain optimal assay sensitivity, since responses can vary diurnally and seasonally *(10,23,24)*.
4. The animals are maintained in groups of 5–10 in separate plastic cages in a thermostatically controlled room at 20–22°C and at a relative humidity of 50 ± 10%. The room is artificially illuminated on a time schedule of 14 h light and 10 h dark. The animals are provided with food and water *ad libitum* 4–7 d prior to and during the assay to prevent dehydration and to avoid stress-induced corticosteroid production, which may result in a diminished inflammatory response.
5. Ear thickness is measured at the tip of the pinna with a spring-loaded micrometer at different time intervals after elicitation of the inflammation. Thickness measurements with calipers are subject to operator error, and care must be taken not to leave the calipers in contact with the ear for too long because it is possible to squeeze substantial amounts of edema fluid out of the ear tissue. To minimize variation due to technique, measurements throughout any one experiment are performed by a single investigator.

References

1. Chang, J. Y. and Lewis, A. J., eds. (1989) *Pharmacological Methods in the Control of Inflammation*, Alan R. Liss, New York.
2. Morgan, D. W. and Marshall, L. A., eds. (1999) *In Vivo Models of Inflammation*, Birkhäuser Verlag, Basel, Boston, Berlin.
3. Gábor, M. (2000) *Mouse Ear Inflammation Models and their Pharmacological Applications*, Akadémiai Kiadó, Budapest, Hungary.
4. Gábor, M. and Rázga, Zs. (1992) Anti-oedematous effects of the H1-receptor antagonist dimethindene maleate. *Agents Actions (Spec. Conf. Issue)* C444–C447.
5. Blazsó, G. and Gábor, M. (1997) Evaluation of the anti-oedematous effects of some H1-receptor antagonists and methysergide in rats. *Pharmacol. Res.* **35,** 65–71.
6. Blazsó, G., Rázga, Zs., and Gábor, M. (1999) Effects of cinnarizine on different experimentally induced oedemas. *Fundam. Clin. Pharmacol.* **13,** 91–95.
7. Blazsó, G. and Gábor, M. (1994) Anti-oedematous action of some H1-receptor antagonists. *Agents Actions* **42,** 13–18.
8. Procopiou, P. A., Biggadike, K., English, F. A., Farrel, R. M., et al. (2001) Novel glucocorticoid antedrugs possessing a 17β-(γ-lactone) ring. *J. Med. Chem.* **44,** 602–612.
9. Young, J. M., Wagner, B. M., and Spires, D. A. (1983) Tachyphylaxis in 12-0-tetradecanoylphorbol acetate-and arachidonic-acid induced ear edema. *J. Invest. Dermatol.* **80,** 48–52.

10. Young, J. M. and De Young, L. M. (1989) Cutaneous models of inflammation for the evaluation of topical and systemic pharmacological agents, in *Pharmacological Methods in the Control of Inflammation* (Chang J.Y. and Lewis, A.J., eds.), A.R. Liss, New York, pp. 215–231.
11. Swingle, K. F., Reiter, M. J., and Schwartzmiller, D. H. (1981) Comparison of croton oil and cantharidin-induced inflammations of the mouse ear and their modification by topically applied drugs. *Arch. Int. Pharmacodyn.* **254,** 168–176.
12. Boris, A. and Hurley, J. F. (1977) Assessment of topical anti-inflammatory activity in rats with cantharidin-induced inflammation. *J. Invest. Dermatol.* **68,** 161–164.
13. Inoue, H., Asaka, T., Nagata, N., and Koshihara, Y. (1997) Mechanism of mustard oil-induced skin inflammation in mice. *Europ. J. Pharmacol.* **333,** 231–240.
14. Brattsand, R., Thalén, A., Roempke, K., Källström, L., and Gruvstad, E. (1982) Influence of 16α, 17α-acetal substitution and steroid nucleus fluorination on the topical to systemic activity ratio of glucocorticoids. *J. Steroid. Biochem.* **16,** 779–786.
15. Gábor, M. and Rázga, Zs. (1990) Effects of non-steroidal antiphlogistics on mouse ear edema induced with dithranol. *Acta Physiol. Acad. Sci. Hung.* **75,** 287–291.
16. Blazsó, G. and Gábor, M. (1995) Effects of prostaglandin antagonist phloretin derivatives on mouse ear edema induced with different skin irritants. *Prostaglandins* **50,** 161–168.
17. Young, J. M., Spires, D. A., Bedord, C. J., Wagner, B., Ballaron, S. J., and De Young, L. M. (1984) The mouse ear inflammatory response to topical arachidonic acid. *J. Invest. Dermatol.* **82,** 367–371.
18. Gábor, M. and Rázga, Zs. (1992) Development and inhibition of mouse ear edema induced with capsaicin. *Agents Actions* **36,** 83–86.
19. Erdö, F., Török, K., Arányi, P., and Székely, J. I. (1993) A new assay for antiphlogistic activity: Zymosan-induced mouse ear inflammation. *Agents Actions* **39,** 137–142.
20. Tsuji, F., Miyake, Y., Enomoto, H., Horiuchi, M., and Mita, S. (1998) Effects of SA6541, a leukotriene A4 hydrolase inhibitor, and indomethacin on carrageenan-induced murine dermatitis. *Europ. J. Pharmacol.* **346,** 81–85.
21. Huguet, A.-I., Recio, M. C., Manez, S., Giner, R.-M., and Rios, J.-L. (2000) Effect of triterpenoids on the inflammation induced by protein kinase C activators, neuronally active irritants and other agents. *Europ. J. Pharmacol.* **410,** 69–81.
22. Viluksela, M. and Kosma, V.-M. (1991) Dithranol (anthralin)-induced skin irritation in C57BL/6, NMRI and SENCAR mice. *Pharmacol. Toxicol.* **69,** 96–104.
23. Soliman, K. F. A., Soliman, M. R. J., Owasoyo, J. O., and Walker, C. A. (1983) Diurnal variation in the phlogogenic response of rats to inflammatory agents. *J. Pharm. Pharmacol.* **35,** 388–389.
24. Labreque, G., Bureau, I.-P., and Reinberg, A. E. (1995) Biological rhytms in the inflammatory response and in the effects of non-steroidal anti-inflammatory drugs. *Pharmac. Ther.* **66,** 285–300.

16

Migration of Specific Leukocyte Subsets in Response to Cytokine or Chemokine Application In Vivo

Mauro Perretti and Stephen J. Getting

1. Introduction

The host inflammatory response is a complex process characterized by several different steps (or phenomena) all contributing to the well-known macroscopic symptoms of this condition, which are pain, fever, redness, swelling, and, in the case of chronic inflammation (such as rheumatoid arthritis), loss of function (*see* **Chapters 1** and **12**). These symptoms are the consequence of a series of local (i.e., at the site of the inflammatory insult) and systemic changes. Locally, arterioles, capillaries, and venules dilate with consequent increase in permeability and blood flow; this leads to exudation of fluid and proteins (*humoral response*); finally, leukocytes also migrate into the inflammatory site (*cellular response*). The latter process is by far the most important because "...the accumulation and subsequent activation of leukocytes are central events in the pathogenesis of virtually all forms of inflammation." (*1*). For this reason, the acquisition of information regarding the molecular mechanisms responsible for leukocyte accumulation during inflammation can, on one hand, increase our knowledge of the etiology of inflammatory pathologies and, on the other hand, lead to the discovery of novel targets for antiinflammatory therapy.

Cytokines [e.g., tumor necrosis factor and interleukin 1 (IL-1)] and chemokines [e.g., interleukin-8 (IL-8) and monocyte chemoattractant protein-1 (MCP-1)] are instrumental in the development of the cellular response that characterizes inflammation (*2,3*), and that must be targeted for effective antiinflammatory drug development. In addition, recent interest in chemokines derives from the possibility to understand, for the first time, the reason why certain pathologies are characterized by the accumulation of a selective leukocyte subtype (for instance, eosinophils accumulate in asthma, whereas neutrophils accumulate during the acute phases of rheumatoid arthritis or chronic obstructive pulmonary disease) *(3,4)*.

The availability of simple experimental systems that mimic some aspects of the pathology of interest is vital to the design and development of novel therapeutics. We will provide here examples on the use of the mouse air-pouch and peritoneal cavity to study cytokine- or chemokine-induced leukocyte recruitment. These models are a simplified version of the more complex experimental reactions elicited by carrageenan or zymosan (*see* **Chapters 13–15** and **20**), hence, they could be of help for the identification and characterization of selective antagonists to cytokine and chemokine receptors. In our opinion, models of cytokine- or chemokine-induced leukocyte migration should be used as a first in vivo screening assay to develop selective receptor antagonists. Candidate molecules should then be tested in more complex experimental inflammatory reactions (e.g., the one elicited by carrageenan or zymosan, **Chapters 13–15** and **20**) or described by Dawson et al. *(5)*.

2. Materials

1. Cytokine and chemokine storage: as with other proteins produced by recombinant techniques, the cytokines such as interleukin 1β (IL-1β) or tumor necrosis factor-α (TNF-α) must be prepared as a concentrated solution, at least 1 mg/mL, in sterile phosphate-buffered saline (PBS) supplemented with 0.1% low-endotoxin bovine serum albumin (BSA; Sigma Aldrich Poole, UK). The same applies to IL-8 and MCP-1. These stock solutions can be stored at –80°C for many years. In view of their tertiary structure *(6)* chemokines are more stable than cytokines, and sometimes working solutions can also be stored at +4°C (e.g., for in vitro experiments). However, we recommend the preparation of fresh working solutions for each in vivo experiment.
Cytokines and chemokines can be obtained from several commercial sources, including R&D Systems Ltd. Europe (Abingdon, UK) or Peprotech EC Ltd. (London, UK), Serotec Ltd (Oxford UK).
A precaution that must be considered when developing one of these models with new cytokines/chemokines is the presence or absence of species specificity. For IL-1β, for instance, either the human or the murine species are active in producing neutrophil influx into the mouse air-pouch.
2. Vehicle for cytokine solution: different studies have used various vehicles. We recommend the use of sterile PBS for experiments of peritonitis, and of low-density carboxy methyl cellulose (CMC; BDH, Poole, UK) for the air-pouch experiments *(7)*. A CMC solution at 0.5% in sterile PBS is prepared on the day of the experiment.
3. Washing buffer: add ethylene diamine tetra-acetic acid (EDTA), sodium salt (Sigma-Aldrich Ltd), to sterile PBS at a final concentration of 3 mM, and add

heparin at a final concentration of 25 U/mL. This lavage solution can be stored at 4°C for 1 wk.
4. Cell counting: the influx of monocytes and neutrophils can be detected easily by light microscopy. To do so, a solution of Turk's is prepared by dissolving 0.1% crystal violet (Sigma-Aldrich) in 3% acetic acid (prepared in sterile water). There is no need to stir, but a vigorous shake of the bottle is sufficient to dissolve crystal violet to a sufficient level to clearly stain monocytes and neutrophils *(8)*.

3. Methods
3.1. Air-Pouch Experiment
3.1.1. Air-Pouch Formation

1. On day 0, mice are injected with 2.5 mL of air subcutaneously on the dorsal area. Usually, the site of injection is at the base of the neck, pushing the air into the dorsal area towards the tail.
2. On day 3, a second injection is performed to reinflate the air-pouch (*see* **Note 1**).
3. On day 6, the air-pouch is ready for experimentation. A lining of tissue 3 to 6 cells deep has formed under the skin of the air-pouch *(9)*. This has the advantage of having a tissue structure with resident cells (mainly macrophage- and fibroblast-like). In addition, the lining tissue will reduce the absorption of the cytokine helping to generate a local response.

3.1.2. Induction of Inflammation

1. Prepare CMC solution by sprinkling 250 mg of CMC onto 50 mL of sterile PBS under continuous stirring at room temperature. It will take approx 30 min to obtain full dissolution. Centrifuge the CMC solution at 1200 rpm (400*g*) for 10 min in a centrifuge to remove lumps that may have been formed. Store on ice.
2. Take an aliquot of the cytokine/chemokine of interest. Dilute it down in sterile PBS to a 11-fold more concentrated solution than required.
3. Calculate on the basis of 0.5 mL of inflammogen solution per mouse. Therefore, for a group of 10 mice, take 5 mL of CMC solution and add 0.5 mL of cytokine/chemokine. Final doses for IL-1β are in the range of 5–10 ng (that means that the 11X solution was 110–220 ng/mL in PBS), whereas an active dose for IL-8 is 0.5–1 µg for an initial 11X solution of 11–22 µg/mL.
4. Anesthetize the mouse (a light halothane anesthesia in sufficient) and inject 0.5 mL of inflammogen into the air-pouch.

3.1.3. Lavage of the Air-Pouch and Cell Counting

1. Air-pouches are washed with 1 mL of buffer. Mice are killed by exposure to carbon dioxide, and a small incision is made in the top part of the air-pouch (near the base of the neck). Inject 1 mL of buffer for lavage with a Gilson™ pipet, wash and resuspend with a 1-mL plastic Pasteur pipet. There is no dead volume if the air-pouch has been prepared correctly, so collect approx 1 mL of lavage fluid,

and add it into a 15-mL tube containing another mL of buffer for lavage. In total each sample will be approx 2 mL. Keep on ice.
2. Centrifuge tubes at 400g for 15 min at 4°C. Take supernatants out, and store them at –20°C for potential future biochemical determinations.
3. Tip the bottom of each tube to make the cell pellet less hard. Add 2 mL of lavage buffer to each tube, and resuspend cell pellets by vigorous vortexing.
4. Take 0.1 mL of cell suspension and add it to 0.9 mL of Turk's solution into an Eppendorf tube. Vortex.
5. Place 10 µL into a Neubauer chamber, and count cells in the central area. Neutrophils are easily identified by their dark blue coloration and the polylobate nucleus consisting, usually, of two or three parts. Monocytes give a pale blue coloration, and have a single, often kidney-shaped, nucleus. A cytoplasm, translucent, is often seen in monocytes by focusing the microscope, and this can be quite large in the case of a macrophage. Lymphocytes produce an intense dark blue coloration, but they have a small rounded nucleus with no visible cytoplasm, so they can be immediately distinguished from the neutrophils.

3.1.4. Data Calculation

1. Calculate the total number of cells which have migrated using the following formula:
$$Y \text{ (Cells/mL)} = N \times 10 \times 10^4$$
where N is the number of cells counted in the Neubauer chamber, 10 is the dilution factor in Turk's solution, and 10^4 is the factor of the chamber.
2. Data can be expressed as number of neutrophils per mL, or as number of neutrophils per mouse (alas, air-pouch). In the latter case, the value Y must be multiplied by 2, because 2 mL of washing buffer were used to resuspend the cell pellets.

3.2. Peritonitis Experiment (see Note 2)

The experimental procedure for the mouse peritonitis is relatively similar to one used for the air-pouch with a few distinctions. The peritoneal cavity is highly vascularized and it is larger. There is, therefore, a higher risk of producing a blood contaminated sample (slight touch to the liver or to other peritoneal tissues during the intraperitoneal injection of inflammogen or of the washing buffer may cause the discard of the sample). Also, there is a much larger "dead volume," so only a portion of the washing buffer will be retrieved. Technically, the following points distinguish the peritonitis from the air-pouch.

3.2.1. Induction of Inflammation

1. Dilute the cytokine/chemokine of interest in sterile PBS to produce the wanted dose in 0.5 mL of PBS volume.
2. Anesthetize the mouse (a light halothane anesthesia in sufficient) and inject 0.5 mL of inflammogen into the peritoneal cavity, taking care not to inject into the intestine.

3.2.2. Lavage of the Peritoneal Cavity and Cell Counting

1. Peritoneal cavities are washed with 3 mL of washing buffer. Mice are killed by exposure to carbon dioxide, and a small incision is made along the median line (i.e., at the middle of the abdomen). Inject 3 mL of washing lavage with a syringe, again making sure that the fluid does not go into the intestine. Gentle massage (30 s) of the mouse abdomen will assure that cells loosely adherent to the peritoneal wall and/or other organs will detach. There is at least 0.5 mL of dead volume in the mouse peritoneal cavity, so use a plastic Pasteur pipet to collect approx 2-mL of lavage fluid into a 15-mL tube. Keep on ice.
2. Once at the microscope, vortex tubes thoroughly and add 0.1 mL of lavage fluid to 0.9 mL of Turk's solution into an Eppendorf tube. Vortex.
3. Place 10 µL into a Neubauer chamber, and count cells as in **Subheading 3.1.3.**

3.2.3. Data Calculation

1. Calculate the total number of cells which have migrated from the following formula:

$$Y \text{ (Cells /mL)} = N \times 10 \times 10^4$$

where N is the number of cells counted in the Neubauer chamber, 10 is the dilution factor in Turk's solution, and 10^4 is the factor of the chamber.
2. Data can be expressed as number of a specific leukocyte per mL, or as number of neutrophils per mouse. In the latter case, the value Y must be multiplied by 3, because 3 mL of washing buffer were used to lavage the peritoneal cavities.

4. Notes

1. It is crucial that the second injection of air *goes into* the first air-pouch. Creation of a second air-pouch will invalidate the determination (the leukocyte response will not be accurate; it will also be difficult to properly wash the air-pouch).
   Fig. 1A gives an example of the role that the vehicle plays in determining the extent of the neutrophil response to IL-1β, whereas in **Fig. 1B**, a comparison of the use of different cytokines to produce neutrophil migration into the mouse air-pouch can be seen. Table 1 provides an example of the importance of the air-pouch age in delivering a good influx on neutrophils in response to specific chemotactic stimuli. As highlighted by Edwards et al. *(9)*, the presence of the lining tissue is crucial for achieving a good cellular response. In addition, there is no basement membrane in an established (e.g., 6-d-old) air-pouch, and, therefore, the process of leukocyte migration can occur at higher intensity.
2. An advantage of the peritoneal cavity is that it is much easier to produce an influx of monocytes and eosinophils in response to selective chemokines. For instance, whereas IL-8 produces neutrophil accumulation into the air-pouch *(10)* as well as in the peritoneal cavity, MCP-1 and eotaxin produce monocyte and eosinophil influx, respectively, only in the peritoneal cavity but not in the air-pouch. The reason for this is unclear, but it is likely to be dependent on the type and/or extent of resident cells present. In the case of eotaxin, mast cell replenishment is necessary to produce a reasonable influx of eosinophils into the air-pouch *(11)*.

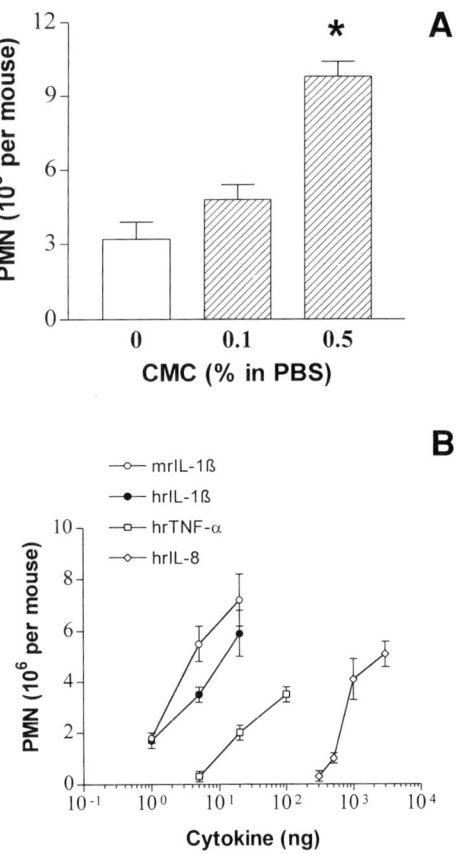

Fig. 1. Use of the mouse air-pouch to study cytokine/chemokine induced neutrophil migration. (**A**) Human recombinant (hr) IL-1β (10 ng) was dissolved in 0.5 mL of PBS alone or with the reported concentration of CMC. Air-pouches were washed 4 h later and cell accumulation in the lavage fluids quantified by differential counting. Values (mean ± s.e.) are from n=6 mice per group. *p<0.01 vs the group without CMC. (**B**) Either hrIL-1β, mouse recombinant (mr) IL-1β, hrTNF-α or hrIL-8 were injected in 0.5 mL CMC (0.5% in PBS) and neutrophil accumulation determined 4 h later. Values are mean ± s.e. of n =5–7 mice per group, and have been corrected for the migration induced by CMC alone (2.2 × 10^6 neutrophils per mouse).

In line with this "refractory" aspect of the mouse air-pouch to produce a cell influx rather than for neutrophils, several days (>6) are required to measure a significant monocyte accumulation into the mouse air-pouch in response to 10 mg zymosan *(5)*, whereas 16–24 h are sufficient to produce a significant monocyte influx (useful for studying putative inhibitors) after 1 mg zymosan injection into the mouse peritoneal cavity *(12)*. Finally, IL-β-induced neutrophil migration

Table 1
Effect of the Age of the Air-Pouch on Neutrophil Recruitment Induced by Several Stimuli

Stimulus Applied	Neutrophils (10^6 per mouse)	
	6-d-old Air-Pouch	10-min-old Air-Pouch
Vehicle	2.3 ± 0.3 (4)	0.05 ± 0.03 (4)
hrIL-1β (20 ng)	8.5 ± 1.4 (4)	0.50 ± 0.10 (4)
hrTNF-α (100 ng)	4.7 ± 0.5 (4)	0.35 ± 0.05 (4)
hr IL-8 (100 ng)	3.6 ± 0.7 (4)	0.17 ± 0.10 (4)
FMLP (1 μg)	2.8 ± 0.5 (4)	0.10 ± 0.04 (4)

Agents were dissolved in 0.5 mL of vehicle (CMC 0.5% w:v in PBS) and injected into 6-d-old air-pouches or into newly formed air-pouches (2.5 mL of air injected sc immediately before challenge with the stimulus). Air-pouches were washed 4 h later and the number of neutrophils accumulated quantified by staining in Turk's solution. Values are mean ± s.e. of (n) mice per group.
FMLP: formyl-Met-Leu-Phe (Sigma-Aldrich); hr, human recombinant

Table 2
Comparison of MCP-1 Induced Monocyte Accumulation Into the Mouse Peritoneal or Air-Pouch Cavities

Stimulus Applied	Leukocyte (10^6 per mouse)		
	Neutrophils	Monocytes	Lymphocytes
Air-Pouch			
CMC	1.2 ± 0.3 (6)	2.4 ± 0.5 (6)	0.2 ± 0.1 (6)
MCP-1	1.1 ± 0.2 (6)	2.0 ± 0.6 (6)	0.3 ± 0.1 (6)
Peritoneal Cavity			
PBS	0.6 ± 0.3 (5)	3.6 ± 0.6 (5)	0.3 ± 0.1 (5)
MCP-1	0.5 ± 0.2 (5)	6.6. ± 0.4 (5)*	0.2 ± 0.1 (5)

Murine recombinant MCP-1 (1 μg) was dissolved in 0.5 mL of vehicle (CMC 0.5% w:v in PBS) and injected into 6-d-old air-pouches or in 0.5 mL PBS and injected into the mouse peritoneal cavity. Leukocyte influx was measured in the 4 h lavage fluids by staining in Turk's solution. Monocyte values refer to a combined counting for monocytes and macrophages, with the latter cell type representing a large percentage (>90%) of the value for PBS in the peritonitis. Data are mean ± s.e. of (n) mice per group. * $P < 0.05$ vs corresponding PBS group.

into the air-pouch is not followed by a time-dependent influx of monocytes (7). **Table 2** provides an example of the monocyte accumulation elicited by MCP-1 in the mouse peritoneal cavity in comparison to its lack of effect after injection into 6-d-old air-pouches.

References

1. Gallin, J. I., Goldstein, I. M., and Snyderman, R. (1992) Overview, in *Inflammation: Basic Principles and Clinical Correlates* (Gallin J. I. and Goldstein I. M., eds.), Raven, New York, pp. 1–4.
2. Mantovani, A., Bussolino, F., and Introna, M. (1997) Cytokine regulation of endothelial cell function: from molecular level to the bedside. *Immunol. Today* **18,** 231–240.
3. Zlotnik, A. and Yoshie, O. (2000) Chemokines: a new classification system and their role in immunity. *Immunity* **12,** 121–127.
4. Baggiolini, M. (1998) Chemokines and leukocyte traffic. *Nature* **392,** 565–568.
5. Dawson, J., Sedgwick, A. D., Edwards, J. C. W., and Lees, P. (1991) A comparative study of the cellular, exudative and histological responses to carrageenan, dextran and zymosan in the mouse. *Int. J. Tissue Reac.* **XIII,** 171–185.
6. Baggiolini, M., Dewald, B., and Moser, B. (1994) Interleukin-8 and related chemotactic cytokines - CXC and CC chemokines. *Adv. Immunol.* **55,** 97–179.
7. Perretti, M. and Flower, R. J. (1993) Modulation of IL-1-induced neutrophil migration by dexamethasone and lipocortin 1. *J. Immunol.* **150,** 992–999.
8. Getting, S. J., Flower, R. J., and Perretti, M. (1997) Inhibition of neutrophil and monocyte recruitment by endogenous and exogenous lipocortin 1. *Br. J. Pharmacol.* **120,** 1075–1082.
9. Edwards, J. C., Sedgwick, A. D., and Willoughby, D. A. (1981) The formation of a structure with the features of synovial lining by subcutaneous injection of air: an in vivo tissue culture system. *J. Pathol.* **134,** 147–156.
10. Perretti, M., Harris, J. G., and Flower, R. J. (1994) A role for endogenous histamine in interleukin-8-induced neutrophil infiltration into mouse air-pouch: investigation of the modulatory action of systemic and local dexamethasone. *Br. J. Pharmacol.* **112,** 801–808.
11. Das, A. M., Flower, R. J., and Perretti, M. (1998) Resident mast cells are important for eotaxin-induced eosinophil accumulation in vivo. *J. Leukoc. Biol.* **64,** 156–162.
12. Ajuebor, M. N., Flower, R. J., Hannon, R., Christie, M., Bowers, K., Verity, A., et al. (1998) Endogenous monocyte chemoattractant protein-1 recruits monocytes in the zymosan peritonitis model. *J. Leukoc. Biol.* **63,** 108–116.

17

Inflammatory Joint Disease

Clinical, Histological, and Molecular Parameters of Acute and Chronic Inflammation and Tissue Destruction

Nancy L. McCartney-Francis, James Chan, and Sharon M. Wahl

1. Introduction

Peptidoglycan-polysaccharide complexes from Group A streptococcal cell walls (SCW) induce a biphasic inflammatory response in rats that resembles rheumatoid arthritis (RA) in humans *(1–3)*. Initiation of synovitis is dependent on the dissemination, deposition, and persistence of the SCW in the synovium. The subsequent infiltration of leukocytes into the synovial tissue coincides with the development of an acute inflammatory response. The clinical acute phase is transient and as the erythema and swelling subside, mononuclear cells are recruited into the synovial tissue as the chronic, erosive arthritis evolves. Similar to RA, susceptibility to the development of SCW-arthritis is gender-biased *(4)* and under genetic control with neuroendocrine and hormonal influences *(5–7)*. Moreover, the mechanisms responsible for the development of SCW-arthritis are susceptible to regulation by pharmacologic agents and biological response modifiers and as such, this model is considered a valid preclinical model of RA.

2. Materials
2.1. Arthritis Induction

1. Lewis rats (LEW/N), female, 80–100 g, virus and pathogen-free (Charles River Breeding Laboratories, Wilmington, MA) (*see* **Note 1**).

2. Peptidoglycan-polysaccharide polymers of sonicated cell walls from *Streptococcus pyogenes*, Group A, D58 strain (Lee Laboratories, Grayson, GA). The SCW is supplied as a sterile 0.85% saline solution with a rhamnose concentration between 3–6 mg/mL and is stored at 4°C (*see* **Note 2**).
3. Sterile saline (0.85% NaCl) or phosphate-buffered saline (PBS).
4. One milliliter syringes and 23-gauge needles.
5. Weighing scale.

2.2. Clinical Evaluation of Arthritis

1. Calipers for measuring ankle diameter (optional).
2. Plethysmometer (optional) (Stoelting Co., Wood Dale, IL).
3. X-ray machine (Faxitron, Faxitron X-Ray Corp., Buffalo Grove, IL).

2.3. Histological Evaluation of Arthritis

2.3.1. Tissue Fixation

1. 10% aqueous buffered zinc formalin (Z-Fix, Anatech, LTD, Battle Creek, MI) or 4% paraformaldehyde in PBS.
2. 2-Methylbutane (Sigma, St. Louis, MO). Stored at 4°C.

2.3.2. Histological Stains

1. Mayer's Hematoxylin (Sigma).
2. Eosin Y/phloxine B (Sigma).
3. Masson's Trichrome staining kit (Sigma).
4. Safranin O (Sigma).

2.3.3. Immunohistochemical Staining

1. Xylene, absolute ethanol (Sigma).
2. Triton X-100 (Research Products International Corp., Mount Prospect, IL).
3. Digest-All Kit (Zymed Laboratories, South San Francisco, CA).
4. Primary antibodies: See listing of available monoclonal mouse anti-rat antibodies to cell surface and MHC antigens *(8)*.
5. Vector ABC kit (blocking serum, biotinylated secondary antibody, ABC reagent conjugated with horseradish peroxidase or alkaline phosphatase) (Vector Laboratories, Burlingame, CA). Stored at 4°C.
6. Peroxidase substrate: diaminobenzidine (DAB) plus nickel chloride or 3-amino-9-ethylcarbazole (AEC); alkaline phosphatase substrate: Vector Red (Vector Laboratories). Stored at 4°C.
7. Counterstains: methyl green or hematoxylin (Sigma).
8. Mounting solutions: glycerol vinyl alcohol (GVA, Zymed), Permount (Fisher Scientific, Fair Lawn, NJ).

Inflammatory Joint Disease 149

2.4. Molecular Evaluation of Arthritis

2.4.1. RNA Isolation

1. Freezer mill (SPEX CertiPrep, Metuchen, NJ).
2. Liquid nitrogen.
3. Guanidinium isothiocyanate lysis buffer (TRIzol, Life Technology/Invitrogen). Stored at 4°C.
4. Chloroform, isopropanol, absolute ethanol. Stored at room temperature.
5. 75% ethanol. Stored at –20°C.
6. DEPC-treated water (1 mL of diethylpyrocarbonate, Fluka Chemical, added to 1 L of double-distilled water and autoclaved).

2.4.2. Northern Analysis

1. RNA samples. Stored at –70°C.
2. Agarose (SeaKem GTG agarose, FMC Bioproducts, Rockland, ME).
3. 10X MOPS buffer: 0.2 M MOPS, 0.05 M Na acetate, 0.01 M ethylene diamine tetraacetic acid (EDTA).
4. RNA loading dye: 10X is 50% glycerol, 1 mM EDTA, 0.4% bromophenol blue, 0.4% xylene cyanol. Stored at 4°C.
5. Ethidium bromide (10 mg/mL, Invitrogen). Stored at room temperature.
6. Turboblotter transfer system (Schleicher & Schuell, Keene, NH).
7. Prehybridization solution: 5X SSC (20X stock solution, Invitrogen), 50% deionized formamide (stored at –20°C), 5X Denhardt's (100X is 2% Ficoll 400, 2% polyvinyl pyrrolidone, 2% BSA), 0.05 M NaPO$_4$, pH 6.5, 0.1% sodium dodecyl sulfate (SDS), 0.1 mg/mL sheared salmon sperm DNA. Stored at 4°C.
8. Hybridization buffer: 5X SSC, 50% deionized formamide, 1X Denhardt's, 0.02 M NaPO$_4$, pH 6.5, 0.1 mg/mL sheared salmon sperm DNA, 10% dextran sulfate, 0.1% SDS (nitrocellulose) or 1% SDS (nylon). Stored at 4°C.
9. Random-priming DNA-labeling kit (Invitrogen). Stored at –20°C.
10. [^{32}P]dCTP (3000 Ci/mmol, Amersham Pharmacia).
11. Washing solutions: 2X SSC, 0.1% SDS; 1X SSC, 0.1% SDS.

2.4.3. Semiquantitative Reverse Transcriptase-PCR (RT-PCR)

1. RNA samples. Stored at –70°C.
2. Oligo dT (Invitrogen). Stored at –20°C.
3. Ribonuclease inhibitor (RNasin, Promega, Madison, WI). Stored at –20°C.
4. 10X PCR buffer (AmpliTaq buffer, Perkin-Elmer, Norwalk, CT). Stored at –20°C.
5. Moloney murine leukemia virus RT (Invitrogen). Stored at –20°C.
6. Deoxynucleotides (dNTP) (Perkin-Elmer). Stored at –20°C.
7. AmpliTaq DNA polymerase (Perkin-Elmer). Stored at –20°C.

2.4.4. RNase Protection

1. RNA samples. Stored at –70°C.
2. Riboquant multiprobe RNase protection kit (BD Pharmingen, San Diego). Stored at –20 and –70°C.
3. RNase-free G50 spin columns (5-Prime 3-Prime, Boulder, CO).
4. [α-^{32}P]UTP (3000 Ci/mmol, 10 mCi/mL, Amersham Pharmacia).

2.5. Protein Analysis

2.5.1. Protein Isolation

1. Lysis buffer: 25 mM Tris-HCl, pH 7.4, 150 mM NaCl, 1% Nonidet P-40 (NP40), 1 mM EDTA, pH 8.0, 1 mM EGTA, pH 8.0. Stored at 4°C. Add proteinase inhibitors (1 mM PMSF, 1 mM Na$_3$VO$_4$, 5 µg/mL aprotinin, 5 µg/mL leupeptin, and 5 µg/mL 4-(2-aminoethyl)-benzene sulfonylfluoride-HCl) just before use.
2. Protein assay kit (Bio-Rad DC Protein Assay, Bio-Rad, Hercules, CA). Stored at room temperature.

2.5.2. Western Blotting

1. Protein samples. Stored at –70°C.
2. Electrophoresis sample buffer (4X): 0.2 M Tris-HCl, pH 6.8, 4% SDS, 20% glycerol, 5% β-mercaptoethanol, 0.005% bromophenol blue. Alternative: 2X Tris-glycine SDS sample buffer (Novex/Invitrogen).
3. Tris-glycine-acrylamide gels (Novex/Invitrogen).
4. Tris-glycine buffer (10X, Novex/Invitrogen).
5. Nitrocellulose (Schleicher and Schuell).
6. Washing buffer (TBS-T): 20 mM Tris-HCl, pH 7.4, 137 mM sodium chloride, 0.1 % Tween-20.
7. Blocking buffer: 5% nonfat dry milk in TBS-T.
8. Super Signal luminol detection system (Pierce, Rockford, IL).
9. Film (Kodak BioMax, Eastman Kodak Co., Rochester, NY).

2.5.3. Electrophoretic Mobility Shift Assay

1. Cellular extract buffer: 20 mM Tris-HCl, pH 7.6, 120 mM NaCl, 1% NP-40, 10% glycerol, 10 mM NaPPi, 100 mM NaF. Stored at 4°C. Add the proteinase inhibitors (2 mM sodium orthovanadate, 1 mM 4-(2-aminoethyl)-benzenesulfonyl fluoride, 5 µg/mL leupeptin) just prior to use.
2. Protein assay kit (Bio-Rad).
3. Double-stranded oligonucleotide (i.e., NF-κB consensus double-stranded oligonucleotide, Promega Corp.).
4. T4 polynucleotide kinase (PNK, 10 U/µL) and 10X PNK buffer (Invitrogen). Stored at –20°C.
5. [γ-^{32}P]ATP, 10 mCi/mL (3000 Ci/mmol, Amersham Pharmacia).

6. G25 spin column (5-Prime 3-Prime).
7. Binding buffer: 10 mM Tris-HCl, pH 7.5, 1 mM dithiothreitol (DTT), 1 mM EDTA, 4% glycerol, 0.08 mg/mL salmon sperm DNA, with a final adjusted concentration of 80 mM NaCl. Alternative: 5X gel shift binding buffer (Promega).
8. 6% polyacrylamide gel.
9. Tris borate EDTA (TBE, 10X stock, Quality Biological, Gaithersburg, MD).

3. Methods
3.1. Arthritis Induction

1. Weigh rats and calculate the volume of SCW to inject (30 µg of rhamnose/g body weight). Vortex the SCW preparation for 30 s prior to injection.
2. Carefully inject the SCW intraperitoneally into the lower left quadrant of the abdomen using a 1-mL syringe and 23-gauge needle so as to avoid internal organs.
3. Control rats receive an equal volume of sterile saline or PBS.
4. Immunomodulators may be introduced into rats by several routes [intravenous (iv), intraperitoneal (ip), intramuscular (im), subcutaneous (sc), intraarticular (ia), gavage) *(9–11)*. Dosing regimens depend upon the chemical properties of each molecule.

3.2. Clinical Evaluation of Arthritis

1. Arthritis severity may be assessed visually by scoring the four distal joints on a scale of 0–4 on the basis of swelling, erythema, and distortion (*see* **Note 3**). A score of 0 represents no arthritis, and 4 represents very severe arthritis. The individual scores are summed to determine the articular index (AI), with a possible maximum score of 16. Each animal is evaluated daily for the first week and then every 2–3 d up to 4–8 wk. It is important that the same individual determine the AI scores throughout the experiment to ensure consistency. For statistical evaluation of the arthritis induction and treatment effectiveness, at least six rats per treatment group should be used. Data are reported as the mean AI ± SEM (*see* **Fig. 1**). Statistical significance is determined using the nonparametric Mann-Whitney *U* test, analysis of variance followed by Scheffe's *post hoc* test, or student's *t*-test.
2. Ankle swelling may also be determined with calipers. Maximal lateral ankle diameter should be measured at the start of the experiment to provide a baseline for comparison of the arthritic ankle. Alternatively, paw volume may be measured by a volume displacement method using a plethysmometer, following manufacturer's instructions (Stoelting Co.) *(12)*.
3. Soft and hard tissue involvement may be assessed by radiography using a Faxitron X-ray machine (*see* **Fig. 1D,E**) *(13,14)*. Radiographs are taken with direct exposure on X-omat film using 30 mev, 90-s exposure with the Faxitron.
4. Body weights may be measured throughout the experimental time period or at the beginning and end of the experiment.

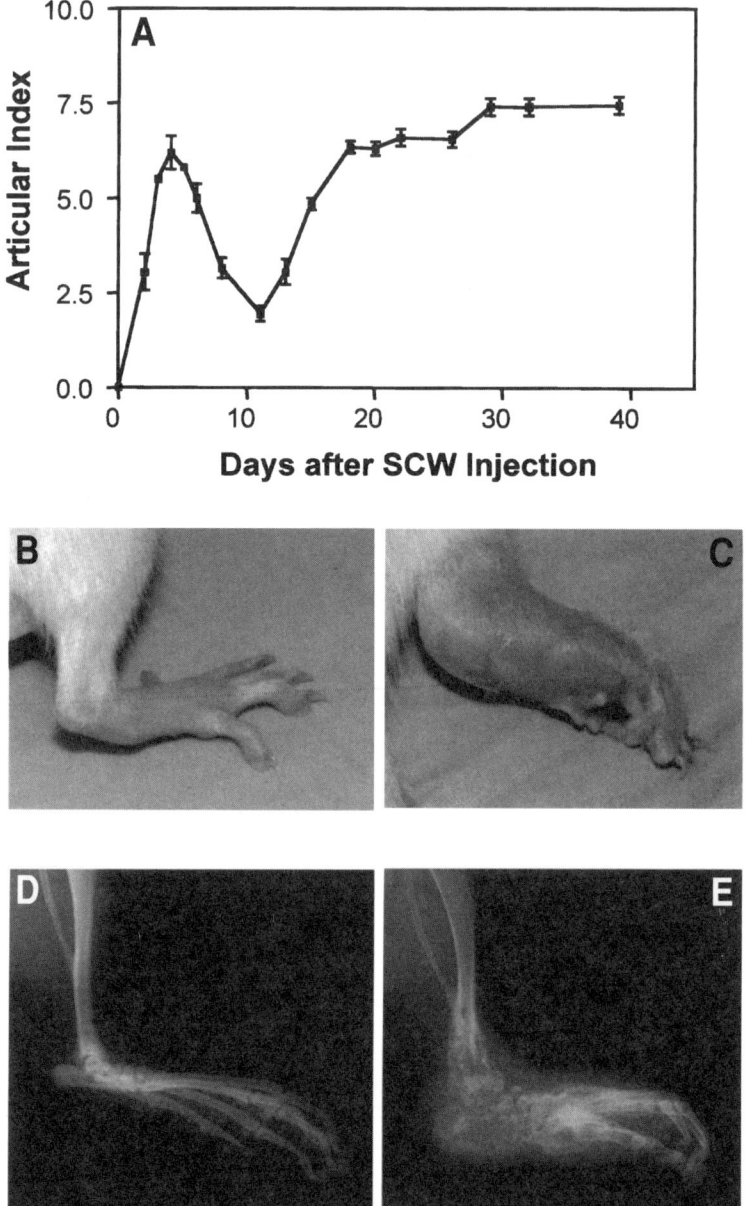

Fig. 1. Induction and clinical evaluation of arthritis. (**A**) A biphasic arthritic response to a single ip injection of SCW (30 µ/g body weight) in female LEW/N rats is monitored clinically by determining the AI, which reflects the degree of joint swelling, erythema, and distortion on a scale of 0 (**B**; normal) to 4 (**C**; severe inflammation)

3.3. Histopathological Evaluation of Arthritis
3.3.1. Tissue Collection and Fixation
1. Euthanize rats with carbon dioxide gas and excise ankle joints.
2. Fix joints in 10% zinc formalin (10 mL) in a 14- or 50-mL Falcon tube (Becton Dickinson, Franklin Lakes, NJ), followed by decalcification in 10% EDTA for 3 d and paraffin embedding.

3.3.2. Histological Staining
1. Stain sections (6 µm) with hematoxylin and eosin for histopathological examination of bone, cartilage, joint space, synovium, pannus formation, and bone marrow (*see* **Note 4**). Masson's trichrome stain is useful to examine collagen (*see* **Fig. 2**) and Safranin O for cartilage.

3.3.3. Immunohistochemical Staining of Cell Surface Antigens
1. Deparaffinize slides by heating to 55°C for 15 min. Submerge slides in xylene twice for 5 min. Rehydrate slides by sequential 5-min incubations in absolute ethanol, 95% ethanol, and 70% ethanol and two 2-min incubations in PBS.
2. Optional antigen retrieval treatment: Pretreat the sections with Triton X-100 (1% in PBS) for 5 min at 37°C. Alternatively, enzyme digest with Digest-All kit using either Ficin (mild digestion), 0.5% Trypsin (medium digestion), or Pepsin (strong digestion).
3. Quench endogenous peroxidase activity by treating sections with 3% hydrogen peroxide in 40% methanol for 10 min.
4. Reduce nonspecific background by incubating sections for 30 min with 10% normal serum (same species in which the secondary antibody is raised) in a humidified chamber.
5. Incubate slides for 1 h with pretitered primary antibody diluted in PBS (*8*).
6. Gently wash slides in PBS for 10 min.
7. Incubate slides with diluted biotinylated secondary antibody for 30 min.
8. Wash for 10 min in PBS and then incubate in ABC reagent for 30 min.
9. Wash again for 10 min and incubate with AEC (3-amino-9-ethylcarbazole) or DAB (3,3'-diaminobenzidine) substrate for horseradish peroxidase or Vector Red for alkaline phosphatase.
10. Counterstain with hematoxylin (AEC, DAB) or methyl green (DAB) and cover slip. AEC reaction product is soluble in organic solvents and must be aqueous mounted (GVA mounting solution), whereas DAB and Vector red stained sections can be cleared with xylene and permanently mounted (Permount).

Fig. 1. *(continued)* for each extremity (maximum total of 16). Each point represents the mean AI ± SEM for each group of animals ($n = 10$). (**D**), (**E**). Radiologic evaluation at 4 wk after SCW injection documents soft tissue swelling and severe bone erosion in a representative arthritic joint (**E**) as compared to a normal joint (**D**).

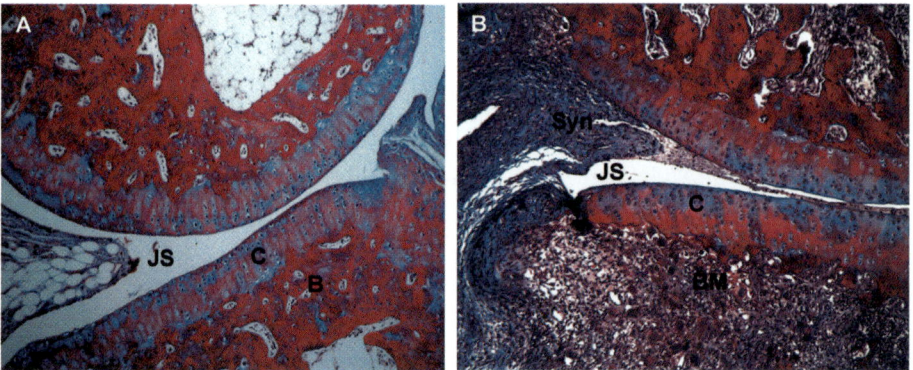

Fig. 2. Histopathological evaluation of arthritis. Joint tissues were excised from a normal (**A**) and arthritic (**B**) rat and processed for histopathology after 4 wk. Masson's trichrome stain reveals decreased collagen (blue stain) in bone and cartilage of arthritic joint due to bone erosion and cartilage degradation. Expansion of the synovial lining (Syn) and pannus formation, narrowing of joint space (JS), mononuclear infiltration, and bone (B) erosion is also evident in the arthritic joint.

3.4. Molecular Evaluation of Arthritis (see Notes 5 and 6)

3.4.1. Tissue Collection and Preparation

1. Excise ankle joints from euthanized rats and place in 14- or 50-mL Falcon tubes. Immediately freeze joints by placing tubes in prechilled 2-methylbutane on dry ice. Store samples at –80°C.
2. Pulverize frozen ankle joints using a freezer mill cooled with liquid nitrogen. Store powdered samples at –80°C.

3.4.2. RNA Isolation

1. Weigh 100-mg joint powder in a 1.5-mL microfuge tube and suspend in 0.75 mL of TRIzol. Vortex samples and proceed with RNA purification steps as outlined by the manufacturer (Invitrogen) or freeze the samples at –20°C for processing at a later date. Dissolve the RNA in DEPC-treated water and heat at 65°C for 10 min to ensure full dissolution of the RNA. Measure the concentration ($A_{260/280}$ ratio approx 2.0) and store RNA at –80°C.

3.4.3. Northern Analysis

1. Electrophorese RNA samples (5 µg in 50% deionized formamide, 2 M formaldehyde, 1X MOPS buffer, 1X RNA loading buffer) in a 1% agarose/1.23 M formaldehyde gel containing ethidium bromide (1 µg/mL) and transfer to a nylon or nitrocellulose membrane using the Turboblotter system. Bake the membrane at 80°C under vacuum for 2 h.

2. Prehybridize membrane in a heat-sealed bag (10 mL solution for a 11 × 14 cm membrane) in a shaking waterbath at 42°C for at least 4 h.
3. Radiolabel cDNA (25–50 ng) to a specific activity of >10^8 cpm/µg with [^{32}P]dCTP (50 µCi) using a random-prime labeling kit according to manufacturer's instructions (Invitrogen). Denature the probe by boiling for 5 min. Transfer to ice. Add the probe to 10 mL hybridization buffer.
4. Add hybridization buffer containing probe to the membrane and hybridize overnight at 42°C.
5. Wash the membrane twice at room temperature in 2X SSC, 0.1% SDS for 15 min and once at 65°C in 0.1X SSC, 0.1% SDS for 30 min.
6. Expose the membrane to a phosphor screen and analyze with a phosphorimager (Molecular Dynamics/Amersham Pharmacia Biotech, Chicago, IL) using ImageQuaNT software.

3.4.4. Semiquantitative RT-PCR

1. Reverse transcribe 2 µg total RNA using oligo(dT) as a primer and 50-µL reaction mix (1X PCR buffer, 2 mM DTT, 10 µg/mL oligo dT, 0.2 mM dNTP, 0.05 U RNasin). Incubate RNA mixture at 70°C for 10 min and cool to room temperature for 15 min. Add reverse transcriptase (0.4 U) and incubate for 2 h at 37°C. Terminate reaction by heating to 95°C for 5 min.
2. Amplify the cDNA (2 µL) by PCR in a reaction mixture of 1X AmpliTaq buffer, 0.2 mM dNTP, 0.4 µM of each sense and antisense primer, and 0.002 U *Taq* polymerase. Perform PCR amplification (denaturation, 94°C for 45 s; annealing, 60°C for 45 s; extension, 72°C for 1 min) for predetermined number of cycles which generates a linear response curve for threefold dilutions of a positive RNA sample (ConA-stimulated mouse spenocytes) *(15)*. Housekeeping genes GAPDH (glyceraldehyde-3-phosphate dehydrogenase) or HPRT (hypoxanthine phosphoribosyltransferase) can be assayed on all samples to verify efficient cDNA synthesis and to allow for comparison of RNA species between different samples.
3. Analyze PCR products (10 µL) from ethidium bromide-stained agarose gels (1.8%) using a digital imaging system (Alpha Innotech Corp., San Leandro, CA).

3.4.5. RNase Protection Assay (RPA)

1. Synthesize a ^{32}P-labeled rat cytokine-specific RNA probe using a cytokine multiprobe template according to manufacturer's instructions (BD Pharmingen). Following DNase digestion, centrifuge the reaction mixture through an RNase-free G50 spin column.
2. Hybridize total RNA (10 µg) overnight at 56°C to the radiolabeled RNA probe (8 × 10^5 Cherenkov counts/sample).
3. Treat samples with RNase cocktail supplied with the RPA kit for 45 min at 30°C. Ethanol precipitate the protected RNA-RNA hybrids, wash with 70% and 90% ethanol and air dry.

4. Resuspend the RNA hybrids in loading buffer and electrophorese in a 6% denaturing acrylamide gel (>40 cm in length). After drying, expose the gel to a phosphor screen and quantify radioactivity by a phosphorimager.

3.5. Protein Analysis
3.5.1. Protein Isolation

1. Weigh 100-mg joint powder and suspend in protein lysis buffer. Incubate 10 min on ice and centrifuge for 10 min at 4°C at 17,900g. Store 50-µL aliquots of supernatant fluid at −70°C. Measure protein concentration of the supernatant fluid using BioRad DC Protein assay.

3.5.2. Western Blot Analysis

1. Boil lysate samples (100 µg) for 5 min in electrophoresis sample buffer.
2. Electrophorese samples in a SDS-acrylamide gel with Tris-glycine buffer and transfer to nitrocellulose. The percentage of acrylamide will depend on the size of the protein to be studied.
3. Incubate membrane overnight at 4°C on a rotary platform in 5% nonfat dry milk in TBS-T.
4. Incubate membrane for 3 h at room temperature or overnight at 4°C with primary antibody diluted in 5% milk/TBS-T.
5. Wash membrane in TBS-T once for 15 min and twice for 10 min at room temperature.
6. Incubate membrane for 1–3 h with diluted HRP (horseradish peroxidase)-conjugated secondary antibody and repeat washes.
7. Shake membrane vigorously for 60 s in HRP substrate (SuperSignal luminol detection system) and immediately expose to film.

3.5.3. Electrophoretic Mobility Shift Assay (EMSA)

1. Dissolve 100 mg powdered joint tissue in 0.3 mL nuclear protein lysis buffer and homogenize with a polytron for 10 s. Centrifuge at 10,600g for 10 min at 4°C. Store 50-µL aliquots of the supernatant fluid at −70°C. Determine total protein concentration using BioRad DC Protein assay.
2. Incubate the double-stranded consensus oligonucleotide (approx 100 ng) with [γ-^{32}P]ATP (50 µCi) and T4 polynucleotide kinase (10 U) in 1X PNK buffer for 30 min at 37°C. Apply sample to a G25 spin column and centrifuge for 4 min according to manufacturer's instructions (5-Prime 3-Prime).
3. Mix cellular extract (5 to 10 µg) with the radiolabeled probe in binding buffer for 30 min at room temperature. Optional: To block binding, preincubate extract with unlabeled, annealed oligonucleotide (10- to 50-fold excess) for 30 min on ice. To supershift the binding complex, preincubate the extract with 1 µL transcription factor antibody (Santa Cruz Biotechnology, Santa Cruz, CA) for 30 min on ice.

4. Electrophorese the binding protein complex in a 6% polyacrylamide gel containing 0.25 M Tris-borate-EDTA.
5. Dry the gel under vacuum, expose overnight to a phosphor screen, and analyze with a phosphorimager.

4. Notes

1. Previous studies have shown that genetic factors play an important role in disease susceptibility *(2,16)*. Female Lewis (LEW/N) rats develop SCW-induced polyarthritis with virtually 100% incidence. In contrast, male Lewis rats, MHC-compatible male and female Fisher (F344/N), and other strains such as WKY and BUF are relatively resistant and develop milder or no disease following exposure to SCW *(16,17)*. Whereas susceptibility to arthritis induction is under polygenic control, a defect in the hypothalamic-pituitary-adrenal axis in the LEW/N rats, as compared to the F344, results in reduced corticosteroid production and thus unabated inflammation *(5,6)*. Age (6–8 wk) and size (100–150 g) of the rats are also critical parameters to effective arthritis induction. Because infection and stress can also affect arthritis induction, it is important to maintain a pathogen-free environment and avoid overcrowded cages to minimize stress. The vendor source of LEW/N rats for experimental autoimmune disease induction also appears critical *(18)* (J. Chan, unpublished), suggesting that genetic changes may occur within colonies. It may be appropriate to perform a pilot study based on vendor prior to initiating larger studies.
2. Critical to the successful induction of arthritis is the preparation of the SCW. Typical dosages range from 10 to 60 µg/g body weight. Low doses (<10 µg/g body weight) may result in a decreased incidence of disease and excess SCW may induce toxicities. Also critical to arthritis induction is size of the SCW particles. In general, particles between 5 to 500×10^6 Da stimulate the typical arthritis profile. Excess sonication generates smaller ($< 5 \times 10^6$ Da) fragments which are highly arthritogenic but generate only acute arthritis. In contrast, particles $>500 \times 10^6$ Da exhibit a low incidence of arthritis induction. Recent commercial preparations of SCW have necessitated a reduction in dosage (15 µg/g body weight as compared to 30 µg/g body weight), increased body size (150 g rat as compared to 80–100 g rat), as well as changing commercial suppliers of LEW/N rats (*see* **Note 1**), in order to induce chronic arthritis. Depending on the source of SCW, it may be necessary to alter the dose/concentration of SCW and utilize different sized animals from different suppliers to maximize arthritis incidence and severity. With recent changes in vendors of SCW and/or animals, the reproducibility and reliability of this experimental model utilized so effectively during the past three decades have been compromised.
3. A single intraperitoneal injection of SCW results in the development of a biphasic inflammatory response that can be monitored noninvasively by quantification of the AI. The acute response develops by days 2–5, followed by a remission phase (days 6–12), after which the chronic, destructive phase ensues (> day 12).

Whereas the maximum AI score may vary between experiments, the pattern of the inflammatory response is consistent (*see* **Fig. 1**) and is highly reproducible. This experimental model of arthritis is particularly useful for studying the pathogenesis of joint inflammation and for evaluating various therapeutic agents.
4. Histological analysis of joint tissue provides a key measurement of the degree and type of inflammation by identification and quantitation of the cellular infiltrate and visualization of the tissue damage and bone erosion. Whereas neutrophil infiltration into the synovium is characteristic in the acute response, monocytes and lymphocytes are the predominant infiltrating cells during the chronic tissue erosive response. Immunohistochemistry can be used to phenotype inflammatory cell populations by their cell surface markers, as well as localize cytokine/mediator production in the inflamed joint *(11)*.
5. Molecular evaluation of the inflammatory events within the joint and the impact of interventional strategies provides important insight. In particular, cytokine analysis within treated and untreated joint tissues can be measured at the RNA level by Northern analysis, RT-PCR, and RNase protection assay *(10,11)*. Protein expression of selected cytokines and inflammatory mediators can also be monitored by Western blot. Because many of the mediators are transcriptionally regulated, cellular lysates can also be analyzed for transcription factor expression and activity via Western blot and gel retardation assays, respectively.
6. Evaluation of this in vivo model of arthritis by multiple parameters including cellular and molecular components of the disease process provides insight into potential mechanisms for therapeutic modulation. The ability to impact the arthritic process through the exogenous administration of specific cytokines or cytokine antagonists links these products to synovial pathogenesis *(9–14)*. Understanding the pathogenesis of synovial inflammation and joint destruction is critical to the design and targeting of therapeutic agents.

References

1. Cromartie, W. J., Craddock, J. G., Schwab, J. H., Anderle, S. K., and Yang, C. H. (1977) Arthritis in rats after systemic injection of streptococcal cells or cell walls. *J. Exp. Med.* **146**, 1585–1602.
2. Wilder, R. L., Allen, J. B., Wahl, L. M., Calandra, G. B., and Wahl, S. M. (1983) The pathogenesis of group A streptococcal cell wall-induced polyarthritis in the rat. Comparative studies in arthritis resistant and susceptible inbred rat strains. *Arthritis Rheum.* **26**, 1442–1451.
3. Hines, K. L., Christ, M., and Wahl, S. M. (1993) Cytokine regulation of the immune response: An in vivo model. *Immunomethods* **3**, 13–22
4. Allen, J. B., Blatter, D., Calandra, G. B., and Wilder, R. L. (1983) Sex hormonal effects on the severity of streptococcal cell wall-induced polyarthritis in the rat. *Arthritis Rheum.* **26**, 560–563.
5. Sternberg, E. M., Hill, J. M., Chrousos, G. P., Kamilaris, T., Listwak, S. J., Gold, P. W., et al. (1989) Inflammatory mediator-induced hypothalamic-pituitary-adre-

nal axis activation is defective in streptococcal cell wall arthritis-susceptible Lewis rats. *Proc. Natl. Acad. Sci. USA* **86,** 2374–2378.
6. Sternberg, E. M., Young, W. S., 3rd, Bernardini, R., Calogero, A. E., Chrousos, G. P., Gold, P. W., et al. (1989) A central nervous system defect in biosynthesis of corticotropin-releasing hormone is associated with susceptibility to streptococcal cell wall-induced arthritis in Lewis rats. *Proc. Natl. Acad. Sci. USA* **86,** 4771–4775.
7. Song, X. Y., Zeng, L., Jin, W., Pilo, C. M., Frank, M. E., and Wahl, S. M. (2000) Suppression of streptococcal cell wall-induced arthritis by human chorionic gonadotropin. *Arthritis Rheum.* **43,** 2064–2072.
8. Puklavec, M. J. and Barclay, A. N. (1999) Monoclonal antibodies to rat leukocyte surface antigens, MHC antigens, and immunoglobulins. *Current Protocols in Immunol.* **4,** A.4C.1–A.4C.12
9. McCartney-Francis, N., Allen, J. B., Mizel, D. E., Albina, J. E., Xie, Q. W., Nathan, C. F., et al. (1993) Suppression of arthritis by an inhibitor of nitric oxide synthase. *J. Exp. Med.* **178,** 749–754.
10. McCartney-Francis, N. L., Song, X. Y., Mizel, D. E., Wahl, C. L., and Wahl, S. M. (1999) Hemoglobin protects from streptococcal cell wall-induced arthritis. *Arthritis Rheum.* **42,** 1119–1127.
11. McCartney-Francis, N. L., Song, X., Mizel, D. E., and Wahl, S. M. (2001) Selective inhibition of inducible nitric oxide synthase exacerbates erosive joint disease. *J. Immunol.* **166,** 2734–2740.
12. Song, X. Y., Gu, M., Jin, W. W., Klinman, D. M., and Wahl, S. M. (1998) Plasmid DNA encoding transforming growth factor-beta1 suppresses chronic disease in a streptococcal cell wall-induced arthritis model. *J. Clin. Invest.* **101,** 2615–2621.
13. Wahl, S. M., Allen, J. B., Costa, G. L., Wong, H. L., and Dasch, J. R. (1993) Reversal of acute and chronic synovial inflammation by anti-transforming growth factor beta. *J. Exp. Med.* **177,** 225–230.
14. Song, X., Zeng, L., Jin, W., Thompson, J., Mizel, D. E., Lei, K., et al. (1999) Secretory leukocyte protease inhibitor suppresses the inflammation and joint damage of bacterial cell wall-induced arthritis. *J. Exp. Med.* **190,** 535–542.
15. McCartney-Francis, N. L., Mizel, D. E., Redman, R. S., Frazier-Jessen, M., Panek, R. B., Kulkarni, A. B., et al. (1996) Autoimmune Sjogren's-like lesions in salivary glands of TGF-beta1-deficient mice are inhibited by adhesion-blocking peptides. *J. Immunol.* **157,** 1306–1312.
16. Wilder, R. L., Calandra, G. B., Garvin, A. J., Wright, K. D., and Hansen, C. T. (1982) Strain and sex variation in the susceptibility to streptococcal cell wall-induced polyarthritis in the rat. *Arthritis Rheum.* **25,** 1064–1072.
17. Wilder, R. L. (1998) Streptococcal cell wall arthritis. *Curr. Protocols in Immunol.* **3,** 15.10.11–15.10.12
18. Swanborg, R. H., Gould, K. E., and Stepaniak, J. A. (1994) Studies of experimental autoimmune encephalomyelitis (EAE). *J. Immunol.* **153,** 2352.

18

The Assessment of Inflammation, Cartilage Matrix, and Bone Loss in Experimental Monoarticular Arthritis of the Rat

Michael P. Seed

1. Introduction

Rheumatic joint disease is commonly treated with nonsteroidal (NSAID) and steroidal antiinflammatory drugs, as well as antirheumatic agents and immunomodulators. These approaches are aimed at reducing the inflammatory processes with the assumption of limiting joint destruction. However, whereas it is clear that these approaches are effective in reducing inflammation and pain, it remains uncertain whether this is translated into an improvement in indices of joint integrity such as bone and cartilage degradation.

Common models of inflammatory joint disease have a heavy reliance on inflammatory or immune indices, and subjective assessments of synovitis and erosion. The erosion of bone rarely features as an end point. There is, thus, a requirement for the rapid and relevant determination of joint inflammation, cartilage and bone damage in a controlled inflammatory environment. The femorotibial joint space of the rat provides a convenient cavity for the induction of inflammation, with ease of induction and relevant biochemical end points. The rat patella provides a unitary source of cartilage and bone that is easily dissectible. Joint diameter can be taken as an index of inflammation and in some cases, synovial fluid volume along with biochemical measures can also be assessed. Patella cartilage matrix proteoglycan content, assayed as glycosaminoglycan (GAG) provides a rapid and simple biochemical end point for cartilage matrix damage, whereas residual bone dry weight indicates bone resorption. The joint space can thus be used just as other models of inflammation such as those induced intra-air pouch, subcutaneously (sc), intra-plantar,

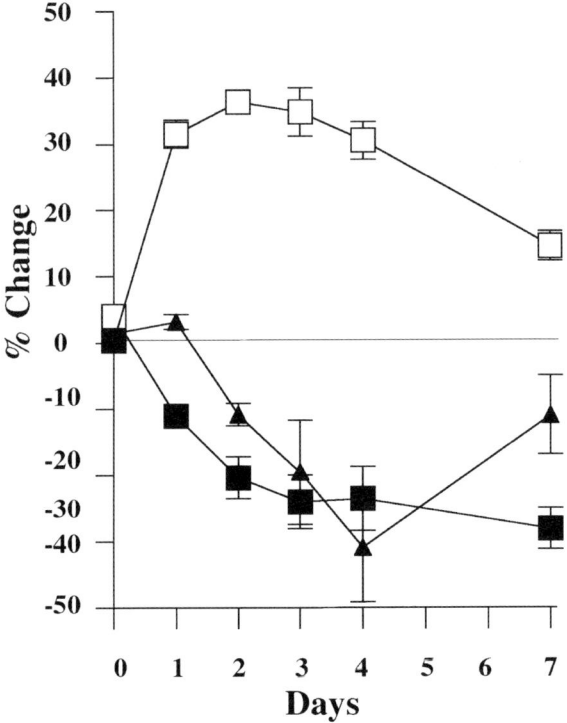

Fig. 1. Time-course for inflammation, patellar bone and cartilage GAG loss for the M.tb. Data are % change in inflammation (mm, □), patellar GAG content (μg, ▲), and bone dry mass (mg, ■) compared to paired saline injected contralateral joints.

or intra-pleurally, for example, to give irritant, delayed-type hypersensitivity, foreign body, arthus, and cytokine-induced inflammation. Each of these may provide a differing pharmacology, and may reveal that a broad link between inflammation and joint destruction cannot be relied upon.

Herein is described the method for inducing heat-killed Mycobacterium tuberculosis (M.tb.), zymosan, and methylated bovine serum albumin(BSA) monoarticular arthritides, with notes on practical experiences with other modes of inflammatory induction. The best described model is the M.tb. monoarticular arthritis of the rat (MAR) *(1)*. This is an intra-articular (ia) granulomatous reaction accompanied by synovial-lining proliferation, joint diameter, patellar GAG, and bone loss peak at 5 d (**Fig. 1**). Antiinflammatory steroids reduce all indices *(2)*, whereas the NSAIDs indomethacin, piroxicam, and naproxen reduce inflammation, and bone loss, but increase cartilage GAG loss *(3–5,* **Table 1**), and tiaprofenic acid and diclofenac do not alter GAG loss. Methotrexate reduces inflammation whereas leaving cartilage GAG and bone loss unchecked. This

Table 1
Illustration of the Use of the M.tb.-Induced Monoarticular Arthritis of the Rat, and the Dislocation of Antiinflammatory and Chondro-Sparing Activities[a]

Drug	Dose mg/kg	(n)	% change in Joint Dia	% change in Patellar GAG	% change in Patellar dry Mass
Cyclosporin	0	(8)	37.4+/–2.8	–27.6+/–3.7	–51.6+/–6.6
	1	(8)	38.2+/–3.4	-22.1+/–2.1	-60.7+/–4.0
	3	(6)	40.2+/–5.1	–19.9+/–3.7	–47.3+/–5.6
	10	(7)	31.8+/–4.5	–7.1+/–3.3**	–20.3+/–2.9**
	30	(8)	24.2+/–2.3**	–6.6+/–2.8**	–24.2+/–5.0*
Methotrexate	0	(9)	41.9+/–2.2	–36.4+/–3.1	–51.9+/–6.3
	0.03	(7)	43.5+/–2.3	–32.9+/–2.0	–65.2+/–5.7
	0.1	(7)	42.1+/–2.1	–31.2+/–2.3	–60.6+/–5.2
	0.3	(8)	39.8+/–4.1	–31.6+/–3.1	–61.1+/–8.9
	1.0	(8)	29.9+/–2.5**	–32.0+/–3.4	–54.6+/–6.6
Naproxen	0	(10)	43.3+/–2.4	-28+/–1.7	–52.7+/–4.0
	1	(6)	38.3+/–2.6	–35.7+/–1.8*	–57.1+/–5.4
	3	(6)	35.8+/–1.1*	–32.2+/–4.5	–48.5+/–4.2
	10	(6)	32.0+/–1.8*	–41.8+/–3.1**	–28.8+/–2.8**
	30	(6)	27.0+/–2.0**	–38.1+/–3.7*	–28.5+/–2.5**

(n) = number of animals in group, *$p < 0.05$ ANOVA with F-test, **$p < 0.01$.
[a]Rats were dosed with drugs suspended in 1% acacia for 1 h prior to the ia injection of 200 μg of heat-killed M.tb. into one stifle joint and saline in the other. Results are calculated as % change in joint diameter (mm), patellar GAG (μg/patella), and patella bone mass (mg) in the arthritic knee compared to the control.

model also responds to low-dose irradiation at levels that reduce inflammatory arthritis in the clinic with a reduction in joint inflammation and increase in bone resorption (6). Both cyclosporin and anti-T-lymphocyte serum (1) reduce inflammation, but this is prior to the development of a positive M.tb. skin test. Developing the reaction into the chronic phase, the joint inflammation develops into a fibrous pannus with angiogenesis and erosion into cartilage. The patellar bone develops osteophytes (see **Fig. 2**) and chondrophytes. A secondary loss of GAG density occurs as the animals become sensitized to the antigen. Zymosan MAR results in less patellar GAG loss (**Fig. 3**), but this is more susceptible to the potentiative effects of NSAIDs and the suppressive effects of antiinflammatory steroidal therapy (7). Low dose X-ray irradiation reduces all three parameters (6). The assessment of GAG uses the method of Farndale et al. (8) modified for use with a microplate reader (9).

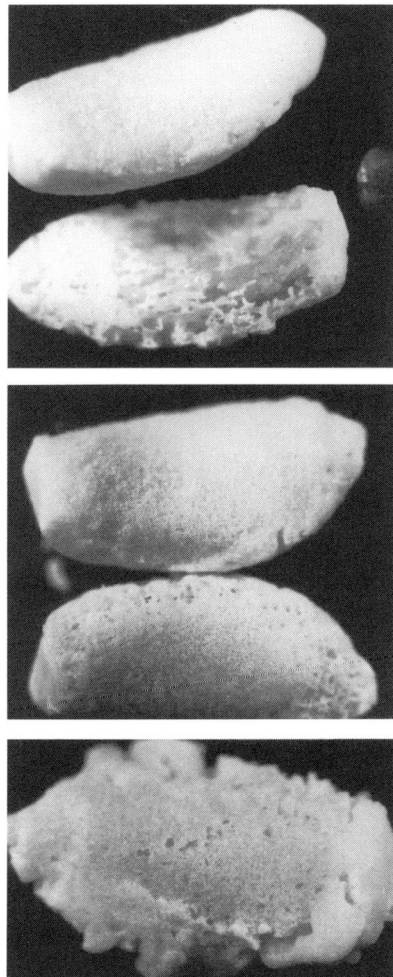

Fig. 2. Patellar bone erosion and subsequent osteophyte formation in rat M.tb. MAR. Protection against resorption is illustrated through the administration of dexamethasone. (**A**) Left (eroded, arthritic, bottom) and right (saline control, top) patellae day 5. (**B**) Dexamethasone (0.1 mg/kg). As A. (**C**) Day 21 arthritic patella illustrating osteophyte formation.

2. Materials
2.1. Animals

The animals used for published work were male Wistar CFHB (130–150 g, Charles River), housed at a maximum of four per cage on wood shavings with free access to food and water. *See* **Note 1** for guidance on animal strains.

Assessment of Inflammation

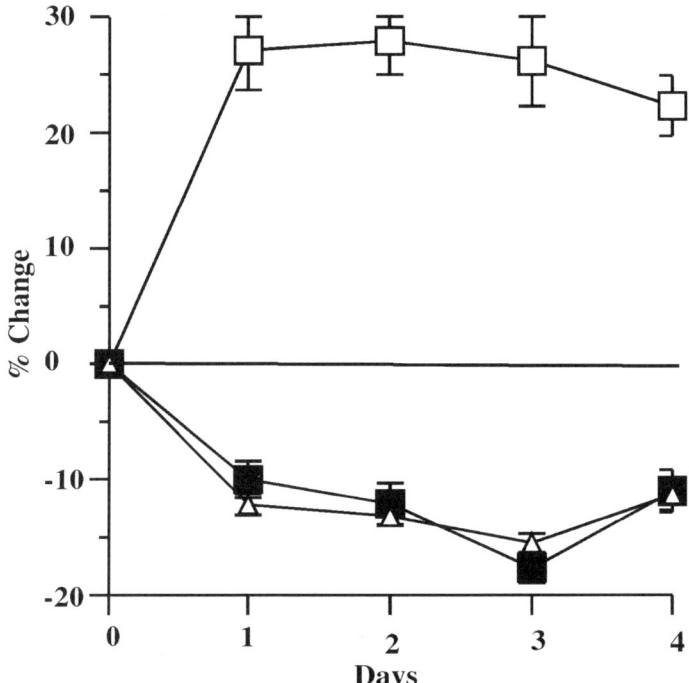

Fig. 3. Time-course for inflammation, patellar bone and cartilage GAG loss for the zymosan (4 mg) MAR. Data are % change in inflammation (mm, □), patellar GAG content (µg, △), and bone dry mass (mg, ■) compared to paired saline injected contralateral joints.

2.2. Preparation of Arthritic Stimuli (see Note 2)

1. Heat-killed *Mycobacterium tuberculosis* (Ministry of Agriculture Fisheries and Food, strain C, DT, PN. Other suppliers include Difco and Sigma). Using an agate mortar and pestle washed in 70% ethanol, 80 mg of M.tb. is ground finely and 10 mL pyrogen free saline added slowly, followed by brief sonication to give 200 µg/25 µL for ia injection.
2. Zymosan, an 80 mg/mL solution is ground as aforementioned into a viscous paste to give 4 mg/50 µL for ia injection. This is not sonicated.
3. Methylated bovine serum albumin (mBSA). This binds to cartilage providing an antigenic focus at the cartilage surface for the delayed-type hypersensitivity reaction.
    a. Sensitization dose: 200 mg mBSA is dissolved in sterilized distilled water, and NaCl added to make 9% saline. 10 mL Freund's complete adjuvant is added and the mixture emulsified by probe sonication or several passages through a white 10-gauge syringe needle until it does not spread when dropped onto water.

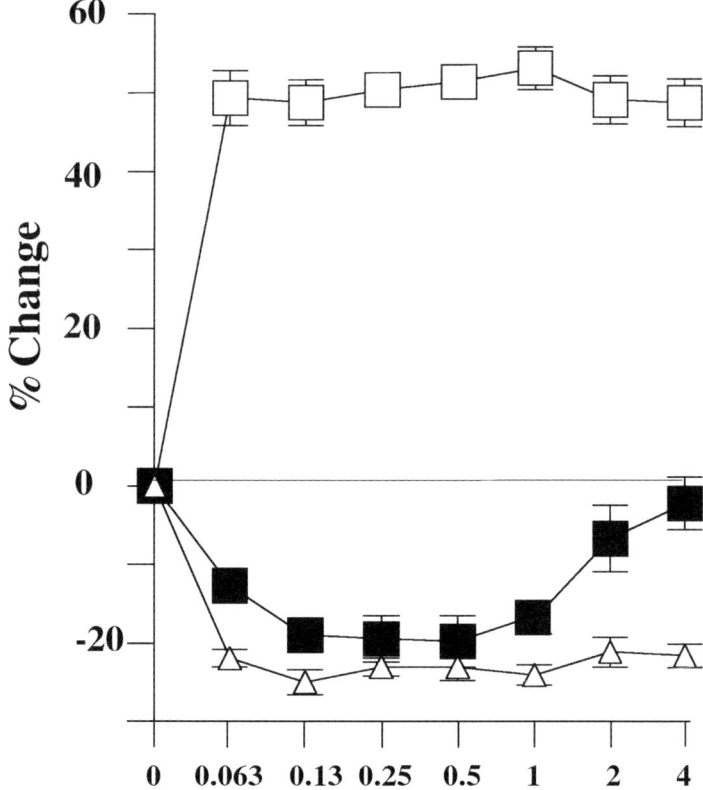

Fig. 4. The effect of mBSA sensitization dose on the mBSA MAR illustrating the importance of protocol characterization (in the Wistar CFHB rat 1 mg sensitization dose is the standard dose for skin test and paw edema inflammation). Data are % change in inflammation (mm, □), patellar GAG content (μg, ■), and bone dry mass (mg, △) compared to paired saline-injected contralateral joints.

b. Challenge dose: Prepare mBSA in distilled water to 40 mg/mL and add NaCl to make 9% saline (1 mg/25 μL) for ia injection.

2.3. Digestion

1. Digestion Buffer: 20 mM disodium hydrogen orthophosphate, 1 mM ethylenediamine tetraacetic acid (EDTA), 2 mM dithiothreitol (DTT). This can be stored for 2 wk at 4°C.
2. Papain: Sigma catalog number P3125.
3. 1,9-dimethylmethylene blue (DMB) solution: Dissolve 40 mg 1,9-dimethylmethylene blue in 5 mL methanol and add this to 1 L distilled water. Mix in 24 mL of 1N hydrochloric acid, 7.6 g glycine, and 5.9 g sodium chloride. Stir until dissolved, with heat if necessary, but do not boil. Make the volume up to 2.5 L

Table 2
Summary of Sensitization and Challenge Protocols for Rat Monoarticular Arthritises

Inflammation	Sensitization Dose	Challenge Dose	GAG Endpoint After Challenge
M.tb. (see **Note 5**)	None	200 µg/25 µL	4 d
Zymosan	None	4 mg/50 µL	3 d
MBSA (antigen-induced, see **Note 6**)	0.25–0.5 mg/0.2 mL	1 mg/25 µL	4 d
r.ratIL-1β (see **Note 7**)	None	1 µg	4 d
rhIL-1β (see **Note 7**)	None	10–50 ng	SF vol 4h
M.tb. (antigen-induced, see **Note 5**)	0.4 mg	20–30 µg	4 d

and store at room temperature in a smoked glass bottle. The solution is stable for 6 mo. Do not use when warm.

4. Chondroitin sulfate standards: Chondroitin sulfate (Sigma catalog number C3254) standards are prepared to give final concentrations between 10 and 300 µg/mL in digestion buffer. When papain digested samples are used, standards are prepared in the appropriate blank.

3. Methods
3.1. Induction of MAR (see Note 3)

Wistar or Lewis rats (150–180 g) are lightly anesthetized under gaseous halothane anesthesia through an anesthetic box. The procedure is fast enough that a nose cone should not be required. The animals are laid on their backs and the joint held by the free hand pointing proximal-distally. The index finger nail is used to locate the femorotibiochondylar groove distal to the patella. The other hand injects the stimulus dose through the patellar ligament into the joint using a dispensing microsyringe set at 25–50 µL and fitted with a 30-gauge stainless steel needle. The contralateral knee is injected with saline or appropriate control vehicle. Between groups, the syringe and needles are sterilized in 70% ethanol. The baseline control group is injected with vehicle into both knees. For general comments on mice, see **Note 4**.

3.2. Sensitization and Stimulus Dose Schedules

For MAR of differing atiologies see **Table 2**. Patellar GAG end points are for the Wistar CFHB strain (see **Note 1**). For other reactions, see **Note 15**.

3.3. End Points

1. Rats are culled by CO_2 suffocation. The skin covering the stifle joints is parted and the joint diameters assessed using a micrometer (or callipers), and the ani-

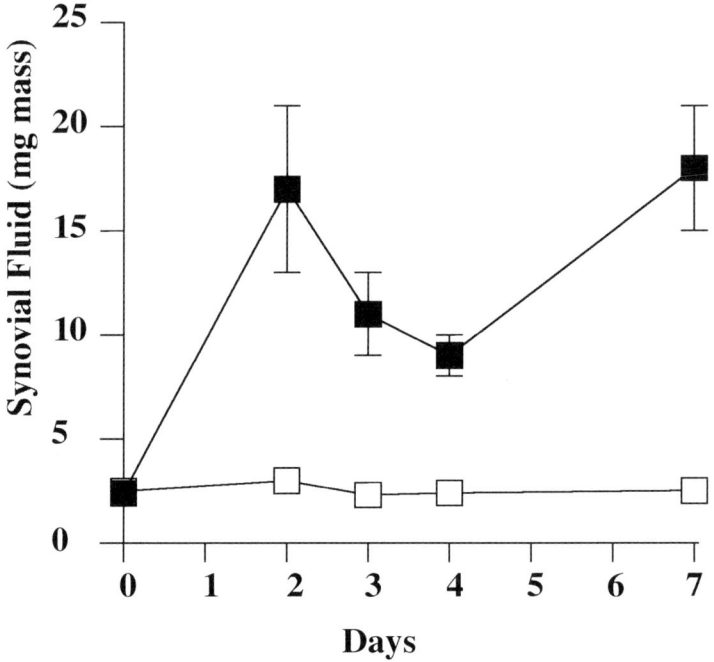

Fig. 5. Demonstration of changes in synovial fluid volume (mg mass) in the zymosan MAR. Data are saline injected (open squares) and zymosan (4 mg, closed squares) injected contralateral joints.

mals weighed. The patellae are dissected free of tendon and other tissue (*see* **Note 8**) and assayed for GAG content. The residual patellar bones are dried in an oven (70°C overnight) and weighed (*see* **Note 9**).
2. Synovial fluid may be sampled using preweighed triangles of filter paper inserted into the joint (*see* **Fig. 5** and **Note 10**) and the volume calculated as difference in mass.

3.4. Patellar Cartilage Proteoglycan Assay (see Note 11)

Proteoglycan GAG is assayed as chondroitin sulfate equivalents through 1,2-DMB binding assay. The binding of DMB to the sulfate moieties of chondroitin sulfate results in a metachromatic shift that is detected at 525 nm *(8,10)* and is adapted for use on a microplate reader *(9)* as follows.

1. Rat patellae are digested in 1 mL digestion buffer and 20 µL papain added to each sample in screw capped tubes. The mixture is heated in a water bath at 65°C for 3 h with the occasional mix.
2. The assay of large numbers of samples is achieved by using a 96-well plate reader to measure the absorbance at 525 nm (peak) and subtracting the absorbance at

690 nm (530 nm and 450 nm can be used depending on filters available) in order to control for nonspecific scattering and absorbance by the plates. Samples are zeroed against blank wells and the GAG content interpolated from a standard curve on each plate. 10 µL samples are placed in each well, with duplicate blanks, and CS standards ranging from 0.25 to 2 µg/well (equivalent to 25–200 µg/mL incubation medium and 50–400 µg/patella. Once the plate is loaded with samples and standards, 200 µL DMB solution is added quickly and smoothly across the plate using a multichannel pipet. The plate is equilibrated for 1 min and then read immediately. The results can be interpolated by linear regression or by curve fitting.
3. Calculations are made as follows: % change in parameter, $p = 100 \times [(p$ treated knee$-p$ untreated knee)/(p untreated knee)].

Patellar GAG can be measured as µg GAG/patella, µg GAG/mg wet mass per whole patella, or µg GAG/mg patellar wet mass–bone mass (i.e., /mg cartilage) (*see* **Note 12**).

3.5. Experimental Design (see Note 13) and Statistics

Animals should be dosed with vehicle, and both positive and negative controls included. Body mass should be assessed. Weight gain in MAR animals is normal, excepting M.tb. MAR when adjuvant disease may appear sporadically in the chronic phase (>day 20). Groups of 8 or above. Analysis by ANOVA followed by F-test, Dunn's Post-hoc test, or Newman-Keul's test should be adequate.

4. Notes

1. The choice of strains is important. Each Laboratory has experience with its own strains. For nonimmune acute inflammation, standard out-bred strains may be used. However, the M.tb. MAR requires strains sensitive to the induction of adjuvant arthritis (such as the Lewis rat). For immune reactions use those strains that have proven susceptibility. As with all in vivo pharmacology, the first experiments should be a time-course followed by a dose-response curve because these have been found to vary from strain to strain. For example, GAG loss induced by M.tb. in the Charles River Lewis rat (UK) appears to peak at 2 d as opposed to 4 d for the Wistar CFHB. *See* **Fig. 4** for a typical characterisation experiment.
2. Preparation of solutions. M.tb. should be ground dry, then saline added slowly while grinding in a circular fashion to make a smooth paste. The final suspension should be tested to pass through the 30-gauge needle (or other needle) without clogging. This requires practice. Care should be taken during injections because the suspension settles. Zymosan: 400 mg/5 mL zymosan is treated as for M.tb. However, this forms a sticky suspension that should be completely dissolved. mBSA is soluble if prepared in distilled water, and saline added slowly last (to prevent bubble formation, swirl, do not shake). If the solution clouds, it should be prepared as fresh. MBSA: when making up mBSA solutions, the solution may

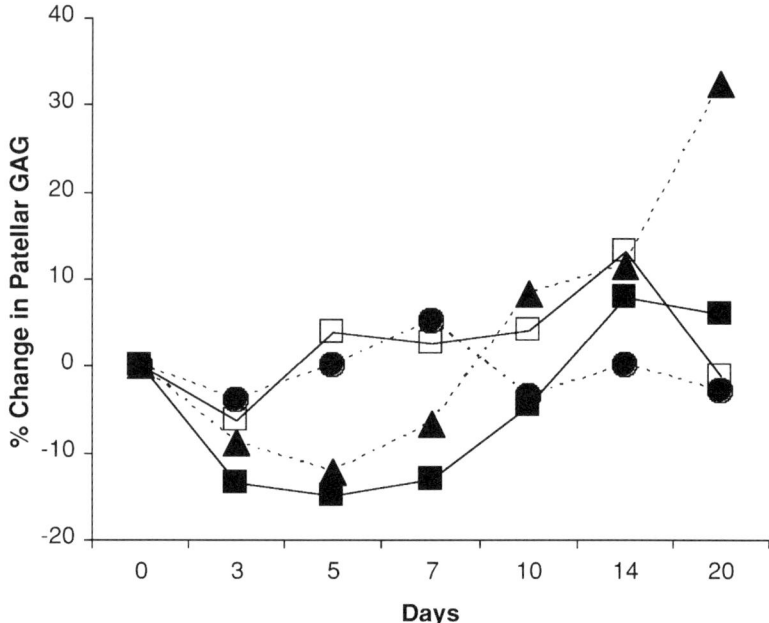

Fig. 6. Time-course for patellar GAG content of patella from mBSA MAR illustrating the effect of treatment with a NSAID (tiaprofenic acid) and immunomodulator (cyclosporine-A). All animals received a sensitization dose of 1 mg mBSA in either Freund's incomplete (negative control) or Freund's complete adjuvant (positive control and drug treatments) and were challenged 2 wk later with 0.5 mg mBSA ia in the left and saline in the contralateral stifle joint. Treatment groups are: negative control (p.o. drug vehicle, circles, dashed lines); positive control (p.o. drug vehicle, triangles, dashed lines); tiaprofenic acid (p.o., 5 mg/kg, closed squares); cyclosporine-A (p.o., 20 mg/kg, open squares).

cloud on the addition of NaCl and must be discarded. Oversonication of the emulsion can result in mBSA precipitation and the preparation should be discarded.
3. Intra-articular (ia) injection. This is best practiced on fresh cadavers using a dilute solution of ink. Often the correct injection is felt as a "pulse" or "filling" through the fingers holding either side of the knee. Moving the skin immediately after injection seals the needle track. This can be seen as a track of dye in practice. In place of 30-gauge stainless steel needles, modern 40-gauge disposable insulin needles may be used, but care must be taken to ensure that particles do not block them, or are filtered out. Drugs may be injected once a day in a volume of 10 µL using a dispensing microsyringe. Increased numbers ($n = 18$ per group) should be used to allow exclusion of animals found to possess inflammation in the control knees due to infection.

4. Mice do not require anesthetising if two people are present. One scruffs the mouse and inverts it, holding one leg. The other injects using a microstepping microsyringe (max. 10 µL per shot) fitted with a brown 26-gauge needle. Paradoxically, the larger gauge needle seals well around the joint. The author finds that tracking of the injectate can occur with fine needles. The needle is pressed into the F-T groove and "clicks" into the joint (a movement of <1 mm). Pressing the dispenser button provides a "puff" of hair movement around the needle and joint to indicate joint filling. Lack of this evidence indicates an sc/peri-articular injection. As in the rat, this will be easily seen at postmortem. Sometimes fluid may be seen coming from the needle track indicating a poor injection (this is never seen after a good injection). Removal of the needle and flexing the skin seals the needle track. Practice on fresh cadavers.
5. M.tb. antigen induced MAR: Rats are sensitized with 0.1 mL (0.4 mg M.tb. in FIA) of the sensitizing emulsion subcutaneously at the back of the neck to avoid the induction of adjuvant arthritis. The tail base should not be used in those strains that are susceptible to adjuvant arthritis, unless in a 1:1 0.4 mg M.tb./FIA:saline emulsion. The sensitizing and challenge doses should be adapted for each rat strain and source of M.tb. A challenge dose of 20 µg M.tb. does not give a response in unsensitized animals, whereas 30 µg may give a small reaction that should be controlled for.
6. mBSA antigen-induced MAR: Rats are sensitized with 0.1 mL (1 mg mBSA) of the sensitizing emulsion subcutaneously at the base of the tail. Rats are challenged 2 wk later with 25 µL 40 mg/mL mBSA solution (1 mg) ia into one knee, and saline into the other. The sensitizing and challenge doses should be adapted for each strain (for example, *see* **Fig. 4**), and nonsensitized (Freund's incomplete adjuvant/mBSA) controls injected with mBSA should be used as negative controls since protein injected into joints can alter patellar GAG levels. Results for GAG loss are best calculated as mg GAG/mg cartilage (wet tissue mass–bone mass).
7. Interleukin-1 (IL-1): High doses of rhIL-1β (1–1000 ng) result in no change in joint diameter, and no GAG loss. Joint effusion can be easily measured at 50 ng. The use of rat rIL-1 (1 µg) results in good GAG loss, but no change on bone mass. Care should be taken with increasing doses of IL-1β to avoid systemic absorption and cytokine-induced hyperaemia.
8. Patellar Dissection: Using sharp pointed small surgical scissors, cut across the distal patellar tendon, leaving a portion attached to the patella. Using a mosquito clamp, grip the residual tendon on the patella, and cut around and behind the patella with the sharp small scissors. Fine iris scissors are helpful. This can be done in one smooth action, taking care not to cut into the bone and not to leave residual tissue, finishing with cutting the patella tendon attached to the clamp. Heavily degraded patellae require special care because the cartilage can par and the bone can fragment. Patellae should be weighed immediately since moisture evaporates rapidly with a reduction in wet mass.

9. Patellar bones. Some bones from the arthritic joint can be particularly fragile (*see* **Fig. 2A**). In these cases, a pointer with "bluetac" on the tip may be helpful. Bones can be dried and stored conveniently in 96-well plates.
10. Synovial fluid sampling (*see* **Fig. 5**): The preweighed filter papers can be inserted into the joint, point first, after the tendon has been clamped and one side incision made, and the joint closed over it. Papers should be weighed immediately (a result of evaporation). Care should be taken to measure fluid from the joint space. For example, the mBSA antigen-induced and M.tb. MAR inflammatory tissue is very oedematous, and can give a falsely raised reading if care is not taken. Thus zymosan and Il-1β-induced MAR (as well as carageenan and arthus reactions) are more appropriate for this end point. The papers can then be used for the assay of enzymes and so on, even in the mouse.
11. GAG plate reader assay: The author prefers the modified method of Farndale et al. *(8)*, but the previous method of Farndale can equally be used. Dithiothreitol should be fresh. Batches of raw materials: DMB should be batch tested for chromatic shift and the DMB solution can be kept as stock in brown glass winchesters at room temperature in the dark, and "matures" with age to increase sensitivity. Papain must be added and mixed just before incubation because it is inhibited by product. Flat-bottomed plates must be used, and plates should be tested (using DMB solution and the appropriate filters) for homogeneity of absorbance before bulk purchase. The samples are placed in the 96-well plate at the bottom edge where the DMB will be introduced. Thus instilling the DMB solution at the side of the well, inducing a swirl and giving complete mixing. 1 min has been shown to develop homogeneity throughout the plate. The color develops quickly and should be read within 3 min as the solution deteriorates when the GAGs and DMB precipitate.
12. Expression of patellar GAG. GAG content can be assessed on a unitary basis for the acute loss. However, osteophyte/chondrophyte formation after about day 5 requires measurement as a unit of wet mass minus bone mass to give an index of GAG density. This can also heighten the sensitivity of the assay in those models where GAG loss is less severe such as the zymosan and mBSA antigen-induced MAR.
13. Experimental design: The advantage of monoarticular models is that direct comparisons can be made between the treated and untreated joints within the same animal, thus drug effects can be isolated to the inflammatory process. Comparisons between control and inflamed joints of vehicle-treated and drug-treated MA animals can also be made to investigate drug effects on normal joint tissues. It is important to include vehicle-treated negative and positive controls, if only to determine the effect of the procedure and drugs on body growth, and thus patellar size (*see* **Note 14**) and joint width. In antigen-induced MAR control antigen-free sensitized animals should be used.
14. The epiphyses of rats do not close. It is thus important to assess the procedure and drug effects on control body mass and patellar indices. Reduced growth as a

result of drug action/toxicity results in smaller patellae. If this occurs, comparisons can still be made within animals.
15. Other reactions: Carageenan and reverse passive arthus (utilizing antirat serum albumin) have been tested, and provide joint swelling and increased synovial fluid volumes, but patellar cartilage GAG in the inflamed joint may be *raised*, perhaps because of exudate plasma protein mediated metalloproteinase inhibition.

Acknowledgment

The author would like to thank Dr. C. P. Gardner and A. Bowden (Roussel Laboratories Ltd, Swindon, UK) for expert and technical assistance, and Dr. P. R. Colville-Nash and Dr. D. Gilroy, Experimental Pathology, Saint Bartholomew's and the Royal London School of Medicine and Dentistry, London, for the provision of up-to-date experiences are gratefully acknowledged.

References

1. Seed, M. P., Hambleton, P. H., Bowden, A. R., Clements, Jewery S. C. J., and Gardner, C. R. (1993) Rapid quantitation of joint destruction in irritant monoarticular arthritis induced by heat-killed *Mycobacterium tuberculosis. Eur. J. Rheumatol. Inflamm.* **13,** 27–33.
2. Seed, M. P., Parker, S., Johns, S., Curnock, A. P., Bowden, A., and Gardner, C. R. (1991) Mycobacterium tuberculosis-induced monoarticular arthritis in the rat, a new *in vivo* model for the assessment of anti-rheumatic drugs. *Clin. Rheumatol.* **10,** 461–462.
3. Willoughby, D. A., Colville-Nash, P. R., and Seed, M. P. (1993) Inflammation and loss of function. *J. Lipid Mediat.* **6,** 287–293.
4. Seed, M. P., Bowden, A., Parker, F. P., Johns, S., Curnock, A., and Gardner, C. R. (1995) Chondrodestructive and chondrosparing properties of non-steroidal anti-inflammatory drugs in a model of destructive monoarticular arthritis. *Br. J. Rheumatol.* **34(S2),** 15.
5. Gilroy, D. W., Tomlinson, A., Greenslade, K., Seed, M. P., and Willoughby, D. A. (1998) The effects of cyclooxygenase-2 inhibitors on cartilage erosion and bone loss in a model of mycobacterium tuberculosis-induced monoarticular arthritis in the rat. *Inflammation* **22,** 509–519.
6. Trott, K., Parker, R., and Seed, M. P. (1995) The effects of X-rays on the experimental arthritis in rats. *Strahlentherapie und Onkologie* **9,** 534–538.
7. Seed, M. P., Parker, F. P., Johns, S., Curnock, A. P., Bowden, A., and Gardner, C. R. (1991) A comparison of mycobacterium tuberculosis and zymosan-induced monoarticular arthritides with respect to steroidal and non-steroidal anti-inflammatory therapy. *Int. Congress on Inflamm.* **Abstract** 191.
8. Farndale, R. W., Buttle, D. J., and Barrett, A. J. (1988) Improved quantitation and discrimination of sulfated glycosaminoglycans by use of dimethylmethylene blue. *Biochim. Bipohys. Acta* **883,** 173–177.

9. Clay, K., Seed, M. P., and Clements Jewery, S. C. (1989) Studies on interleukin-1β induced glycosaminoglycan release from rat femoral head cartilage in vitro. *J. Pharm. Pharmacol.* **41,** 503–504.
10. Farndale, R. W., Sayers, C. A., and Barrett, A. J. (1982) A direct spectrophotometric microassay for sulfated glycosaminoglycans in cartilage cultures. *Connect. Tissue Res.* **9,** 247–248.

19

Collagen-Induced Arthritis

Adrian R. Moore

1. Introduction

Collagen-induced arthritis (CIA) is a polyarthritis induced by sensitization of susceptible strains of animals with collagen II (the major collagen of hyaline cartilage). Because the original description of the model in rats by Trentham et al. *(1)*, it has become clear that species including rats, mice, and primates can develop CIA. In this respect, the disease is quite different to adjuvant-induced arthritis, which appears to be a disease restricted to rats.

Both humoral and cellular immune responses to collagen II are seen in sensitized animals. Both components are involved in disease progression. Thus, disease can be transferred from sensitized to naïve animals using serum *(2)* (also specific complement-fixing monoclonal antibodies to collagen II) or immune cells *(3)*.

Many regard collagen II arthritis to be a suitable model of human rheumatoid arthritis (RA). There are certain similarities with the human condition including linkage of disease to genes residing in the histocompatability locus *(4)* and erosion of cartilage and bone by synovial pannus *(5)*. However, periostitis is more marked in rodent forms of collagen II arthritis and immune responses to collagen II, though present in some RA patients, are not a consistent feature of the human disease. Nonetheless, collagen II induced arthritis is a valuable model for assessing both pathogenesis of arthritis and potential therapeutic agents.

This chapter will describe CIA in a rat and a mouse strain. As is often the case with experimental models of inflammation, protocols vary between laboratories and the reader needs to be aware of these differences when comparing their data with the data in the published literature.

2. Materials

All reagents can be purchased from Sigma Chemical Co. (Poole, Dorset, UK) unless otherwise stated.

2.1. Rat Collagen II Arthritis (see Note 1)

1. Bovine type II collagen (*see* **Note 2**) is dissolved overnight at 4 mg/mL in 0.01 M acetic acid on a roller mixer at 4°C.
2. An emulsion is formed with an equal volume of ice-cold Freund's incomplete adjuvant (*see* **Note 3**).
3. Female Lewis rats (Harlan Bicester, Oxfordshire, UK) about 170–190 g are ideal subjects (*see* **Note 3** and **5**). In any individual experiment the weight range should be no more than about 20 g.
4. Rats are anesthetized with a suitable gaseous anesthetic such as halothane or isofluorane.
5. The area at the base of the tail is shaved with clippers.
6. Two intradermal injections of 100 µL, separated by approx 1.5 cm, are made into the shaved area.
7. The animal is allowed to recover from the anesthetic.
8. Symptoms of arthritis develop approx 14 d after sensitization (*see* **Note 6**).

2.2. Quantification of Rat CIA (see Notes 7 and 8)

1. Clinical scores based on the degree of inflammation of the hind paws provide a semi-quantitative measure of inflammation. A normal ankle is scored as 0, an inflamed pad 1, and an additional 1 to 3 added on depending on how swollen the ankle appears.
2. Plethysmometry provides a quantitative measure of hind paw volume (*see* **Note 9**). The author uses a Ugo Basille plethysmometer [Ugo Basille, Comerio (VA), Italy], which measures paw volume by water displacement. Some workers mark the ankles to indicate the level to which the paws should be dipped. Others dip the paw to the level at which hair begins to grow.

3. Methods
3.1. Collagen-Induced Arthritis (CIA) in Mice (see Notes 10 and 11)

1. Chick sternal type II collagen is dissolved overnight at 4 mg/mL in 0.01 M acetic acid on a roller mixer at 4°C.
2. An emulsion is formed with an equal volume of ice-cold Freund's complete adjuvant (4 mg/mL heat-killed *Mycobacterium tuberculosis (M.tuberculosis)* in Freund's incomplete adjuvant).
3. Male DBA/1 mice (Harlan UK) of 18–20 g make ideal experimental subjects (*see* **Note 12**).
4. Mice are anesthetized with a suitable gaseous anesthetic such as halothane or isofluorane.

5. The area at the base of the tail is shaved with clippers.
6. An intradermal injection of 100 µL is made into the shaved area.
7. The animal is allowed to recover from the anesthetic.
8. On day 21 postsensitization mice are boosted by the intraperitoneal injection of 100 µL of 1mg/mL collagen II in 0.01 M acetic acid prepared as described earlier.
9. Symptoms of arthritis develop from approx 25 d after sensitization.

3.2. Quantification of Murine CIA

1. Plethysmometer chambers are available for measuring hind paw volume in mice. However, unlike rats, the disease in mice will affect any limb with almost equal frequency. In addition, digit involvement, sometimes in the absence of gross paw swelling, is more common. Measuring hind paw volume by plethysmometry is, therefore, of questionable value.
2. The literature describes a number of scoring systems for murine CIA. The author favors a system that allows as much clinical information to be gathered as possible, because this can allow the use of alternative scoring systems in order to compare data from other groups. Each involved digit can be scored as 1, hind limbs can score an additional 1; each for swollen pad and ankle swelling. Fore limbs can be scored an additional 1 for wrist involvement. This allows a cumulative score to be determined from each animal. Numbers of involved limbs should also be recorded.

3.3. Other Assays That May Be Applied to CIA

1. It is now accepted that there is not a straightforward relationship between swollen joints and underlying destruction of cartilage and bone. Therefore, measures of joint integrity at the end of an experiment are important. These may take the form of X-rays and/or histological analysis.
2. Serological markers may also be of value. Acute phase proteins, e.g., α 1 acid glycoprotein in rats and serum amyloid protein in mice are elevated as the disease manifests itself although do not remain chronically elevated in the way that the human acute phase protein, c-reactive protein, does in RA.
3. Serological markers of joint destruction are arguably more reliable in animal model systems than in man. Serum cartilage oligomeric matrix protein may have value in reflecting cartilage degradation and serum bone sialoprotein bone degradation (*6*).

4. Notes

1. A disease incidence of 80–100% can be expected with this protocol.
2. The species of collagen II and batches of collagen II can vary widely in their suitability for inducing CIA. The reader is advised to batch test collagen on a small number of animals before committing to a large experiment. The author has recently obtained collagen from Chondrex, Inc., Redmond, WA. Although experience with this company is limited, the material supplied to date has been of excellent quality.

3. When making emulsions with Freund's adjuvants, much is made of producing a thick consistency that will retain its shape when a drop is applied to cold water. In the author's experience, this is not necessary and has the distinct disadvantage that air bubbles are often drawn into syringes along with the thick emulsion. A thinner emulsion is fine, but should be thoroughly mixed each time a syringe is filled.
4. Although Lewis rats are an inbred strain, there do appear to be differences in susceptibility of animals to collagen II induced arthritis between suppliers.
5. Lewis are not the only strain of rat susceptible to CIA. The Dark Agouti rat is favored by many and requires less collagen II in the inoculum.
6. If studies are to be carried out using a therapeutic dosing regime, rats can be moved between cages before dosing begins to produce groups with approximately equal disease severity (this should not be done with mice—see later).
7. Animals should be distress scored every day from the time of disease onset. Disease severity is part of that score, but so too is behavior, grooming, appearance, and weight loss. Objective limits can then be agreed between experimenters and ethical committees or other regulatory authorities to ensure that animals are culled if presenting with an unusually severe form of the disease.
8. When an animal needs to be culled from an experiment owing to severity of the arthritis it is always difficult to know how to handle the data. Some workers will exclude the data from the study, others will carry data over for the remainder of the experiment. One compromise approach is to express data for each animal as area under curve and to divide this by the time the animals were in the study. This gives a weighted mean that can be combined with the weighted means for the other animals.
9. In the author's hands, the model as described will give rise to a disease that manifests itself clinically as swelling of the ankles and pad with little involvement of the digits. The inflammatory component of the disease is, therefore, conveniently quantified by plethysmometry.
10. Many of the notes relating to the rat model in terms of supply of animals, collagen II, preparation of the inoculum, distress scoring and the problems of culling apply equally to the murine model.
11. The mouse model is more protracted than the rat with onset, incidence, and severity being quite variable between experiments.
12. Once groups of mice have been established in their cages they should not then be moved. Mice will, otherwise, become stressed and will fight amongst themselves.

References

1. Trentham, D. E., Townes, A. S., Kang, A. H., and David, J. R. (1978) Humoral and cellular sensitivity to collagen in type II collagen-induced arthritis in rats. *J. Exp. Med.* **146,** 857–868.
2. Stuart, J. M. Cremer, M. A. Townes, A. S., and Kang, A. H. (1982) Type II collagen-induced arthritis in rats: passive transfer with serum and evidence that IgG anticollagen antibodies can cause arthritis. *J. Exp. Med.* **155,** 1–16.

3. Trentham, D. E. Dynesius, R. A., and David, J. R. (1978) Passive transfer by cells of type II collagen induced arthritis in rats. *J. Clin. Invest.* **62,** 359–366.
4. Griffiths, M. M., Eichwald, E. J., Martin, J. H., Smith, C. B., and De Witt, C. W. (1981) Immunogenetic control of experimental type II collagen-induced arthritis. I. Susceptibility and resistance among inbred strains of rats. *Arthritis Rheum.* **24,** 781–789.
5. Stuart, J. M., Watson, W. C., and Kang, A. H. (1988) Collagen autoimmunity and arthritis. *FASEB J.* **2,** 2950–2956.
6. Larsson, E., Mussener, A., Heinegard, D., Klareskog, L., and Saxne, T. (1997) Increased serum levels of cartilage oligomeric matrix protein and bone sialoprotein in rats with collagen arthritis. *Br. J. Rheumatol.* **36,** 1258–1261.

20

Air-Pouch Models of Inflammation and Modifications for the Study of Granuloma-Mediated Cartilage Degradation

Paul Colville-Nash and Toby Lawrence

1. Introduction

Animal models are essential for the study of the pathophysiological basis of disease this particularly holds true for the study of inflammation and inflammatory disease. The inflammatory response in vivo involves multiple interactions between signaling pathways which have developed a high degree of redundancy and synergy. Although it is possible to dissect individual inflammatory events in detail with in vitro studies, the interactions involved in the inflammatory response in vivo are difficult to simulate in vitro. The complex etiology of inflammatory disease has led to the development of many different models of both acute and chronic inflammation that have distinct advantages and limitations *(1)*.

Hans Selye originally described that the injection of air into the dorsal surface of rats provides a cavity in which the inflammatory response may be studied *(2)*. Subsequently, it has been shown that the injection of air over a period of 7 d leads to the development of a lining of granulation tissue consisting of fibroblasts, macrophages, and mast cells *(3)*. The formation of the lining tissue allows a response to inflammatory stimuli and irritants injected into the air pouch to be quantified by virtue of the formation of fluid exudate and the number of infiltrating inflammatory cells *(4,5)*. The air-pouch model has been extensively used for the study of various types of inflammation and inflammatory processes *(6–10)*. This model has distinct advantages over other models of acute inflammation because of the technical ease of the procedure and the ability to perform biochemical analysis of both the exudate and inflammatory cells together with the histological analysis of the air-pouch lining. The air pouch can also be used to study granulomatous inflammation in response to appropriate irritants that has proved of use in studying processes occurring in wound healing *(11–14)* which does not require the development of a lining tissue.

Additionally, modifications to the air pouch have enabled its use to study the effect of acute and granulomatous inflammation on the degradation of juxtaposed cartilage *(15)* and the effects of antirheumatic and other drugs on this process *(16)*. Owing to the variety of models that have been developed, three of these will be described in detail: the murine carrageenan air pouch *(10)*, the murine chronic granulomatous air pouch *(12)*, and the murine granuloma-mediated cartilage degradation model *(15)*.

2. Materials
2.1. Murine Carrageenan Air Pouch

1. 25–28 g female TO mice (*see* **Note 1**).
2. Lambda carrageenan. Stored lyophilized at 4°C.
3. Sterile physiological saline. Stored at 4°C.
4. Sterile Hank's balanced salt solution (HSBB). Stored at 4°C.
5. Trisodium citrate. Stored at room temperature.

2.2. Murine Chronic Granulomatous Air Pouch

1. 25–28 g female TO mice (*see* **Note 1**).
2. Incomplete Freund's adjuvant. Stored at 4°C.
3. *Mycobacterium tuberculosis* (*M. tuberculosis*). Heat-killed; stored at room temperature.
4. Croton oil. Stored at room temperature. NB. Powerful carcinogen, exercise due care.

2.3. Granuloma-Mediated Articular Cartilage Degradation Model
2.3.1. Isolation of Rat Femoral Head Cartilage

1. 110–120 g male rats (*see* **Note 2**).
2. Sterile HBSS, stored at 4°C.
3. Antibiotic/antimycotic solution (final concentration when diluted of 100 µg/mL streptomycin, 100 U/mL penicillin, 2.5 µg/mL amphotericin B). Stored at –20°C as 100X stock concentrate.
4. 70% v/v aqueous ethanol. Prepare fresh.

2.3.2. Wrapping of Cartilage

1. Sterile 5±0.2 mg cotton squares (1 cm × 1 cm). Prepare fresh and autoclave immediately prior to use in sealed borosilicate glass container (*see* **Note 3**).
2. Sterile HBSS, stored at 4°C.
3. Antibiotic/antimycotic solution (final concentration when diluted of 100 µg/mL streptomycin, 100 U/mL penicillin, 2.5 µg/mL amphotericin B). Stored at –20°C as 100X stock concentrate.

2.3.3. Implantation of Cartilage

1. 25–30 g Female mice.
2. 70% v/v Aqueous ethanol. Prepare fresh.

2.3.4. Assessment of Cartilage Destruction

1. Digestive buffer: 0.05 M phosphate buffer, pH 7.0, supplemented with 0.33 g/L N-acetyl cysteine and 12 U/mL papain. Prepare fresh and use immediately.
2. Stock 1,9-dimthylmethylene blue (DMB) solution: 16 mg DMB dissolved in 5 mL ethanol to which is added 95 mL formate buffer (2 g sodium formate and 1.9 mL 90% formic acid made up to 1 L with distilled water). This is stored in the dark at 4°C and diluted 1:9 with formate buffer prior to use in the assay.
3. Chondroitin sulfate. Lyophilized powder stored at 4°C.
4. 4 M aqueous sodium hydroxide. Prepare fresh.
5. 0.47 M aqueous citric acid. Prepare fresh.
6. Chloramine T solution (freshly made): 0.14 g chloramine T solution dissolved in 1 mL propan-2-ol followed by addition of 1 mL distilled water and 8 mL citrate buffer pH 6.0 (10 g citric acid monohydrate, 14.5 g anhydrous sodium acetate, 6.8 g sodium hydroxide in 150 mL distilled water, followed by addition of 2.4 mL glacial acetic acid, pH adjusted, and made up to a final volume of 200 mL. This buffer may be stored at 4°C under toluene for up to 3 mo).
7. Dimethylaminobenzaldehyde (DMAB)/perchloric acid (prepared fresh): 1.7 g DMAB dissolved in 7 mL propan-2-ol followed by addition of 3 mL 60% perchloric acid and kept at 65°C to maintain DMAB in solution.
8. Hydroxyproline. Stored at 4°C.

3. Methods
3.1. Murine Carrageenan Air Pouch

1. Mice are anesthetized with halothane or another suitable anaesthetic protocol.
2. An air pouch is raised by the dorsal subcutaneous injection of 3 mL of air and allowed to recover (*see* **Note 4**).
3. 4 d later, the pouch is reinflated by the injection of a further 1.5 mL air (*see* **Note 5**).
4. 7 d after initial injection of air, 0.5 mL 1% w/v lambda carrageenan in physiological saline is injected into the pouch cavity (*see* **Notes 6** and **7**).
5. Mice euthanazed at time points as appropriate for experimental end points by asphyxiation with carbon dioxide.
6. Inflammatory cells are removed from the cavity by injection of 1 mL ice-cold HBSS supplemented with 0.315% w/v trisodium citrate and the pouch gently massaged. An incision is made into the superior portion of the pouch and fluid in the pouch aspirated with a pastette.
7. Inflammation can be assessed by volume of exudate recovered by weighing the fluid (using the approximation of 1 g equivalent to 1 mL) and counting cells per milliliter of exudate using a Coulter counter. The inflammatory cells separated

by centrifugation at 200g for 10 min at 4°C followed by removal of the cell free exudate. Both of these components can then be further assayed as required (*see* **Note 8**).

3.2. Murine Chronic Granulomatous Air Pouch

1. Mice are anesthetised with halothane or another suitable anaesthetic protocol.
2. An air pouch is raised by the dorsal subcutaneous injection of 3 mL of air and allowed to recover (*see* **Note 4**).
3. 24 h later, 0.5 mL of complete Freund's adjuvant (5 mg/mL *M. tuberculosis* in incomplete Freund's adjuvant) supplemented with 0.1% croton oil is injected into the air pouch (*see* **Notes 9** and **10**).
4. Mice euthanazed at time-points as appropriate for experimental end points by asphyxiation with carbon dioxide.
5. Skin overlying the dorsum of the air pouch is dampened with 100% ethanol and an incision made through the skin approx 5 mm away from the edge of the air pouch. The air pouch can then be dissected free from the underlying dorsal musculature by careful blunt dissection and then subsequently freed from the undersurface of the skin. The fluid exudate in the pouch can be recovered by aspiration with a syringe and 21 gauge needle (*see* **Note 11**). The granuloma can be removed in its entirety for biochemical analysis by draining the fluid content and then scraping the pouch free from the skin with a large scalpel blade that leaves the skin behind. Wet and dry weight can then be ascertained by weighing immediately and after drying for 2 d at 56°C in an oven (*see* **Note 12**).

3.2.1. Isolation of Rat Femoral Head Cartilage

1. Rats euthanazed by asphyxiation with carbon dioxide.
2. Whole body of rat immersed in 70% aqueous ethanol and subsequent procedures carried out using aseptic technique in laminar flow cabinet.
3. Skin flap raised exposing musculature overlying the lower back and hindquarters allowing access to pelvis and hip joints (*see* **Note 13**).
4. Incise musculature overlying femur's greater trochanter and dislocate hip joint exposing the femoral head cartilage.
5. Grasp outer edge of cartilage with bone clippers and remove femoral head cartilage from the head of the femur and place into HBSS supplemented with antibiotic/antimycotic.

3.2.2. Wrapping of Cartilage

1. Wash femoral head cartilages twice by inverting tube containing the cartilages and HBSS several times, aspirating the HBSS and replacing with fresh solution.
2. Place a cotton square into a petri dish and dampen with a small quantity of HBSS supplemented as aforementioned. Place a cartilage into the center of the square and, using forceps, tuck the edges of the cotton into the central cavity.
3. Place each cotton-wrapped cartilage into a well of a 96-well plate for ease of transport and prevention of drying prior to implantation.

3.2.3. Implantation of Cartilage

1. Mice are anesthetized with halothane or another suitable anesthetic protocol.
2. Fur over the lower dorsum is swabbed with 70% aqueous ethanol or other swabbing solution.
3. An incision is made through the lateral skin of the lower dorsum and a pocket created by blunt dissection superiorly, large enough to accept the cotton wrapped cartilage.
4. Following insertion of the wrapped cartilage, air is expelled from the pocket and the skin wound closed using a michel clip. The procedure is repeated for the contralateral flank and the animal allowed to recover from anesthesia (*see* **Note 14**).

3.2.4. Removal of Implants and Analysis of Granuloma Development

1. At appropriate time points, mice are euthanazed by asphyxiation with carbon dioxide and implants removed by incision through the skin away from the implant and dissection of the granuloma and implant from the undersurface of the skin to which it is attached.1
2. The cartilage is removed from the cotton and granuloma by incision with a scalpel blade, being careful to avoid slicing parts from the enclosed cartilage. Granulomas are then weighed wet immediately and when dried after 2 d at 56°C, thus giving an approximation of fluid content (using 1 g equivalent to 1 mL fluid) and dry weight of granuloma (following subtraction of the initial 5 mg of cotton.

3.2.5. Assessment of Cartilage Destruction

1. Cartilages are digested for at least 2 h at 56°C in 1 mL digestive buffer (*see* **Note 15**).
2. Glycosaminoglycan content of the cartilage is determined by addition in duplicate of 10 µL of digest to a well of a 96-well microtiter plate and the addition of 200 µL of DMB solution. A standard curve from 0–200 µg/mL is constructed using digestive buffer and chondroitin sulfate as a reference glycosaminoglycan. Plates are read at 535 nm with a reference wavelength of 450 nm in a plate reader. (*See* **Chapter 18** for additional details [*see* **Note 16**].)
3. Cartilage collagen content is assessed using an assay for hydroxyproline content. Two hundred microliters of digests are evaporated to dryness at 100°C for 12–18 h in borosilicate glass ampules. Residues are redissolved in 200 µL sodium hydroxide solution, the vials sealed and incubated at 120°C for 3 h, opened and the contents again evaporated overnight (*see* **Note 17**).
4. Residues are redissolved in 200 µL distilled water and 200 µL 0.47 M citric acid. 20 µL of this sample in duplicate are added to a well of a 96-well microtiter plate, 100 µL of chloramine T solution added and the plate incubated at room temperature for 20 min.
5. 100 µL of DMAB/perchloric acid solution are added and the plate incubated at 65°C for 15 min. Plates are read at 560 nm and sample hydroxyproline content calculated against a standard curve constructed from hydroxyproline dissolved in distilled water/citric acid treated as above and with a range from 0–160 µg/mL.

4. Notes

1. Age of the mice is also important for the formation of the air pouch. If animals of more than 30 g are used, then the formation of the pouch becomes difficult to control and may distort out of shape. This can result in variation in the surface area of the pouch and as this is the interface between the irritant and the soft tissues where the inflammatory response is initiated, wide variation can be seen in pouch development parameters.
2. Age of the donor animals is critical. Experience shows that the most consistent and highest cartilage initial glycosaminoglycan and collagen contents are found in young male animals. As animals age, contents may both decrease and become more variable. It is, therefore, necessary to specify a close weight range to maintain consistency. It is also important that the subchondral bone is not removed with the femoral head cartilage and this becomes more likely to detach with the cartilage as age increases.
3. Source of cotton. The easiest and most convenient source has been found to be cotton dental rolls which can be readily obtained from medical suppliers. These can be divided in half and the central soft core removed which leaves a convenient sheet of compressed cotton which can be divided into approx 1 cm × 1 cm squares, which can then be trimmed to give the final weight desired. As the weight of cotton will govern to some extent the amount of granuloma development which occurs it is essential that care is taken to obtain cotton squares of very similar weights which should be within 0.2 mg of the desired value.
4. It is important to control the formation of the air pouch with the fingers of the other hand as the pouch is inflated to ensure a round cavity is obtained. The needle for injection should be a 25 gauge with the air injected from the cranial end of the animal at a point between the shoulder blades. The pouch is ideally situated approx 1 cm from the back of the head, but without care, the air can travel along the fascial planes and result in extensions of the pouch that involve the head or the forelimbs. This renders analysis of outcome impossible due to variation in pouch development (see later).
5. It is usual that air pouches will need to be reinflated on the fourth day. However, the volume of air required to reinflate the pouches does vary owing to differing rates of air resorption between animals. The original paper suggests pouches should be reinflated to tension but should not be inflated further otherwise the size of the pouch may be increased, however, the authors have found that inflation with a standard volume of 1.5 mL yields more consistent results.
6. The length of time the pouch is left to develop after the initial inflation and before the injection of carrageenan dictates the size of the response; thus if the pouch is left for shorter periods of time a smaller inflammatory reaction is evident. The maximal response to the irritant is seen when the pouch is left to develop for a 7-d period as detailed above.
7. Lambda carrageenan is best prepared by warming the physiological saline to 37°C then in a large beaker such that there is a large surface area and shallow depth, then carefully layering on the required amount of carrageenan, covering and

allowing this to sit for several hours to fully hydrate. The resultant gel can then be carefully stirred with a magnetic stirrer at slow speed to ensure homogeneity but avoiding air entrapment and finally made up to the required volume to account for any evaporation during the hydration process.

8. It is not practical to try to recover the pouch lining alone as this is very thin in this carrageenan variant of the pouch model, however, full thickness (i.e., skin plus pouch lining) specimens can be taken for cryotomy/fixation and wax embedding for histological analysis.
9. The croton oil batch variation is such that each batch should be tested to ascertain the inflammatory response to this part of the irritant and concentration adjusted as desired to ensure consistency.
10. Injection of the complete Freund's adjuvant/croton oil mix should also be performed with a 25 gauge needle. The *M. tuberculosis* needs to be very finely ground to avoid blocking this, an agate pestle and mortar is suitable for this. It is also important to ensure that the needle is wiped clean before the injection is made to prevent contamination of the injection site and fur with the adjuvant/croton oil as this will result in ulceration at the injection site and possible rupture of the pouch. It is also recommended that the site of the injection is compressed between two fingers as the needle is withdrawn, which also tends to retain the adjuvant/croton oil in the pouch cavity and prevent it being drawn back through the skin on the needle with similar outcome.
11. Because of the presence of large amounts of incomplete Freund's adjuvant and the croton oil in the fluid of the pouch, analysis of the exudate component of the reaction, with the exception of volume, is not practical and if measurements of mediators in the exudate is required, the reader it is suggested that the reader seeks an alternative variant of the air pouch model.
12. For histology of the pouch, experience has shown that it is better to remove a full thickness section from the pouch thus leaving the pouch lining attached to the skin which stabilizes the tissue when freezing/fixing and embedding prior to sectioning.
13. Extraction of the femoral head cartilages can be difficult. To expose the joint, the authors initially lift the hindquarter of the carcass by the femur in a vertical direction relative to the animals usual posture, which raises a pale prominence in the musculature near the pelvis that correlates to the greater trochanter. A single incision with a scalpel blade between this prominence and the pelvis to the bone is then made. If the knee joint is flexed through 90o and the foot rotated medially and the femur pushed vertically at the same time, the hip is dislocated and the cartilage of the femoral head exposed. The teres ligament may additionally need to be severed to allow removal of the cartilage using bone clippers. Freeing the cartilage can be made easier by first lightly encircling the edge of the cartilage with the bone clippers jaws prior to levering the cartilage free from the bony femoral head. It is essential that cartilages are placed immediately into HBSS supplemented with antibiotics and antimycotics and not allowed to dry out as this will kill the cartilage and lead to much faster rates of cartilage destruction and

large differences in the observations subsequently made. It is also important that any adherent soft tissue and ligament is trimmed from the cartilage prior to wrapping and implantation as this will also interfere in the analysis of the outcome.
14. If the effect of the granuloma is to be dissected further, it may be of use to the researcher to implant a nonwrapped femoral head cartilage in the contralateral side. Also other sources of cartilage may be used, for example, bovine nasal cartilage, if so desired.
15. The digest of the femoral head cartilage as described only removes the hyaline cartilage and leaves the mineralized core of the femoral head intact in the resultant digest. If cartilage mineral content and/or total glycosaminoglycan and collagen content is desired to be measured, then digestive buffer can be substituted with an ethylenediaminetetraacetic acid (EDTA) supplemented digestion buffer consisting of 0.5 M phosphate buffer pH 7.0 diluted 1:9 with EDTA solution (75 g disodium EDTA and 7.5 g sodium hydroxide in 400 mL distilled water, pH readjusted to 7.0 and made up to a final volume of 500 mL).
16. On addition of DMB to the digests from the cartilage, plates should be left on the bench for a minute to allow equilibration of color development but should not be left for more than 3 min as the dye in combination with the glycosaminoglycan will precipitate out.
17. It is essential in the hydroxyproline assay that the solutions indicated are made fresh and that both the chloramine T and the DMAB stock reagents are also fresh as these do have a limited shelf life. Further, precipitation may be seen if the DMAB solution and the plate used for the assay are allowed to cool. If this is seen, they may be reincubated at 65°C to solubilize the crystals which will be evident. If degradation of collagen is a particularly desired end point, it should be noted that significant collagen loss is only evident from 2 wk onward and a 4-wk time-point is the author's preferred end point for analysis of this component of the cartilage.

References

1. Sedgwick, A. D. and Willoughby, D. A. (1994) Animal models for testing immunopharmacological agents, in *Textbook of Immunopharmacology*. (Dale, M. M., Foreman, J. C., and Tai-Ping, D. F., eds.), Blackwell, Oxford, U.K., pp. 279–288.
2. Selye, H. (1953) On the mechanism through which hydrocortisone affects the resistance of tissue to injury. *J. Am. Med. Assoc.* **152,** 1207–1213.
3. Edwards, J. C., Sedgwick, A. D., and Willoughby, D. A. (1981) The formation of a structure with the features of synovial lining by subcutaneous injection of air: an in vivo tissue culture system. *J. Pathol.* **134,** 147–156.
4. Sin, Y. M., Sedgwick, A. D., Chea, E. P., and Willoughby, D. A. (1986) Mast cells in newly formed lining tissue during acute inflammation: a six day air pouch model in the mouse. *Ann. Rheum. Dis.* **45,** 873–877.

5. Dawson, J., Sedgwick, A. D., Edwards, J. C., and Lees, P. (1991) A comparative study of the cellular, exudative and histological responses to carrageenan, dextran and zymosan in the mouse. *Int. J. Tissue React.* **13,** 171–185.
6. Sedgwick, A. D., Moore, A. R., Al-Duaij, A. Y., Edwards, J. C., and Willoughby, D. A. (1985) The immune response to pertussis in the 6-day air pouch: a model of chronic synovitis. *Br. J. Exp. Pathol.* **66(4),** 455–464
7. Ferrandiz, M. L., Gil, B., Sanz, M. J., Ubeda, A., Erazo, S., Gonzalez, E., et al. (1996). Effect of bakuchiol on leukocyte functions and some inflammatory responses in mice. *J. Pharm. Pharmacol.* **48,** 975–980.
8. Nickerson-Nutter, C. L., and Medvedeff, E. D. (1996) The effect of leukotriene synthesis inhibitors in models of acute and chronic inflammation. *Arthritis Rheum.* **39,** 515–521.
9. Perretti, M., Ahluwalia, A., Harris, J. G., Harris, H. J., Wheller, S. K., and Flower, R. J. (1996) Acute inflammatory response in the mouse: exacerbation by immunoneutralization of lipocortin 1. *Br. J. Pharmacol.* **117,** 1145–1154.
10. Cronstein, B. N. (1995) The antirheumatic agents sulfasalazine and methotrexate share an anti- inflammatory mechanism. *Br. J. Rheumatol.* **34(Suppl. 2),** 30–32.
11. Kimura, M., Suzuki, J., and Amemiya, K. (1985) Mouse granuloma pouch induced by Freund's complete adjuvant with croton oil. *J.Pharmacobiodyn.* **8,** 393–400.
12. Appleton, I., Tomlinson, A., Colville-Nash, P. R., and Willoughby, D. A. (1993) Temporal and spatial immunolocalization of cytokines in murine chronic granulomatous tissue. Implications for their role in tissue development and repair processes. *Lab. Invest.* **69(4),** 405–414.
13. Colville-Nash, P. R., Alam, C. A., Appleton, I., Brown, J. R., Seed, M. P., and Willoughby, D. A. (1995) The pharmacological modulation of angiogenesis in chronic granulomatous inflammation. *J Pharmacol Exp Ther.* **274(3),** 1463–1472.
14. Vane, J. R., Mitchell, J. A., Appleton, I., Tomlinson, A., Bishop-Bailey, D., Croxtall, J., et al. (1994) Inducible isoforms of cyclooxygenase and nitric-oxide synthase in inflammation. *Proc. Natl. Acad. Sci. USA* **15;91(6),** 2046–2050
15. De Brito, F. B., Moore, A. R., Holmes, M. J., and Willoughby, D A. (1987) Cartilage damage by a granulomatous reaction in a murine species. *Br. J. Exp. Pathol.* **68(5),** 675–686
16. Bottomley, K. M., Griffiths, R. J., Rising, T. J., and Steward, A. (1988) A modified mouse air pouch model for evaluating the effects of compounds on granuloma induced cartilage degradation. *Br. J. Pharmacol.* **93,** 627–635.

21

Quantitative Analysis of Angiogenesis Using the Murine Chronic Granulomatous Air Pouch

Chandan A. S. Alam

1. Introduction

Angiogenesis, the growth of new capillary blood vessels is an integral part of development, repair, and reproduction. Normal tissue growth such as in embryonic development, wound repair, and the menstrual cycle is characterized by dependence on new vessel formation for the supply of oxygen and nutrients, as well as the removal of waste products. Also, a large number of different and nonrelated diseases are associated with angiogenesis, e.g., tissue damage postreperfusion of ischemic tissue *(1,2)*. In several diseases, excessive angiogenesis is part of the pathology, e.g., cancer (both solid and hematological), cardiovascular disease (atherosclerosis), chronic inflammation (rheumatoid arthritis, Crohn's disease), diabetes (diabetic retinopathy), and psoriasis. These diseases may benefit from therapeutic inhibition of angiogenesis *(3,4)*.

The quantification of vascularity in inflammation has been difficult to determine, and the antiinflammatory effects of angiomodulatory therapies have had to be inferred from their known properties or by quantitative histology *(5–7)*. Existing methods include histomorphometry, which is labor intensive, laser Doppler flowmetry *(8)*, and ^{133}Xe clearance *(9)*. However, these methods are unsuitable for routine use in drug discovery, and methods involving blood flow can be influenced by the pharmacological modulation of mediators, of vascular tone and plasma exudation, involved in inflammation, such as histamine and the prostaglandins.

The reader is referred to **Chapter 20** in this book (Please *see* **Subheading 3.** in **Chapter 20**.) A number of published papers deal with the murine chronic granulomatous air pouch *(10–13)*.

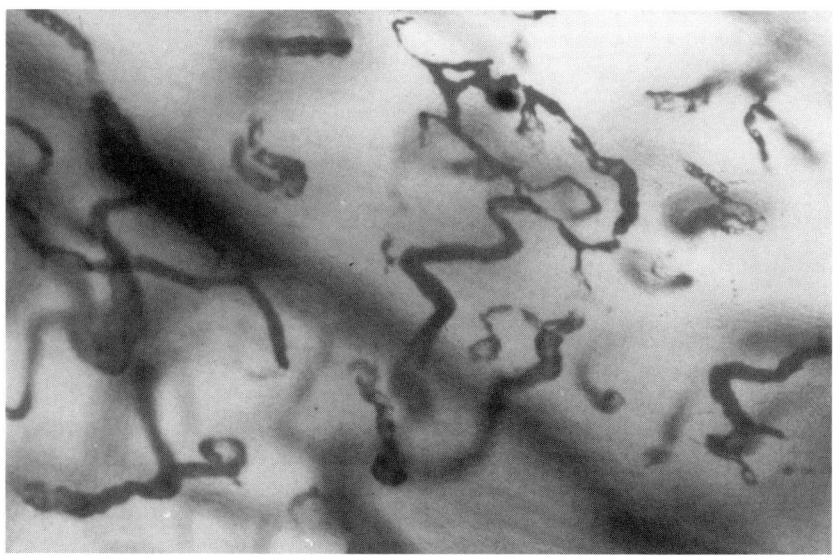

Fig. 1. Photomicrograph of cedar wood oil cleared air pouch vasculature (light microscopy ×400).

2. Materials

1. 25–28 g Female TO mice (*see* **Chapter 20**, **Note 1**).
2. Incomplete Freund's adjuvant. Stored at 4°C.
3. *Mycobacterium tuberculosis*. Heat killed; stored at room temperature.
4. Croton oil. Stored at room temperature. NB: Powerful carcinogen, exercise due care.
5. Carmine (Cat. No. C-1002, Sigma).
6. Gelatine (Cat. No. 44045 4B, BDH/Merck).
7. Hypnorm® (Janssen Pharmaceuticals).
8. Hypnovel® (Roche Pharmaceuticals).
9. Papain (Cat. No. P-3125, Sigma).
10. N-acetyl cysteine (Cat. No. A 7250, Sigma).
11. Digestion buffer: 0.33 g/L N-acetylcysteine, 12 U/mL papain, 0.05 M phosphate buffer pH 7.0.
12. Hank's Buffered Saline Solution (HBSS) may be obtained from Sigma.
13. All other chemicals were of Analar grade and obtained from Merck Ltd. or Sigma Chemical Company UK.

3. Methods

1. Chronic granulomatous air pouches are established in mice, according to the protocol described in **Chapter 20**.

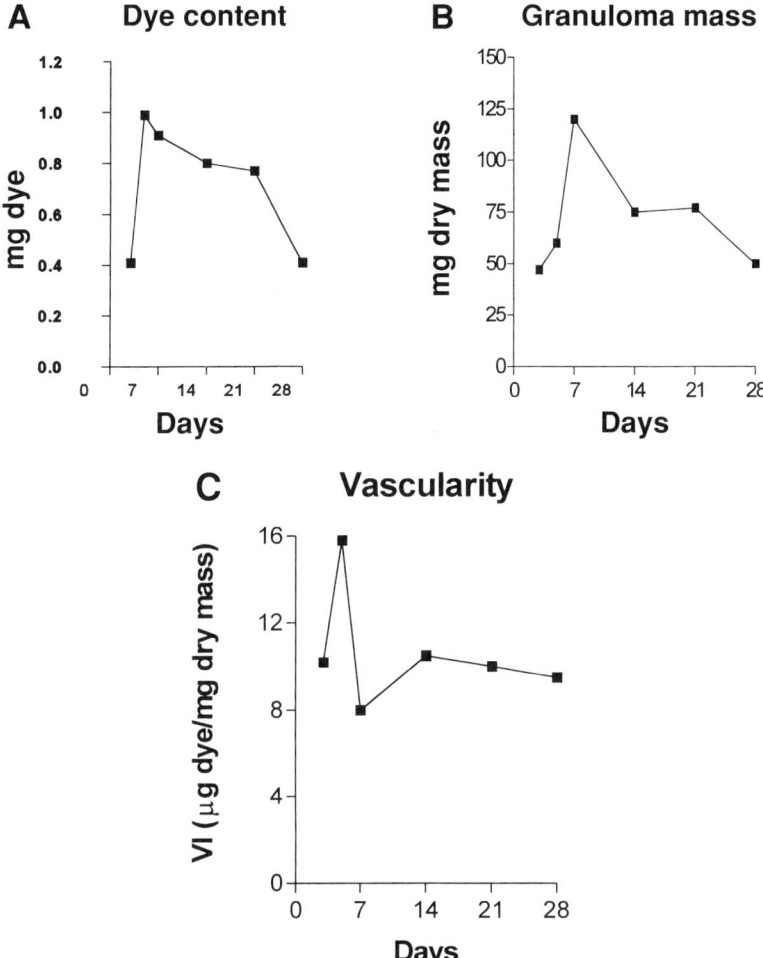

Fig. 2. Four-week time-course of nontreated murine chronic granulomatous air pouch.

2. Mice are anesthetised with Hypnorm®/Hypnovel® and placed on a thermostatically controlled heating pad at 400C (see **Note 1**).
3. 1 mL of 5% carmine/10% gelatine is injected intraveneously (iv) into the tail vein of each mouse (see **Note 2**).
4. The cadavers are chilled at 4°C for 2 h (see **Note 3**).
5. Skin overlying the dorsum of the air pouch is moistened with 100% ethanol and an incision made through the skin approx 5 mm away from the edge of the air pouch. The air pouch can then be dissected free from the underlying dorsal musculature by careful blunt dissection and then subsequently freed from the

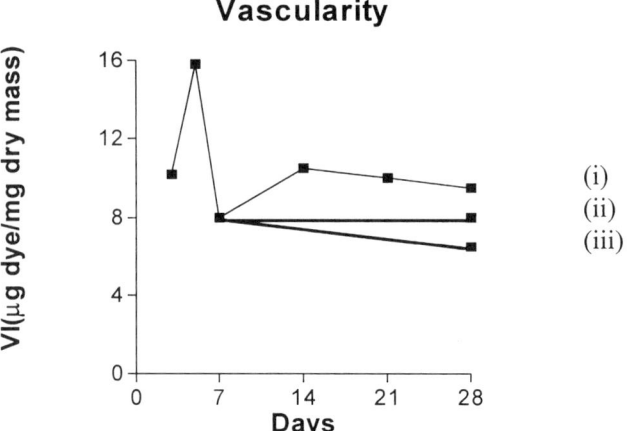

Fig. 3. Prophylactic dosing from day 7 to show i) as control; ii) angiostasis; iii) regression.

undersurface of the skin. The fluid exudate in the pouch may be recovered by aspiration with a syringe and a 21-g needle. The granuloma is removed in its entirety for further assay by draining the fluid content and then scraping the pouch free from the skin with a large scalpel blade which leaves the skin behind. Wet and dry weights can then be ascertained by weighing immediately and after drying to a constant weight, usually 2 d at 56°C in an oven (see **Note 4**).

6. Each dried granuloma tissue is then digested in 9 mL digestion buffer at 56°C for a further 2 d. To the resulting "pink" colored fluid is added 1 mL of 5 M NaOH to solubilize any remaining carmine dye. The digests are then centrifuged at 2000g for 10 min. Each sample is filtered through a 0.22-μm Whatman disposable filter to remove any particulate matter. 200 μL of each sample is then added to duplicate wells of a 96-well microtiter plate. A standard curve is also constructed from 0.1–0.01mg/mL carmine dye in 0.5 M NaOH (see **Note 5**). Samples and standards are read using a microplate reader at a wavelength of 490 nm. From this, the total carmine content of each granuloma is determined. Results are expressed as the ratio of total carmine per gram of tissue–the vascular index.
7. To visualize the vessels of the air pouch, carmine is injected as aforementioned, the dorsal fur shaved, and the skin cleaned with alcohol. The top surface of the pouch is excised and washed in HBSS. The pouch is then "pinned" onto a piece of card and immersed in 10% formol saline for 48 hours (see **Note 6**). Air pouches are then dehydrated through two changes of 70% and 90% absolute alcohol for 48 h each and then "cleared" by immersion in cedar wood oil for 7 d (see **Fig. 1** light microscopy).

3.1. Examples of Published Results

Using this method, the development of the granulomatous tissue has been studied over a period of 28 d in groups of eight animals. Tissue dry mass accumulated rapidly to a maximum of 118 ± 12.0 mg at day 7 and then fell to 75.5 ± 10.5 mg at day 14, and this mass slowly decreased to 50.5 ± 7.0 mg by day 28. The derived vascular index (VI) was 10 ± 1.2 µg dye/mg and peaked on day 5 at 15 ± 0.6 µg/mg, 2 d earlier than the peak in granuloma dry mass. Regression after the acute phase to 8.21 ± 0.04 µg/mg was followed by a second period of vascular development in the wound-healing phase to 10 ± 1.6 µg/mg by day 14 and then decreased to 8.1 ± 0.3 µg/mg by day 28 (*see* **Fig. 2A, B, C**).

This model has been further modified to show regression of existing vasculature *(14)*. A pattern that is continually observed is that the minimum point seen on the vascularity time-course is always at day 7 (*see* **Fig. 3**). When the test compound is administered to the mice from day 7, the resulting vascularity profile can be i) similar to untreated, i.e., the test compound has had no effect; ii) a profile results such that the curve is parallel to the *x*-axis, i.e., the compound is angiostatic or; iii) the resulting curve follows a course which takes it below the day 7 point, i.e., the test compound has a regressive element (*see* **Fig. 3**).

4. Notes

1. Mice were anesthetised with Hypnorm®/Hypnovel® (1:1, added to two parts saline 0.9%), and peripheral vasodilation was raised by placing on a heating pad for 10 min. The induction of peripheral vasodilation in the mice is important in overcoming alterations in peripheral vasomotor tone and tissue perfusion related to anesthesia and ambient temperature that may invalidate the results *(8)*.
2. The carmine/gelatine mixture is kept at 40°C on a hot plate and continually stirred using a magnetic stirrer. Individual, disposable, 1-mL syringes and 25-gauge needles (short) should be used once. The action of injecting the mixture results in the mouse expiring within 10 s. Use a tail vein for the injection site, starting at the tip of the tail and working up toward the base, if necessary. (Carmine is a natural substance - important to use same Lot No.)
3. Sets the gelatine and thereby forms a vascular cast of all the vessels in the mouse. Care must be taken to keep each test group of mice separate and mice should not be placed on top of each other, as this leads to pressure on the pouch and may cause the blood/carmine/gelatine to be squeezed out of the pouch.
4. This stage should be performed by one researcher to maintain continuity and homogeneity in dissection. 24-well plastic culture plates are ideal for storing and drying of the granulomas. *See* **Fig. 4** for an example of the excised air pouch.
5. As soon as the NaOH is added, the color starts to bleach, so time is of the essence. The addition of the NaOH to the digests and the formation of the dilutions for the standard curve is best done simultaneously. At this point, a coresearcher is very useful. If not available, the researcher should make the standard curve while the digests are being centrifuged. (Papain is a natural substance - important to use the same Lot No.)
6. The pouch skin should not be stretched too much as this will cause the carmine/gelatine cast to fracture or may cause the vessels to rupture. Experiments were performed with Evans blue or carmine, with or without gelatine. The cleared

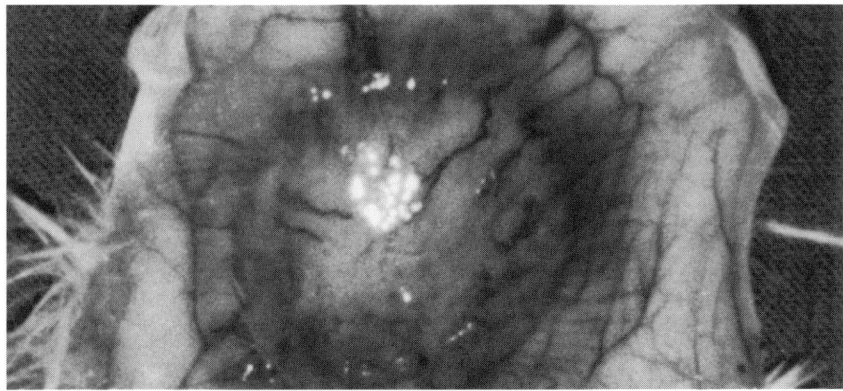

Fig. 4. Excised air pouch.

pouch preparations demonstrated that Evans blue with or without gelatine, was not retained within the vasculature. The dye was found to infiltrate the perivascular space of the tissue as well as the exudate fluid, which was found to be discolored. Additionally, carmine in the absence of gelatine was exuded into the perivascular space, but obvious retention of dye within the vasculature was achieved when it was combined with gelatine to form a vascular cast.

References

1. Carmeliet, P., Ng, Y. S., Nuyens, D., Theilmeier, G., Brusselmans, K., Cornelissen, I., et al. (1999) Impared myocardial angiogenesis and ishemic cardiomyopathy in mice lacking the vascular endothelial growth factor isoforms VEGF 164 VEGF 188. *Nat. Med.* **5,** 495–502.
2. Ferrara, N. and Alitalo, K. (1999) Clinical applications of angiogenic growth factors and their inhibitors. *Nat. Med.* **5,** 1359–1364.
3. Folkman, J. (1995) Angiogenesis in cancer, vascular, rheumatoid and other disease. *Nat. Med.* **1,** 27–31.
4. Hanahan, D. and Folkman, J. (1996) Patterns and emerging mechanisms of the angiogenic switch during tumourigenesis. *Cell* **86,** 353–364.
5. Chandar, C. L., Colville-Nash, P. R., Moore, A. R., Howat, D. W., Desa, F. M., Willoughby, D. A. (1989) The effects of heparin and cortisone on an experimental model of pannus. *Int. J. Tissue React.* **11,** 113–116.
6. Peacock, D. J. and Banquerigo, M. L. (1992) Angiogenesis inhibition suppresses collagen arthritis. *J. Exp. Med.* **175,** 1135–1138.
7. Dunn, C. J. and Galinet, L. A. (1991) Angiostatic cortexone-heparin combination treatment suppresses chronic granulomatous inflammation in mice. *Drug Devel. Res.* **23,** 341–348.
8. Orlandi, C. (1988) Evaluation of angiogenesis in chronic inflammation by laser-Doppler flowmetry. *Clin. Sci.* **74,** 119–121.

9. Andrade, S. P., Fan, T-P. D., Lewis, G. P. (1987) Quantitative studies on angiogenesis in a rat sponge model. *Br. J. Exp. Path.* **68,** 755–766.
10. Kimura, M., Amemiya, K., Yamada, T., and Suzuki, J. (1985) Mouse granuloma pouch induced by Freund's complete adjuvant with croton oil. *J. Pharmacobiodyn.* **8,** 393–400.
11. Appleton, I., Tomlinson, A., Colville-Nash, P. R., and Willoughby, D. A. (1993) Temporal and spatial immunolocalisation of cytokines in murine chronic granulomatous tissue. Implications for their role in tissue development and repair process. *Lab. Invest.* **69(4),** 405–414.
12. Colville-Nash, P. R., Alam, C. A. S., Appleton, I., Brown, J. R., Seed, M. P., and Willoughby, D. A. (1995) The pharmacological modulation of angiogenesis in chronic granulomatous inflammation. *J. Pharmacol. Exp. Ther.* **274(3),** 1463–1472.
13. Vane, J. R., Mitchell, J. A., Appleton, I., Tomlinson, A., Bishop-Bailey, D., Croxtall, J., et al. (1994). Inducible isoforms of cyclooxygenase and nitric-oxide synthase in inflammation. *Proc. Natl. Acad. Sci. USA* **15;91(6),** 2046–2050.
14. Alam, C. A. S., Seed, M. P., and Willoughby, D. A. (1995). Angiogenesis and vascular regression in chronic granulomatous inflammation induced by diclofenac in combination with hyaluronan. *J. Pharm. Pharmacol.* **47,** 407–411.

22

Models of Coronary Artery Occlusion and Reperfusion for the Discovery of Novel Antiischemic and Antiinflammatory Drugs for the Heart

Nicole S. Wayman, Michelle C. McDonald, Prabal K. Chatterjee, and Christoph Thiemermann

1. Introduction

Cardiovascular disease (CVD) is the leading cause of death in the Western world. The American Heart Association estimates that the treatment of CVD in 1999 cost the U.S. more than $286 billion, and when unsuccessful, claimed the lives of more than 1 million U.S. citizens. Thus, in the U.S. every 29 s someone will suffer a coronary event, and every 60 s, someone will die from the consequences of acute myocardial infarction. Thus, there is still a great need to develop novel drugs for the therapy of CVD and particularly, acute myocardial infarction.

The earliest description of the clinical features of angina pectoris resulting from ischemic heart disease dates back to the Egyptian Ebers papyrus (1500 B.C.), the contents of which date back to approx 2500–2000 BC. The term "angina" was found in writings of the Greek physician Hippocrates (460–370 BC). A better understanding of the anatomy of the heart by Da Vinci (1452–1519) and Vasalius (1514–1564), the discovery of the nutritive blood flow of the heart via the coronary arteries (Harvey, 1628) and the characterization of the pathology of coronary arteriosclerosis (Morgagni, 1761) provided the basis for the first pathophysiological concepts for the relationship between clinical symptoms of angina, atherosclerotic plaques of coronary arteries, and impaired coronary blood supply. The finding of an imbalance of coronary blood supply and myocardial oxygen demand can be regarded as the essential pathophysiological

From: *Methods in Molecular Biology, vol. 225: Inflammation Protocols*
Edited by: P. G. Winyard and D. A. Willoughby © Humana Press Inc., Totowa, NJ

explanation of myocardial ischemia and, thus, provided the rationale for the first experimental therapeutic interventions to reduce myocardial tissue injury resulting from the occlusion of a coronary artery in the dog *(1)*. The majority of myocardial infarcts in humans involves the myocardium supplied by a single coronary artery and, hence, results in a regional loss of myocardial function and ultimately, myocardial tissue. When studied postmortem, a majority, but not all, of such infarcts are related to the recent occlusion of a coronary artery usually by thrombosis, superimposed on preexisting atherosclerotic disease. Close serial histological sectioning and reconstruction of occluded segments of coronary arteries established that the thrombotic occlusion of this artery is associated with a ruptured endothelial cell layer, haemorrhage into the atherosclerotic plaque and rupture of plaque, contents into the residual coronary lumen.

The early mortality associated with an acute myocardial infarction is usually a result of ischemia-induced cardiac arrhythmias resulting in ventricular fibrillation, whereas the late mortality following hospitalization can be attributed to pump-failure of the ischaemic/necrotic myocardium resulting in heart failure and potential cardiogenic shock. Both the reduction in ventricular function and the incidence of arrhythmias are directly proportional to the size of the injured area *(2)*. We know today that the degree of cardiac injury is dependent on i) the severity and the duration of ischemia and ii) the degree of reperfusion injury. There is no doubt that reperfusion can increase the apparent severity of tissue injury, but there has been much speculation over whether reperfusion can, *per se*, lethally injure cells. More recent studies suggest that reperfusion is a very real phenomenon, and it is now widely believed that reperfusion injury is not simply a postmortem manifestation of lethal injury suffered during the ischaemic period, and thus, does indeed damage cells that, until the onset of reperfusion, had the potential to be salvaged. There are several pathophysiological events, which in concert may cause reperfusion injury. These include i) ATP depletion below the critical level; ii) cell swelling and membrane rupture, caused by intracellular edema and sodium retention; iii) metabolically induced membrane rupture, (iv) oxygen derived free radical formation; v) calcium overload; and vi) an excessive inflammatory response *(3,4)*.

Clearly, there is still a great need to develop novel therapeutic approaches for ischemia-reperfusion injury of the heart. To evaluate the effects of an experimental drug, we need animal models of myocardial ischemia and reperfusion. The clinical scenario of coronary artery thrombosis followed by reperfusion during thrombolysis is often modeled in animals by ligating a major branch of a coronary artery for a specified period of time, whereas reperfusion is initiated by removal of the snare occluder. The most common species for studies of regional myocardial ischemia and reperfusion in vivo are mice, rats, rabbits, and pigs. The development of murine models of myocardial ischemia is very

eBooks

- Search through hundreds of eBooks and electronic journal articles
- All eBooks are available in Adobe PDF eBook format for immediate download
- **New!** Over 200 eBooks **NOW** available for instant download
- Why wait for delivery? Download eBooks for instant access
- Start downloading your eBook collection today at *humanapress.com*

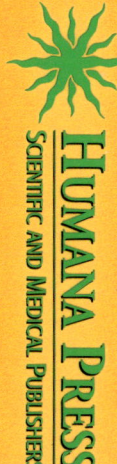

HUMANA PRESS
SCIENTIFIC AND MEDICAL PUBLISHERS

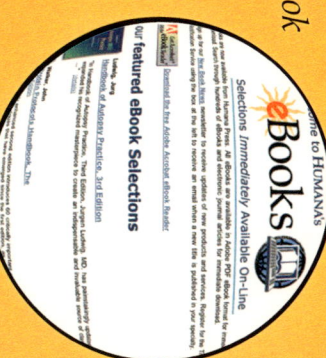

Humana Press Inc. • 999 Riverview Drive, Suite 208 • Totowa, NJ 07512 • USA

Humana's Electronic Journals

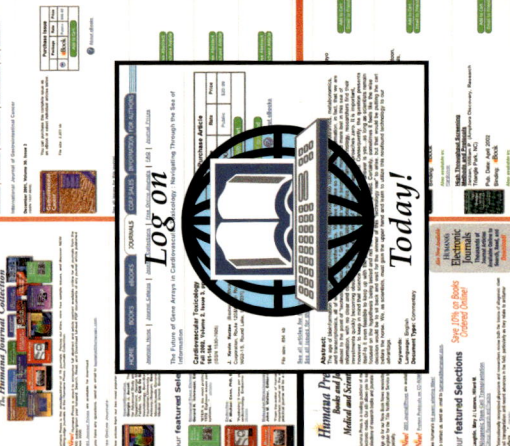

Humana Press is proud to offer . . .

Full abstract and article content available online for all journals from the 2000 subscription year forward.

Thousands of Journal Articles Available Online to Search, Read, and Download!

Visit: www.humanapress.com

Also Now Available

fashionable, as it allows the use of genetically modified animals (knock-out or transgenes) to study the role of a specific protein (or even proteins) in the pathophysiology of ischemia-reperfusion injury of the heart. Rats are quite commonly used to study the effects of novel interventions in regional myocardial ischemia and reperfusion. The determination of infarct size in rats is relatively easy and this species allows the evaluation of the efficacy of a novel drug even if only very small (mg) quantities of these compounds are available. If the investigators wish to evaluate cardiac contractility and/or regional myocardial blood flow distribution, a rabbit model of myocardial ischemia and reperfusion may be more suitable. Finally, a porcine model of regional myocardial ischemia and reperfusion also offers several distinct advantages, namely that the coronary circulation of the pig is similar to the one in humans and also that a drug can be administered locally into the coronary circulation via a catheter. This chapter outlines models of regional myocardial ischemia and reperfusion in the rat *(5)*, rabbit *(5–7)*, and pig *(8)* and specifically highlights some of the differences in surgical approach and/or determination of relevant endpoint in the these different species.

2. Materials

1. *Saline*: Nonpyrogenic saline (0.9% w/v NaCl) obtained from Baxters Health Care Ltd., (Thetford, Norfolk, UK).
2. *Hepsal*: Add 1 mL heparin (25,000 IU/mL), obtained from National Veterinary Supplies (Stoke on Trent, Staffordshire, UK) to 1 L saline (see above) and mix thoroughly by shaking to provide a 25 IU/mL working solution.
3. *Sodium thiopentone* (rat): Intraval® Sodium, obtained from Merial Aminal Health Ltd. (Dublin, Republic of Ireland). Make a solution of 30 mg/mL by adding 300 mg Intraval® Sodium B.P powder to 10 mL saline. Vortex thoroughly. Administer 4 × kg body weight as a bolus ip injection, e.g., if animal weighs 0.3 kg administer 1.2 mL of 30 mg/mL solution.
4. *Hypnorm* (including fentanyl citrate and fluanisone) (rabbit): Obtained from Janssen Pharm. Ltd. (Oxford, UK), containing 0.315 mg/mL fentanyl citrate and 10 mg/mL fluanisone. Administer 0.1 mL/kg im.
5. Sodium pentobarbitone (rabbit, pig): Sagatal® Sodium, obtained from May and Baker (Dagenham, Essex, UK). Pig; 25 mg/kg iv bolus followed by 20 mg/kg/h. Rabbit: 30 mg/kg iv via ear vein.
6. *Ketamine/Xylazine* (pig): Obtained from Sigma Chemical Co. (Poole, Dorset, U.K.). 40 mg/kg and 0.8 mg/kg im, respectively.
7. *Evans blue dye*: Obtained from Sigma Chemical Co. 2% w/v. Add 10 g Evans blue powder to 500 mL distilled water and mix thoroughly by shaking.
8. *p-nitroblue tetrazolium*: Obtained from Sigma Chemical Co. Make up 5 mL per animal of 0.5 mg/mL solution 10 min prior to end of reperfusion phase. Add 2.5 mg *p*-nitroblue tetrazolium powder to 5 mL saline.

9. *Tween-80*: Obtained from Sigma Chemicals Co. 0.01% w/v made up with saline.
10. *2,3,5-triphenyltetrazolium chloride in phosphate buffer*: Obtained from Sigma Chemicals Co. 1.5% w/v dissolved in 20 mM phosphate buffer (pH 7.4, obtained from Sigma Chemical Co.).

3. Methods

The care and use of animals outlined in the following paragraphs are accordance with guidelines published by the UK Home Office (*Guidance in the Operation of the Animals (Scientific Procedures) Act 1986*) (Her Majesty's Stationery Office, London, UK) and also conform to the *Guide for the Care and Use of Laboratory Animals* published by the U.S. National Institutes of Health (N.I.H. Publication No. 85-23, revised 1996). As full details of tracheotomy, cannulation of carotid artery and jugular vein (for the rat) are described in Chapter 23, the remainder of this Chapter will concentrate on models of coronary artery occlusion and reperfusion in different species.

3.1. Coronary Artery Occlusion and Reperfusion in the Rat

1. Male Wistar rats weighing 250–320 g and receiving a standard diet and water *ad libitum*, are anesthetised with thiopentone sodium (Intraval®, 120 mg/kg ip) and maintained by supplementary injections (approx 10 mg/kg iv) (*see* **Note 1**). The rats are tracheotomized, intubated, and ventilated with a Harvard ventilator (inspiratory oxygen concentration: 30%; 70 strokes/min, tidal volume: 8–10 mL/kg).
2. Body temperature is maintained at 38±1°C by means of a rectal probe thermometer attached to a homoeothermic blanket control unit.
3. The right carotid artery is then cannulated and connected to a pressure transducer (Spectramed, P23XL) to monitor mean arterial blood pressure (MAP) and heart rate (HR). MAP and HR are continuously recorded on a 4-channel Grass 7D polygraph recorder (Grass, MA). The pressure rate index (PRI), a relative indicator of myocardial oxygen consumption *(9)*, is calculated as the product of MAP and HR, and expressed in mmHg/min·10^3.
4. The right jugular vein is cannulated for the administration of drugs.
5. A lateral thoracotomy is performed and the heart is suspended in a temporary pericardial cradle. A snare occluder is placed around the left anterior descending coronary artery (LAD).
6. After completion of the surgical procedure, the animals are allowed to stabilize for 15 min before LAD ligation (*see* **Note 2**).
7. The coronary artery is occluded at time 0 by tightening of the occluder.
8. After 25 min of acute myocardial ischemia, the occluder is reopened to allow the reperfusion for 2 h.
9. Determination of area at risk: Following the 2-h reperfusion period, the coronary artery is reoccluded and 1 mL Evans blue dye (2% w/v) is injected into the left ventricle, via the right carotid artery cannula, to distinguish between perfused and nonperfused (area at risk or AAR) sections of the heart (*see* **Note 3**, **Fig. 1**).

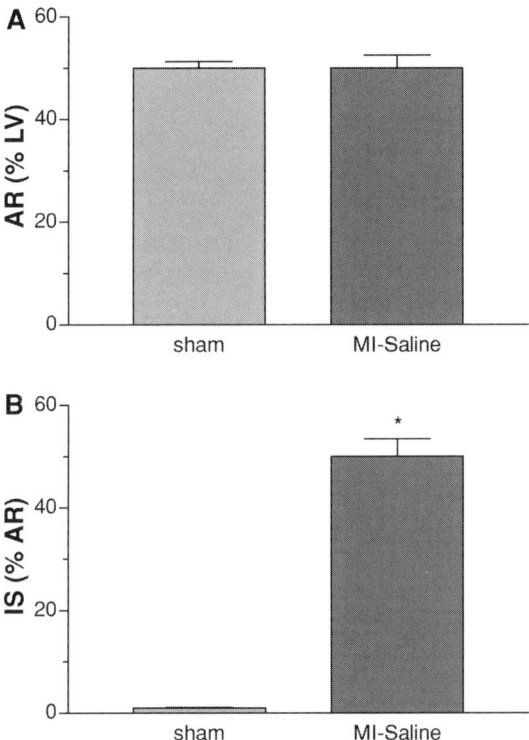

Fig. 1. The figure depicts (**A**) area at risk (AR, nonperfused myocardium) expressed as a percentage of the left ventricle (LV) and (**B**) the infarct size (IS) expressed as a percentage of the area at risk in rats subjected to the surgical procedure alone (sham) or in rats subjected to occlusion of the left-anterior descending coronary artery (for 25 min) and reperfusion (for 2 h), which were treated with vehicle (saline, MI-saline). $*p < 0.05$ when compared to sham by unpaired Student's t-test.

10. The animals are killed with an overdose of anesthetic and the heart is excised.
11. The heart is sectioned into slices of 3–4 mm, the right ventricular wall is removed, and the AAR (pink) is separated from the nonischemic (blue) area.
12. The AAR is cut into small pieces and incubated with p-nitroblue tetrazolium (NBT, 0.5 mg/mL) for 20 min at 37°C (*see* **Note 4**, **Fig. 1**).

3.2. Coronary Artery Occlusion and Reperfusion in the Rabbit

1. Male New Zealand White rabbits weighing 2.0 to 2.8 kg receiving a standard diet and water *ad libitum*, are premedicated with Hypnorm (0.1 mL/kg im containing 0.315 mg/mL fentanyl citrate and 10 mg/mL fluanisone). General anesthesia is then induced using sodium pentobarbitone (30 mg/kg iv via the ear vein) and maintained with supplementary doses of sodium pentobarbitone as required.

2. Following tracheotomy, the animals are intubated and ventilated with room air from a Harvard ventilator (ventilation rate: 36–40 strokes/min, tidal volume: 18–20 mL) (see **Note 5**).
3. Body temperature is monitored and maintained at 38±1°C by means of a rectal probe thermometer attached to a homeothermic blanket control unit.
4. The left femoral vein is cannulated for the administration of drugs and the right femoral artery for the measurement of phasic blood pressure.
5. Another catheter is placed in the right common carotid artery for the measurement of left ventricular systolic pressure (LVSP) and the subsequent injection of microspheres and Evan's blue dye solution.
6. A 2–3-cm left intercostal thoracotomy (fourth intercostal space) is performed and the heart is suspended in a temporary cradle (see **Note 6**).
7. The first anterolateral branch of the left coronary artery (LAL) is occluded at time 0 by tightening the snare occluder. This is associated with the typical electrocardiographic (ST-segment elevation) and hemodynamic (fall in blood pressure) sign of the onset of severe myocardial ischemia.
8. The snare occluder is reopened after 1 h to allow reperfusion of the previously ischaemic myocardium for a further 3 h.
9. Hemodynamic parameters including HR, systolic and diastolic blood pressure, and left ventricular systolic pressure (LVP) are recorded on a 4-channel Grass recorder.
10. A lead II electrocardiogram is continuously recorded using subdermal platinum electrodes on a 7P4H Grass ECG-amplifier attached to a Grass recorder (see **Note 7**).
11. Measurements of regional myocardial blood flow: ^{113}Sn-labeled microspheres can be used to determine regional myocardial blood flow (RMBF) at the end of the 3-h reperfusion period (see **Note 8**) *(10)*.
12. Microspheres of 15±3 μm diameter are suspended in physiological saline solution containing 0.01 % (w/v) Tween-80 (see **Note 9**). To ensure adequate dispersion, the microsphere suspension, prewarmed to 38±1°C is sonicated for 10 s immediately before use.
13. The LAL is then reoccluded and 150,000 to 200,000 microspheres (0.6 mL total volume) are injected into the left ventricle over a period of 30 s. This is followed by the immediate injection of 1 mL of saline solution over 15 s. Concurrently, blood is withdrawn from a catheter placed in the left femoral artery at a rate of 2 mL/min (using a Braun-Melsungen syringe). Blood withdrawal is continued for a period of 90 s.
14. Nonischaemic left ventricular myocardium, AAR, and infracted tissue are blotted dry and placed in separate vials for weighing and scintillation counting. The reference blood sample and radioactive material remaining in the injection syringe or cannula are also counted. Furthermore, both kidneys are removed, cleared of adhering connective tissue, blotted dry, weighed, and counted. Subsequently, renal flow values are used as a control for adequate microsphere dispersion and mixing. All samples are counted in a 1282 LKB gamma counter with a 2" by 2" NaI(Tl) well type detector.

15. Regional myocardial blood flow (RMBF) is calculated by using the reference blood flow method *(11)* according to the following formula: myocardial blood flow (mL/min) = reference blood flow (femoral artery, mL/min) × counts/min in myocardial blood sample / counts/min in reference blood sample. RMBF is expressed as mL/min × 100 g wet weight.

3.3. Coronary Artery Occlusion and Reperfusion in the Pig

1. Adult pigs weighing between 23–30 kg are sedated with Ketamine®/Xylazine® (40 mg/kg and 0.8 mg/kg im, respectively) and subsequently anesthetised with sodium pentobarbital (25 mg/kg iv as a bolus followed by an iv infusion at a rate of 20 mg/kg/h) and ventilated with a Bird-Mark-8 respirator delivering room air (ventilation rate: 16 strokes/min; tidal volume: 400–500 mL). Oxygen is supplied via the respirator as needed (1–2 L/min) in order to maintain arterial blood pO_2 values at approx 100 mmHg and pCO_2 values at approximately 35 mmHg *(8)*.
2. A thoracotomy is performed through the fifth intercostal space, the lungs are retracted, and the heart is suspended in a pericardial cradle.
3. The LAD is freed from adjacent tissue below the first diagonal branch and a thread is placed around the artery for later occlusion.
4. MAP is measured with a catheter-tip manometer placed in a femoral artery and LVP is recorded with another tip-catheter, which is inserted retrogradely from a carotid artery into the left ventricle.
5. HR is calculated from the LVP waveform and the left ventricular end-diastolic pressure (LVEDP) is measured on a high-sensitivity scale. Myocardial contractility (dP/dt_{max}) is measured as the rate of rise of LVP. Hemodynamic data are recorded continuously during the course of the experiment on a MK 260 Brush Gould polygraph (Cleveland, OH).
6. Following a 60-min equilibration period, the LAD is occluded with a snare for 60 min to induce ischemia.
7. Reperfusion is accomplished by releasing the snare placed around the LAD. The duration of reperfusion is usually 180 min. At the end of the reperfusion period, all animals are killed with an overdose of anesthesia and the heart is removed for assessment of infarct size.
8. Determination of infarct size: The isolated heart is then perfused simultaneously with two solutions at the same pressure (100 mmHg). Evans blue (0.5% w/v) is infused retrogradely via the stump of the aorta to determine the anatomic area at risk (nonperfused myocardium) and the nonischemic area. Subsequently, 2,3,5-triphenyltetrazolium chloride (TTC, 1.5% w/v) dissolved in a 20-mM phosphate buffer (pH 7.4) is infused into the LAD just distal to the site of occlusion (*see* **Note 10**).
9. The right ventricle is then removed and the left ventricle plus septum (LV + S) is cut in slices, approx 1-cm thick, from the base of the apex. Each slice is placed in a Petri dish filled with saline and photographed. The area at risk and the infarcted area (in each slice) are determined from the relevant color photographs using

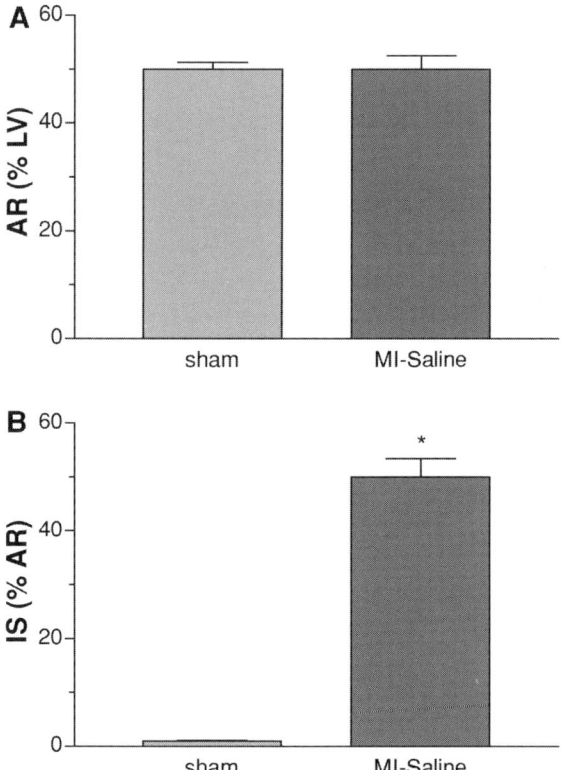

Fig. 2. The figure depicts (**A**) area at risk (AR, nonperfused myocardium) expressed as a percentage of the left ventricle (LV) and (**B**) the infarct size (IS) expressed as a percentage of the area at risk in pigs subjected to occlusion of the left-anterior descending coronary artery (for 1 h) and reperfusion (for 2 h), which were treated with vehicle (saline, MI-control) or 3-aminobenzamide, an inhibitor of the nuclear enzyme poly (ADP-ribose) polymerase. *$p < 0.05$ when compared to MI-control by unpaired Student's *t*-test.

computer-assisted planimetry using specialized computer software (Elas, Leitz, Wetzlar, Germany). The AAR is calculated as percentage of the (LV + S) and the infarcted area as percentage of the AAR (*see* **Fig. 2**).

4. Notes
1. In rats, this anesthetic protocol, which has been approved by the UK Home Office, leads to a long-lasting surgical anesthesia.
2. Study design: In a standard experiment, the following experimental groups are studied: i) LAD-occlusion (25 min) and reperfusion (2 h) plus administration of vehicle (e.g., saline, 1 mL/kg iv bolus), starting 1 min prior to reperfusion and maintained throughout the reperfusion period (at 1 mL/kg/h) ($N=8–12$). ii) LAD-

occlusion and reperfusion plus administration of the test drug (iv bolus injection 1 min prior to reperfusion followed by an infusion of 0.1 mg/kg/h, $N=8-12$). iii) Sham-operation (no LAD-occlusion) and infusion of vehicle ($N=6-8$). iv) Sham-operation (no LAD-occlusion) and infusion of saline ($N=6-8$).
3. The Evan's blue dye stains the perfused myocardium, whereas the occluded vascular bed remains uncolored.
4. In the presence of intact dehydrogenase enzyme systems in the viable myocardium, NBT forms a dark blue formazan, whereas areas of necrosis lack dehydrogenase activity and therefore fail to stain *(12)*. Pieces are separated according to staining and weighed to determine the infarct size as a percentage of the weight of the AAR *(12)*.
5. Arterial blood gases and pH should be checked periodically, e.g., on a Corning 168 pH blood gas analyser. When necessary, the ventilation rate and or oxygen flow rate (if additional oxygen is supplied) are adjusted to maintain physiological blood gas values (pO_2: 90–130 mmHg, pCO_2: 30–35 mmHg, and pH 7.38–7.42).
6. A snare occluder is placed around the first anterolateral branch of the left coronary artery (LAL) 1 cm distal from its origin. In contrast to other species, the LAL of the rabbit supplies most of the left ventricular myocardium including most of the septum and apex *(14)*. Care should be taken not to include any veins draining blood from this area. Upon completion of the surgical procedure, fluid loss is replaced by injection of 3 mL of physiological saline solution. The animals are then allowed to stabilize for 30 min before LAL-occlusion.
7. R-wave and Q-wave amplitude together with ST-segment changes are calculated as absolute differences with respect to the J-point of the QRS complex of a least 10 cardiac cycles and expressed as ΔmV. The HR is calculated and the PRI is calculated as the product of MAP and HR and used as a relative marker for myocardial oxygen consumption.
8. Details of this procedure have been described elsewhere *(11)* and validated for the rabbit, cat, and minipig *(10,13)*.
9. As myocardial ischemia is associated with a pronounced dilation of the coronary vascular bed, smaller microspheres may not be trapped in the microcirculation and, hence, may produce inaccuracies in flow determinations in the rabbit *(13)*.
10. In the presence of intact dehydrogenase enzyme systems (normal myocardium), TTC forms a brick-red color, whereas areas of necrosis lack dehydrogenase activity and therefore do not stain. Thus, the viable areas located within the area at risk were stained red, whereas the necrotic myocardium (within the area at risk) remained unstained (pale yellowish color) if infarcted.

References

1. Maroko, P. R., Kjekshus, J. K., Sobel, B. E., Watanabe T., Covell, J. W., Rose, J. et al. (1971) Factors influencing infarct size following experimental coronary artery occlusion. *Circulation* **43**, 67–82.
2. Roberts, R., Husain, A. H., Ambos, H. D., Oliver, G. C., Cox, J. R., and Sobel, B. E. (1975) The relationship between infarct size and ventricular arrhythmia. *Br. Heart J.* **37**, 1169–1175.

3. Romson, J. L., Hook, B. G., Kunkel, S. L., Abrams, G. D., Schork, M. A., and Lucchesi, B. R. (1983) Reduction of the extent of ischaemic myocardial injury by neutrophil depletion in the dog. *Circulation* **67,** 1016–1023.
4. Mullane, K. M., Read, N., Salmon, J. A., and Moncada, S. (1984) Role of leukocytes in the acute myocardial infarction in anaesthetised dogs: relation to myocardial salvage by anti-inflammatory drugs. *J. Pharmacol. Exp. Ther.* **228,** 510–522.
5. McDonald, M. C., Zacharowski, K., Bowes, J., Cuzzocrea, S., and Thiemermann, C. (1999) Tempol reduces infarct size in rodent models of regional myocardial ischemia and reperfusion. *Free Rad. Biol.* **27,** 493–503.
6. Thiemermann, C., Thomas, G. R., and Vane, J. R. (1989) Defibrotide reduces infarct size in a rabbit model of experimental myocardial ischemia and reperfusion. *Br. J. Pharmacol.* **97,** 401–408.
7. Thiemermann, C., Bowes, J., Myint, F., and Vane, J. R. (1997) Inhibition of the activity of poly(ADP ribose) synthetase reduces ischemia-reperfusion injury in the heart and skeletal muscle. *Proc. Natl. Acad. Sci. USA* **94,** 679–683.
8. Bowes, J., Ruetten, H., Martorana, P. A., Stockhausen, H., and Thiemermann, C. (1998) Reduction of myocardial reperfusion injury by an inhibitor of poly (ADP-ribose) synthetase in the pig. *Eur. J. Pharmacol.* **359,** 143–150.
9. Baller, D., Bretscheneider, H. J., and Hellige, G. (1981) A critical look at currently used indices of myocardial oxygen consumption. *Basic. Res. Cardiol.* **76,** 163–181.
10. Maxwell, M. P., Hearse, D. J., and Yellon, D. M. (1987) Species variation in the coronary collateral circulation during regional myocardial ischemia: a critical determinant of the rate of evalution and extent of myocardial infarction. *Cardiovasc. Res.* **21,** 737–746.
11. Heymann, M. A., Payne, B. D., Hoffmann, J. I. E., and Rudolph, A. M. (1977) Blood flow measurements with nucleotide-labelled particles. *Prog. Cardiovasc. Dis.* **20,** 55–79.
12. Nachlas, M. M. and Shnitka, T. K. (1963) Macroscopic identification of early myocardial infarct by alterations in dehydrogenase systems. *Am. J. Pathol.* **43,** 379–405.
13. Hof, R. P., Wyler, F., and Stadler, G. (1980) Validation studies for the use of the microsphere method in cats and young minipigs. *Basic Res. Cardiol.* **75,** 747–756.
14. Flores, N. A., Davies, R. L. I., Penny, W. J., and Sheridan, D.S. (1984) Coronary microangiography in the guinea pig and ferret. *Int. J. Cardiol.* **6,** 459–471.

23

Assessment of Anticolitic Drugs in the Trinitrobenzene Sulfonic Acid (TNBS) Rat Model of Inflammatory Bowel Disease

Brendan J. R. Whittle, Maryan Cavicchi, and Dominique Lamarque

1. Introduction

The pathogenesis of the inflammatory bowel diseases (IBD), which include ulcerative colitis and Crohn's disease, is still not fully understood. It is likely that proinflammatory cytokine release and derangement of the immune response play a role in the inflammatory processes *(1,2)*, whereas the roles of a wide range of proinflammatory mediators are currently under investigation. In addition, the release of more ephemeral cytotoxic species such as reactive oxygen species or nitric oxide (NO) and other nitrogen species may also be involved in creating epithelial and microvascular injury *(3–8)*. The expression of the inducible calcium-independent isoform of nitric oxide synthase (iNOS) can be considered as a marker of the inflammatory response in the gut. Thus, the quantities of NO produced by iNOS, either by inflammatory cells or the gut tissue, particularly the epithelium, may be involved in both initial cell injury along with oxygen radical such as superoxide, which forms the injurious peroxynitrite, as well as in the subsequent healing of the tissue injury *(3–8)*.

There is a continuing major interest in novel therapeutic approaches to the control of colitis, from pathophysiological, clinical, and pharmaceutical perspectives. Thus, experimental models have been developed for the investigation of the pathological processes in the colon leading to colitis, and for the screening and assessment of potential antiinflammatory agents *(9)*. Although in common with all models of inflammation, the various models on colitis based on initial colonic challenge have limitations in their chronicity and origin, one model has been used extensively since its preliminary description by Professor

Gerald Morris et al. some 16 yr ago, with publication of a subsequent fuller paper *(10)*. This model is the colitis induced by a single intracolonic challenge with a solution of the hapten, 2, 4, 6-trinitrobenzene sulfonic acid (TNBS) in rats *(10–12)*. This model produces an intense local inflammatory response that reaches its nadir after 2 to 3 d, which can last up to 10–21 d, depending on the severity of the challenge.

The inflammatory response is considered to reproduce many of the macroscopic, histological, and immunological hallmarks of Crohn's disease *(13–16)*. Thus, open ulceration may be produced, with transmural inflammation and thickening of the bowel wall. Histological features include distorted crypt architecture, crypt atrophy, granulomata, giant cells, basal lymphoid aggregates, and the presence of an inflammatory infiltrate *(10–16)*. The model has therefore been used and validated for studying colonic inflammation and, therefore, to address aspects of the pathogenesis of IBD *(17–29)*. Expression of iNOS can be detected in the inflamed colonic tissue, and it's modulation can affect the progress of the colitis *(6,30–32)*. In addition, inflammatory cell infiltration is a notable feature, as estimated by histological evaluation and by the determination of myeloperoxidase (MPO) as an index of polymorphonuclear cells (PMN) accumulation *(33)*. Thus, the TNBS model of colonic inflammation in the rat has been extensively used for the evaluation of a wide range if therapeutic approaches and potential anticolitic agents *(34–62)*.

2. Materials
2.1. Challenging Agent
1. The 2,4,6-trinitrobenzene sulfonic acid (TNBS), also known as picrylsulfonic acid is obtained from Fluka Chemie AG, Buchs, Switzerland, Germany, or from the Sigma Chemical Company.

2.2. The iNOS Assay
1. [^{14}C]-L-arginine-monochloride for the assay is from Amersham Pharmacia Biotech., Buckinghamshire, UK. All other reagents and chemicals can be purchased from Sigma Chemical Company.
2. Homogenization buffer: 10 mM N-[2-hydroxyethyl]piperazine-N'-[2-ethanesulfonic acid] (HEPES, 32 mM), sucrose, 1 mM dithiotreitol (DTT), 0.1 mM ethylenediamine tetraacetic acid (EDTA), 10 µg/mL soybean trypsin inhibitor, 10 µg/mL leupeptin, and 2 µg/mL aprotinin.
3. Assay buffer: 50 mM KH$_2$PO$_4$, 1.5 mM MgCl$_2$, 50 mM L-valine, 0.3 mM CaCl$_2$, 1 mM DTT, 1 mM L-citrulline, 15.5 nM L-arginine, 30 µM flavin adenine dinucleotide (FAD), 30 µM flavin mononucleotide (FMN), 30 µM tetrahydro-L-biopterin dihydrochloride (BH$_4$), 450 µM β-nicotinamide adenine dinucleotide phosphate (β-NADPH), 12 pM of [^{14}C]-L-arginine monohydrochloride.

2.3. Western Blotting

1. Tris-mannitol buffer: 2 mM Tris-HCl 7.0–9.0, 50 mM mannitol, 100 µM phenyl methyl sulfonyl fluoride, 2 µM leupeptin, 0.5 µg/mL aprotinin, 0.5% Triton X-100.
2. Denaturing buffer: 20 mM Tris-HCl pH 7.0–9.0, 3 mM EDTA, 2% sodium dodecyl sulfate (SDS), 10% β-mercaptoethanol, 20% glycerol.
3. Blocking buffer: PBS (pH 7.4), 0.25% Tween-20 (v/v), and 5% nonfat dried milk,
4. The anti-iNOS polyclonal antibody is from Santa Cruz Biotechnology; Inc., Santa Cruz, CA.
5. The horseradish peroxidase-conjugated anti-rabbit antibody is from Jackson Immuno research Inc., West Grove, PA.
6. *Bis*-acrylamide solution (19:1) and protein weight markers are from the Sigma Chemical Company.
7. The nitro-cellulose membranes (Hybond ECL) are from Amersham, Pharmacia Biotech., Buckinghamshire, UK.

3. Methods
3.1. Induction of Colitis

1. Male Wistar rats (approximate body weight of 220–260 g) are allowed free access to water and food during experiments, and are assigned to groups of at least five per treatment, depending on the experimental design.
2. Under transient ether-induced anesthesia, 2,4,6-trinitrobenzene sulfonic acid (TNBS; 10–30 mg in 50% ethanol, v/v) is administered intrarectally through an 8-cm-long soft plastic catheter, in a volume of 0.25 mL (*see* **Notes 1** and **2**).
3. The animals are sacrificed by cervical dislocation at different time points as required. As the maximal extent of colonic damage is seen 2 to 3 d after challenge, this is the usual period for the initial study of the actions of potential anti-colitic drugs, but studies on the more-chronic time-course is valuable at subsequent stages of development (*see* **Notes 3–8**).

3.2. Macroscopic Assessment of Severity of Colitis

1. The distal 8-cm portion of the colon is excised, gently rinsed ice-cold PBS at pH 7.4 and cut longitudinally.
2. The extent of macroscopically visible damage, involving regions of haemorrhagic necrosis, is determined in a randomized manner from photographs via computerized planimetry (such as Summa Sketch III; SigmaScan V3-92).
3. The area of mucosal damage is calculated as the percentage of the total colonic segment area that shows macroscopically visible damage.
4. A section of the colon from the overtly inflamed and noninflamed tissue can be taken for histological evaluation if required.
5. The inflamed region of the distal colon is then divided in a number of segments to determine inflammatory markers. These can include myeloperoxidase (MPO) activity, iNOS protein expression, and iNOS enzyme activity.

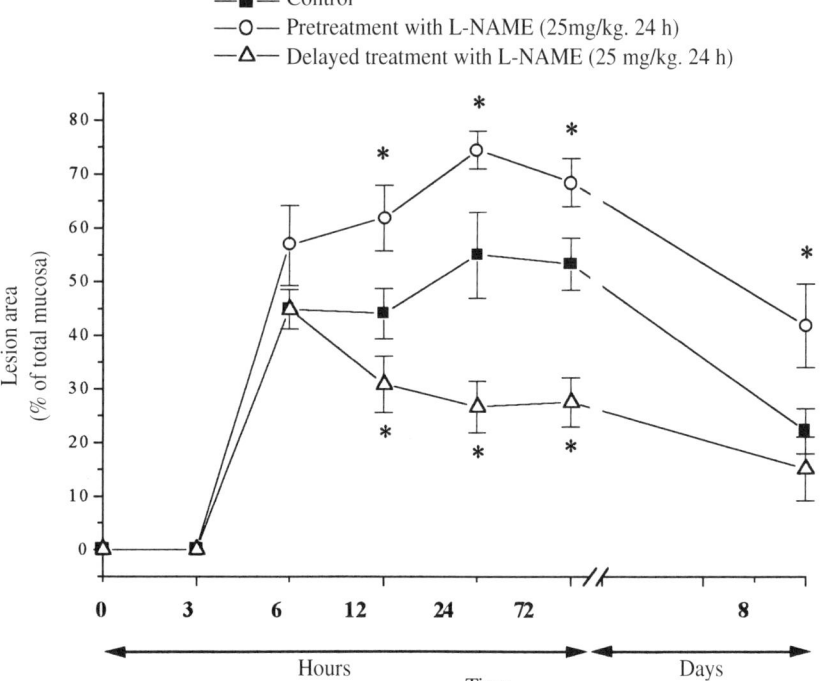

Fig. 1. Inflammatory injury to the colonic mucosa following challenge with trinitrobenzene sulfonic acid (TNBS; 30 mg in 0.25 mL of 50% ethanol). Rats were treated with N^G-nitro-L-arginine methyl ester (L-NAME) added in a dose of 25 mg/kg^{-1} per 24 h to drinking water commencing 48 h prior to challenge (○), or commencing 6 h following challenge (△) or in the control group, with saline (■). Data are shown as the mean ± S.E. of 6–15 experiments, where * indicates significant difference from control ($P < 0.05$). Data are adapted from Kiss et al. 1997 *(31)*.

3.3. MPO Activity (see Notes 9–11)

1. The MPO activity is assessed using a modification of the method described by Bradley et al. *(33)*, as described here:
2. Colonic segments are homogenized in ice-cold phosphate buffer (50 mM, pH 6.0) containing 0.5% hexadecyltrimethylammonium-bromide, freeze-thawed three times and spun (15,000g; 15 min; 4°C).
3. Then, 12 µL of the supernatant are mixed with 280 µL phosphate buffer (50 mM, pH 6.0) containing 0.167 mg/mL O-adenosine dihydrochloride and the reaction started with 10 µL 0.0005% hydrogen peroxide.
4. The reaction product is assayed spectrophotometrically (λ = 490 nm) after 90 s shaking. MPO activity is expressed as mU/g wet tissue.

3.4. iNOS Activity: L-Arginine Conversion Assay (see Notes 12–16)

1. Nitric oxide synthase activity is determined by quantifying the conversion of [^{14}C]-radiolabeled L-arginine to citrulline *(31)*.
2. A segment of colon is homogenized (Ultraturrax T25; 13,500 s^{-1}; 2 × 30 s) in the homogenization buffer.
3. Homogenates are spun for 20 min at 10,000g at 4°C.
4. Samples (40 µL) are incubated for 10 min at 37°C in 100 µL of assay buffer.
5. The reaction is terminated by the addition of 0.5 mL of 1:1 (v/v) suspension of ice-cold Dowex (Na$^+$-form) in distilled water. The mixture is resuspended by the addition of 850 µL of ice-cold distilled water. Aliquots of the supernatant (970 µL) are removed after allowing mixture to settle for 30 min and the radioactivity determined by scintillation counting.
6. Calcium-dependency of the NOS activity is determined by the addition of 10 µL of ethylene glycol-*bis* (β-aminoethyl ether) tetraacetic acid (EGTA; 1 mM). NOS activity is confirmed by its inhibition by N^G-monomethyl-L-arginine (L-NMMA, 300 µM). The iNOS activity is defined as the citrulline formation that is inhibited by L-NMMA but not inhibited by EGTA.
7. The constitutive NOS activity is calculated from the difference between citrulline formation which was inhibited by EGTA and the total activity. As the nature of the constitutive isoform (eNOS or nNOS) was not determined in this method, this activity is referred to as cNOS. NOS activity expressed as pmol min^{-1} mg^{-1} protein.

3.5. Western Blotting

1. Colonic tissue is homogenized in ice-cold Tris-mannitol buffer.
2. Homogenates are spun for 20 min at 12,000g at 4°C. Aliquots of 25 µg of total cellular protein are denatured by mixing and boiling v/v with the denaturing buffer.
3. The samples are electrophoresed (100V, 25 mA/gel) on 7.5% SDS-polyacrylamide gel, and transferred (100V, 50 mA/gel, 2 h) to nitrocellulose membrane.
4. Equivalent protein loading is determined by staining the blot with 0.1% Ponceau red in 5% acetic acid.
5. Two hours after blocking with the blocking buffer, membranes are probed with anti-iNOS polyclonal antibody (1/2000, 1 h) at room temperature, washed three times with PBS-Tween-20 and then incubated with horseradish peroxidase-conjugated anti-rabbit antibody (1/2000) or iNOS for 1 h at room temperature.
6. Membranes are developed using an enhanced chemiluminescence system (ECL+Plus, Amersham Pharmacia Biotech.) and exposed to Hyperfilm (Biomax light-1, Eastman Kodak Co., Rochester, NY).
7. Films are analyzed using the ImageQuant Software (Amersham Pharmacia Biotech.) after scanning it with GelAnalyst 3.01 Software (Iconix, Toronto, Canada).

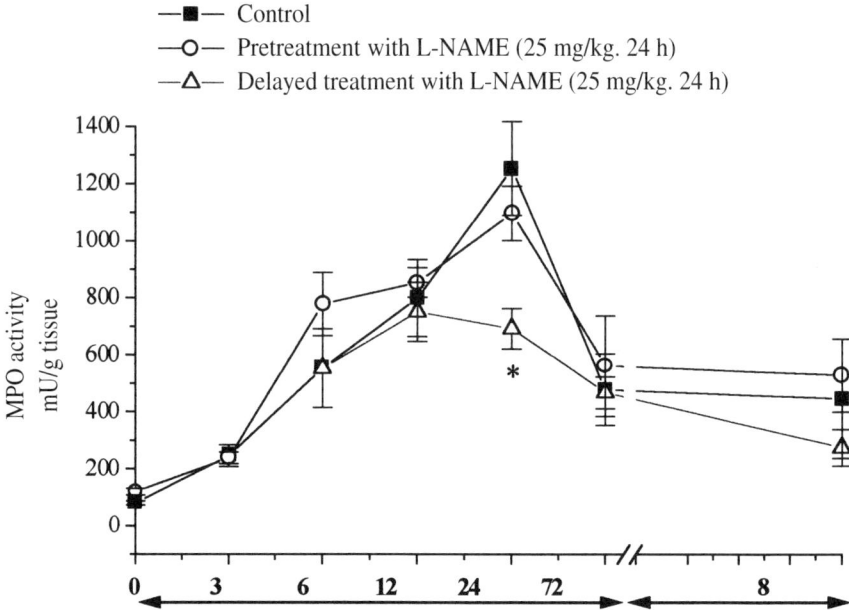

Fig. 2. MPO activity in the colon following challenge with trinitrobenzene sulfonic acid (TNBS; 30 mg in 0.25 mL of 50% ethanol). Rats were treated with N^G-nitro-L-arginine methyl ester (L-NAME) added in a dose of 25 mg/kg^{-1} per 24 h to drinking water commencing 48h prior to challenge (○), or commencing 6 h following challenge (△) or in the control group, with saline (■). Data, shown as the mU g^{-1} wet tissue, are means ± S.E. of 7–10 experiments, where * denotes significant difference from control ($P < 0.05$). Data are adapted from Kiss et al. 1997 *(31)*.

3.6. Administration of Anticolitic Drugs

1. The protocol that is adopted for the evaluation of anticolitic drugs will depend on the pharmacodynamic and pharmacokinetic characteristics of the agents under consideration.
2. Thus, agents can be administered by oral gavage or in the drinking water, the latter approach only being possible if the agent or its suspending or solubilizing vehicle is palatable to the rat.
3. Compounds can be administered by subcutaneous (sc) injection or by use of sc depot form, including use of the osmotic minipump or similar devices.
4. It is not recommended that compounds being evaluated for potential anticolitic activity be given by the intraperitoneal route to avoid any direct interference with gut function and motility, which could obscure their activity in the model.
5. It is, however, feasible to administer a locally acting compound by intrarectal

instillation, but care must be taken that there is no physicochemical interaction with the challenging agent.
6. Compounds that have a slow onset of action can be administered prior to challenge with TNBS; thus studies have reported where agents have been administered for 3 d prior to challenge.
7. For agents with a relatively short chemical or biological half-life, the compound can be administered up to three times a day. Moreover, the compounds can be administered throughout the study period following challenge.

3.7. Data Presentation and Statistical Analysis

1. Data are shown as means ± S.E.M. of at least five animals in each group. Data can also be expressed as median and semiquartile ranges.
2. Western blot is usually from three independent experiments.
3. Statistical significance between group is assessed by Student's t-test where $p < 0.05$ was taken as significant, by analysis of variance or by nonparametric data analysis.

4. Notes
4.1. Macroscopic Damage after TNBS Challenge

1. Challenge with TNBS causes macroscopic hemorrhagic and necrotic lesions of the colon, that became evident 6 h after TNBS administration (*see* **Fig. 1**).
2. The ethanol (50% v/v) included in the challenge instillate is required to cause initial superficial disruption to the colonic epithelial barrier, allowing the TNBS to reach subepithelial layers and, hence, set up the more-chronic inflammatory response. The concentration of ethanol has been found optimum for this purpose in this laboratory, but could be varied in order to modify the extent of colonic injury. Higher concentrations of ethanol, however, could cause more-extensive direct acute cellular and necrotic injury, which would, hence, confound the observation of the more-gradual development of the inflammatory injury.
3. The maximal level of damage occurs between 2 and 3 d after challenge reaching some 60% of the total colonic area following intracolonic challenge with TNBS at a concentration of 30 mg instilled in a volume of 0.25 mL (*see* **Fig. 1**).
4. The macroscopic injury starts to decline from day 6 after TNBS challenge reaching some 25% of the total colonic area at 10 d.
5. The extensive macroscopic mucosal injury with this concentration of TNBS may be difficult to modulate with some potential anticolitic agents. Thus, challenge with TNBS (10 mg in 0.25 mL) may also be used, which produces a consistent but lower extent of mucosal injury involving some 30–35% of the colonic area under investigation, determined 3 d after challenge.
6. It is important that vehicle control groups are always included in the experimental design when evaluating the activity of novel compounds, as some of solubilising agents such as DMSO may themselves have pharmacological activity in this model.

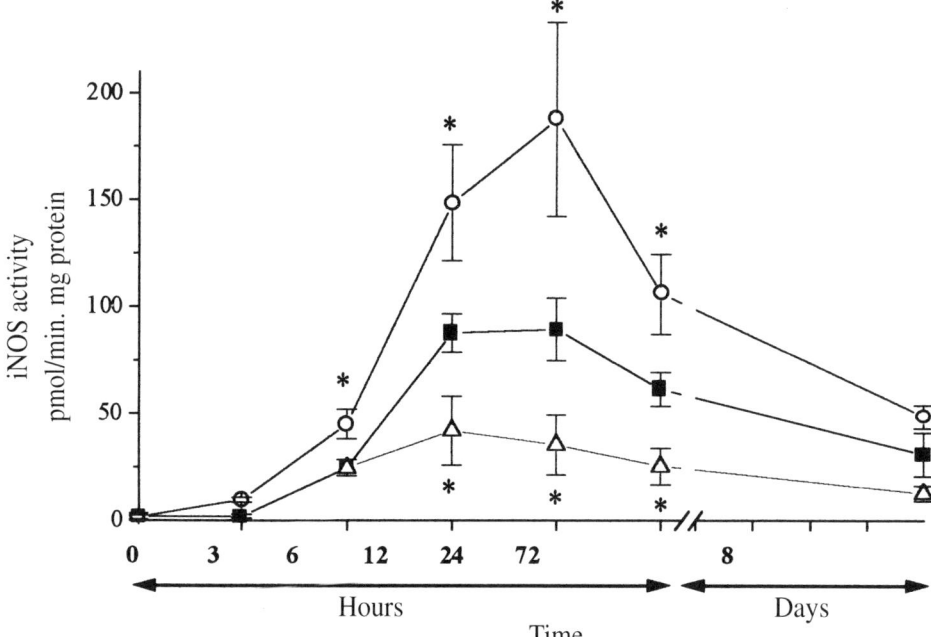

Fig. 3. Activity of iNOS in the colon following challenge with trinitrobenzene sulfonic acid (TNBS; 30 mg in 0.25 mL of 50% ethanol). Rats were treated with N^G-nitro-L-arginine methyl ester (L-NAME) added in a dose of 25 mg/kg^{-1} per 24 h to drinking water commencing 48h prior to challenge (○), or commencing 6 h following challenge (△) or in the control group, with saline (■). Data shown as the Ca^{2+}-independent activity (pmol/min^{-1}/mg^{-1} protein), are means ± S.E. of 7–10 experiments, where * denotes significant difference from control ($p < 0.05$). Data are adapted from Kiss et al. 1997 *(31)*.

7. Multiple dosing of the potential anticolitic agent by the intra-colonic route that involves viscous substances or vehicles is not recommended as it may obscure the development of the lesions following challenge, by acting as a physical barrier for the TNBS.
8. The model can thus be adapted to study the effects of agents that can prevent the development of colitis by pretreatment schedule, whereas it can also indicate the ability of an agent to ameliorate the colitis if administered after the instillation of the TNBS.

4.2. Myeloperoxidase Activity After TNBS Challenge

9. In TNBS-challenged animals, colonic MPO activity increases progressively from 3 h to 2 d, as shown in **Fig. 2**.
10. This activity then decreases to basal level during the 10 d after TNBS instillation (*see* **Fig. 2**).
11. The activity of MPO in the colonic tissue may fall more rapidly toward the basal level than the degree of gross macroscopic injury after such challenge.

4.3. Determination of iNOS Expression and Activity After TNBS Challenge

12. The iNOS protein in colonic tissue is faintly detectable by Western blot analysis from 6 h after TNBS administration and peaks at 2 d. This iNOS expression remains detectable at day 6, then declines over the 10-d period following TNBS administration, no longer being expressed at day 10.
13. The iNOS enzyme activity follows a similar time-course to protein expression. Basal iNOS activity is very low and increases from 6 h after TNBS challenge to reach its maximal level at 2 d (*see* **Fig. 3**).
14. The iNOS activity then decreases to basal levels over the 10-d experimental period (*see* **Fig. 3**).
15. Thus, the expression of iNOS activity follows a similar pattern to the changes in MPO, as a marker of PMN infiltration into the inflammatory site after intracolonic challenge with TNBS.
16. However, as can be seen from the data, the effectiveness of certain potential anticolitic agents can be schedule-dependent. In the study shown in **Figs. 1–3**, inhibition of constitutive NOS by pretreatment with a nonselective NOS inhibitor aggravated the colonic injury and inflammation, whereas delayed administration until a time of known iNOS expression attenuates such colonic damage.

Acknowledgment

This work was supported in part by a grant from the William Harvey Research Foundation, London, UK.

References

1. Kappeler, A. and Mueller, C. (2000) The role of activated cytotoxic T cells in inflammatory bowel disease. *Histol. Histopathol.* **15,** 167–172.
2. Papadakis, K. A. and Targan, S. R. (2000). Role of cytokines in the pathogenesis of inflammatory bowel disease. *Ann. Rev. Med.* **51,** 289–298.
3. Boughton-Smith, N. K., Evans, S. M., Hawkey, C. J., Cole, A. T., Balsitis, M., Whittle B. J. R., et al. (1993) Nitric oxide synthase activity in ulcerative colitis and Crohn's disease. *Lancet* **342,** 338–340.
4. Dijkstra, G., Moshage, H., van Dullemen, H. M., de Jager-Krikken, A., Tiebosch, A. T., Kleibeuker, J. H., et al. (1998) Expression of nitric oxide synthases and

formation of nitrotyrosine and reactive oxygen species in inflammatory bowel disease. *J. Pathol.* **186,** 416–421.
5. Singer, I. I., Kawka, D. W, Scott, S., Weidner, J. R., Mumford, R. A., Riehl, T. E., et al. (1996) Expression of inducible nitric oxide synthase and nitrotyrosine in colonic epithelium in inflammatory bowel disease. *Gastroenterology* **111,** 871–885.
6. Boughton-Smith, N. K., Evans, S. M., Whittle, B. J. R., and Moncada, S. (1993) Induction of nitric oxide synthase in rat intestine and its association with tissue injury. *Agents Actions* **38,** C125–126.
7. Whittle, B. J. R. (1997) Nitric oxide-a mediator of inflammation or mucosal defence. *Eur. J. Gastroenterol. Hepatol.* **9,** 1026–1032.
8. Kubes, P. (2000) Inducible nitric oxide synthase: a little bit of good in all of us. *Gut* **47,** 6–9.
9. Sartor, R. B. (1997) Review article: How relevant to human inflammatory bowel disease are current animal models of intestinal inflammation? *Aliment. Pharmacol. Ther.* **11,** 89–96.
10. Morris, G. P., Beck P. L., Herridge, M. S., Depew, W. T., Szewczuk, M. R., and Wallace, J. L. (1989) Hapten-induced model of chronic inflammation and ulceration in the rat colon. *Gastroenterology* **96,** 795–803.
11. Boughton-Smith, N. K., Wallace, J. L., Morris G. P., and Whittle, B. J. R. (1988) The effect of anti-inflammatory drugs on eicosanoid formation in a chronic model of inflammatory bowel disease in the rat. *Br. J. Pharmacol.* **94,** 65–72
12. Boughton-Smith, N. K. and Whittle, B. J. R. (1988). Laboratory methods for studying the role of eicosanoids in inflammatory bowel disease. In *Advances in Eicosanoid Research-Eicosanoids and the Gastrointestinal Tract* (Hiller, K., ed.), MTP, Lancaster, PA, pp. 12–45.
13. Grisham, M. B., Volkmer, C., Tso, P., and Yamada, T. (1991) Metabolism of trinitrobenzene sulfonic acid by the rat colon produces reactive oxygen species. *Gastroenterology* **101,** 540–547.
14. Yamada, Y, Marshall, S., Specian, R. D., and Grisham, M. B. (1992) A comparative analysis of two models of colitis in rats. *Gastroenterology* **102,** 524–534.
15. Torres, M. I., Garcia-Martin, M., Fernandez, M. I., Nieto, N., Gil, A., and Rios, A. (1999) Experimental colitis induced by trinitrobenzenesulfonic acid: an ultrastructural and histochemical study. *Dig. Dis. Sci.* **44,** 2523–2529.
16. Neurath, M., Fuss, I., and Strober W. (2000) TNBS-colitis. *Int. Rev. Immunol.* **19,** 51–62.
17. Hoffmann, P., Zeeh, J. M., Lakshmanan, J., Wu, V. S., Procaccino, F., Reinshagen, M., et al. (1997) Increased expression of transforming growth factor alpha precursors in acute experimental colitis in rats. *Gut* **41,** 195–202.
18. Jacobson, K., McHugh, K., and Collins, S. M. (1997) The mechanism of altered neural function in a rat model of acute colitis. *Gastroenterology* **112,** 156–162.
19. Miampamba, M. and Sharkey, K. A. (1998) Distribution of calcitonin gene-related peptide, somatostatin, substance P and vasoactive intestinal polypeptide in experimental colitis in rats. *Neurogastroenterol. Motil.* **10,** 315–329.
20. Stein, J., Ries, J., and Barrett, K. E. (1998) Disruption of intestinal barrier func-

tion associated with experimental colitis: possible role of mast cells. *Am. J. Physiol.* **274,** G203–209.
21. Sans, M., Panes, J., Ardite, E., Elizalde, J. I., Arce, Y., Elena, M., et al. (1999) VCAM-1 and ICAM-1 mediate leukocyte-endothelial cell adhesion in rat experimental colitis. *Gastroenterology* **116,** 874–883.
22. Ballinger, A., El-Haj, T., Perrett, D., Turvill, J., Obeid, O., Dryden, S., et al. (2000) The role of medial hypothalamic serotonin in the suppression of feeding in a rat model of colitis. *Gastroenterology* **118,** 544–553.
23. Hoffmann, P., Reinshagen, M., Zeeh, J. M., Lakshmanan, J., Wu, V. S., Goebell, H., et al. (2000) Increased expression of epidermal growth factor-receptor in an experimental model of colitis in rats. *Scand. J. Gastroenterol.* **35,** 1174–1180.
24. Chang, Q., Soper, B. D., Yacyshyn, B. R., and Tepperman, B. L. (2000) Alterations in protein kinase C isoforms in experimentally-induced colitis in the rat. *Inflamm. Res.* **49,** 27–35.
25. Lin, C. L., Moniz, C. and Chow, J. W. (2000) Treatment with fluoride or bisphosphonates prevents bone loss associated with colitis in the rat. *Calcif. Tissue Int.* **67,** 373–377.
26. Ardite, E., Sans, M., Panes, J., Romero, F. J., Pique, J. M., and Fernandez-Checam J. C. (2000) Replenishment of glutathione levels improves mucosal function in experimental acute colitis. *Lab. Invest.* **80,** 735–744.
27. Sun, F. F., Lai, P. S., Yue, G., Yin, K., Nagele, R. G., Tong, D. M., et al. (2001) Pattern of cytokine and adhesion molecule mRNA in hapten-induced relapsing colon inflammation in the rat. *Inflammation* **25,** 33–45.
28. Hoffmann, J. C., Peters, K., Henschke, S., Herrmann, B., Pfister, K., Westermann, J., et al. (2001) Role of T lymphocytes in rat 2,4,6-trinitrobenzene sulfonic acid (TNBS) induced colitis: increased mortality after gamma delta T cell depletion and no effect of alpha beta T cell depletion. *Gut* **48,** 489–495.
29. Sans, M., Salas, A., Soriano, A., Prats, N., Gironella, M., Pizcueta, P., et al. (2001) Differential role of selectins in experimental colitis. *Gastroenterology* **120,** 1162–1172.
30. Seo, H. G., Takata, .I, Nakamura, M., Tatsumi, H., Suzuki, K., Fujii, J., et al. (1995) Induction of nitric oxide synthase and concomitant suppression of superoxide dismutases in experimental colitis in rats. *Arch. Biochem. Biophys.* **24,** 41–47.
31. Kiss, J., Lamarque, D., Delchier, J. C. and Whittle, B. J. R. (1997) Time-dependent actions of nitric oxide synthase inhibition on colonic inflammation induced by trinitrobenzene sulfonic acid in rats. *Eur. J. Pharmacol.* **336,** 219–224.
32. Yue G., Lai, P. S., Yin, K., Sun, F. F., Nagel, R. G., Liu, X., et al. (2001) Colon epithelial cell death in 2,4,6-trinitrobenzenesulfonic acid-induced colitis is associated with increased inducible nitric-oxide synthase expression and peroxynitrite production. *J. Pharmacol. Exp. Ther.* **297,** 915–925
33. Bradley, P. P., Priebat, D. A., Christensen, R. D., and Rothstein, G. (1982) Measurement of cutaneous inflammation: estimation of neutrophil content with an enzyme marker. *J. Invest. Dermatol.* **78,** 206–209.
34. McCafferty, D. M., Sharkey, K. A., and Wallace, J. L. (1994) Beneficial effects

of local or systemic lidocaine in experimental colitis. *Am. J. Physiol.* **266**, G560–567.
35. Palmen, M. J., Dijkstra, C. D., van der Ende, M. B., Pena, A. S., and van Rees, E. P. (1995) Anti-CD11b/CD18 antibodies reduce inflammation in acute colitis in rats. *Clin. Exp. Immunol.* **101**, 351–356.
36. Veljaca, M., Lesch, C. A., Pllana, R., Sanchez, B., Chan, K., and Guglietta, A. (1995) BPC-15 reduces trinitrobenzene sulfonic acid-induced colonic damage in rats. *J. Pharmacol. Exp. Ther.* **272**, 417–422.
37. Tatsumi, Y. and Lichtenberger, L. M. (1996) Molecular association of trinitrobenzenesulfonic acid and surface phospholipids in the development of colitis in rats. *Gastroenterology* **110**, 780–789.
38. Yue, G., Sun, F. F., Dunn, C., Yin, K., and Wong, P. Y. (1996) The 21-aminosteroid tirilazad mesylate can ameliorate inflammatory bowel disease in rats. *J. Pharmacol. Exp. Ther.* **276**, 65–70.
39. Peterson, T. C. and Davey, K. (1997) Effect of acute pentoxifylline treatment in an experimental model of colitis. *Aliment. Pharmacol. Ther.* **11**, 575–580.
40. Ribbons, K. A., Thompson, J. H., Liu, X., Pennline, K., Clark, D. A., and Miller, M. J. (1997) Anti-inflammatory properties of interleukin-10 administration in hapten-induced colitis. *Eur. J. Pharmacol.* **323**, 245–254.
41. Miampamba, M., Parr, E. J., McCafferty, D. M., Wallace, J. L., and Sharkey, K. A. (1998) Effect of intracolonic benzalkonium chloride on trinitrobenzene sulfonic acid-induced colitis in the rat. *Aliment. Pharmacol. Ther.* **12**, 219–228.
42. Eliakim, R., Karmeli, F., Rachmilewitz, D., Cohen, P., and Fich, A. (1998) Effect of chronic nicotine administration on trinitrobenzene sulfonic acid-induced colitis. *Eur. J. Gastroentero. Hepatol.* **10**, 1013–1019.
43. Zingarelli, B., Cuzzocrea, S., Szabo, C., and Salzman, A. L. (1998) Mercaptoethylguanidine, a combined inhibitor of nitric oxide synthase and peroxynitrite scavenger, reduces trinitrobenzene sulfonic acid-induced colonic damage in rats. *J. Pharmacol. Exp. Ther.* **287**, 1048–1055.
44. Kim, Y. S., Son, M., Ko, J. I., Cho, H., Yoo, M., Kim, W. B., et al. (1999) Effect of DA-6034, a derivative of flavonoid, on experimental animal models of inflammatory bowel disease. *Arch. Pharm. Res.* **22**, 354–360
45. Tozaki, H., Fujita, T., Odoriba, T., Terabe, A., Okabe, S., Muranishi, S., et al. (1999) Validation of a pharmacokinetic model of colon-specific drug delivery and the therapeutic effects of chitosan capsules containing 5-aminosalicylic acid on 2,4,6-trinitrobenzenesulfonic acid-induced colitis in rats. *J. Pharm. Pharmacol.* **51**, 1107–1112.
46. Sykes, A. P., Bhogal, R., Brampton, C., Chander, C., Whelan, C., Parsons, M. E., et al. (1999) The effect of an inhibitor of matrix metalloproteinases on colonic inflammation in a trinitrobenzenesulfonic acid rat model of inflammatory bowel disease. *Aliment. Pharmacol. Ther.* **13**, 1535–1542.
47. Gulluoglu, B. M., Kurtel, H., Gulluoglu, M. G., Aktan, A. O., Yegen, B. C., Dizdaroglu, F., et al. (1999) Bombesin ameliorates colonic damage in experimental colitis. *Dig. Dis. Sci.* **44**, 1531–1538.

48. McCafferty, D. M., Smith, C. W., Granger, D. N., and Kubes, P. (1999) Intestinal inflammation in adhesion molecule-deficient mice: an assessment of P-selectin alone and in combination with ICAM-1 or E-selectin. *J. Leuko. Biol.* **66,** 67–74.
49. Tozaki, H., Fujita, T., Odoriba, T., Terabe, A., Suzuki, T., Tanaka, C., et al. (1999) Colon-specific delivery of R68070, a new thromboxane synthase inhibitor, using chitosan capsules: therapeutic effects against 2,4,6-trinitrobenzene sulfonic acid-induced ulcerative colitis in rats. *Life Sci.* **64,** 1155–1162.
50. Padol, I., Huang, J. Q., Hogaboam, C. M., and Hunt, R. H. (2000) Therapeutic effects of the endothelin receptor antagonist Ro 48-5695 in the TNBS/DNBS rat model of colitis. *Eur. J. Gastroenterol. Hepatol.* **12,** 257–265.
51. Peterson, T. C., Cleary, C. E., Shaw, A. M., Malatjalian, D. A., and Veldhuyzen van Zanten, S. J. (2000) Therapeutic role for bismuth compounds in TNBS-induced colitis in the rat. *Dig. Dis. Sci.* **45,** 466–473.
52. Kennedy, R. J., Hoper, M., Deodhar, K., Kirk, S. J., and Gardiner, K. R. (2000) Probiotic therapy fails to improve gut permeability in a hapten model of colitis. *Scand. J. Gastroenterology* **35,** 1266–1271.
53. Galvez, J., Garrido, M., Merlos, M., Torres, M. I., and Zarzuelo, A. (2000). Intestinal anti-inflammatory activity of UR-12746, a novel 5-ASA conjugate, on acute and chronic experimental colitis in the rat. *Br. J. Pharmacol.* **130,** 1949–1959.
54. Girgin, F., Karaoglu, O., Erkus, M., Tuzun, S., Ozutemiz, O., Dincer, C., et al. (2000). Effects of trimetazidine on oxidant/antioxidant status in trinitrobenzenesulfonic acid-induced chronic colitis. *J. Toxicol. Environ. Health. A.* **59,** 641–652.
55. D'Argenio, G., Grossman, A., Cosenza, V., Valle, N. D., Mazzacca, G. and Bishop, P. D. (2000). Recombinant factor XIII improves established experimental colitis in rats. *Dig. Dis. Sci.* **45,** 987–997.
56. Reinshagen, M., Rohm, H., Steinkamp, M., Lieb, K., Geerling, I., Von Herbay, A., et al. (2000) Protective role of neurotrophins in experimental inflammation of the rat gut. *Gastroenterology* **119,** 368–376.
57. Kitani, A., Fuss, I. J., Nakamura, K., Schwartz, O. M., Usui, T., and Strober, W. (2000) Treatment of experimental (Trinitrobenzene sulfonic acid) colitis by intranasal administration of transforming growth factor (TGF)-beta1 plasmid: TGF-beta1-mediated suppression of T helper cell type 1 response occurs by interleukin (IL)-10 induction and IL-12 receptor beta2 chain downregulation. *J. Exp. Med.* **192,** 41–52.
58. Zeeh, J. M., Zorlu Riley, N. E., Hoffmann, P., Ruwe, M., Goebell, H., Gerken, G., et al. (2001) Mycophenolate mofetil reduces tissue damage and inflammation in an experimental model of colitis in rats. *Scand. J. Gastroenterol.* **36,** 66–70.
59. Armstrong, A. M., Foulkes, R., Jennings, G., Gannon, C., Kirk, S. J., and Gardiner, K. R. (2001) Tumour necrosis factor inhibitors reduce the acute-phase response in hapten-induced colitis. *Br. J. Surg.* **88,** 235–240.
60. Nakase, H., Okazaki, K., Tabata, Y., Uose, S., Ohana, M., Uchida, K., et al. (2001) An oral drug delivery system targeting immune-regulating cells ameliorates

mucosal injury in trinitrobenzene sulfonic acid-induced colitis. *J. Pharmacol. Exp. Ther.* **297,** 1122–1118.
61. Guo, X., Ko, J. K., Mei, Q. B., and Cho, C. H. (2001) Aggravating effect of cigarette smoke exposure on experimental colitis is associated with leukotriene B4 and reactive oxygen metabolites. *Digestion* **63,** 180–187.
62. Yoshida, N., Yoshikawa, T., Yamaguchi, T., Naito, Y., Tanigawa, T., Murase, H., et al. (2001) A novel water-soluble vitamin E derivative protects against experimental colitis in rats. *Antioxid. Redox Signal.* **1,** 555–562.

24

An In Vivo Model of Ischemia/Reperfusion and Inflammation of the Kidneys of the Rat

Prabal K. Chatterjee and Christoph Thiemermann

1. Introduction

Renal failure is defined as the cessation of kidney function. Acute renal failure (ARF) involves the failure of the kidney over a period of hours or days and is potentially reversible, whereas chronic renal failure (CRF) develops over months or years and involves the irreversible destruction of kidney tissue by progressive renal disease(s) leading to endstage renal disease (ESRD).

Despite significant advances in critical care medicine, ARF still remains a major clinical problem and the mortality associated with ARF has not decreased significantly over the last 50 yr *(1,2)*. Additionally, ARF is frequently implicated in the etiology of other life-threatening complications including sepsis and multiorgan failure *(3,4)*. ARF may be classified as i) prerenal; ii) renal; or iii) postrenal, which involves, respectively: i) failure of the kidney to receive an adequate blood supply as a result of a fall in renal blood flow caused by, e.g., renal ischemia (cessation of blood flow to the kidney); ii) intrinsic damage to the kidney tissue caused by, e.g., nephrotoxins; or iii) impairment of urinary flow because of obstruction caused by, e.g., bladder cancer. Overall, ARF is caused by several factors, either directly affecting the kidney or interfering with its circulation and involves sudden deterioration of renal function characterized by rapidly rising serum levels of urea (uremia) and creatinine. Previous interventions against ARF have proved to be largely negative and to date, dialysis still remains the only effective therapy *(2)*.

The etiology of CRF involves one or more progressive renal diseases ranging from polycystic kidney disease to glomerulonephritis, with diabetes and hypertension accounting for the vast majority of patients suffering CRF and associated ESRD *(5,6)*. Dialysis or transplantation remain the only viable treatments for CRF, which, if left untreated, leads to ESRD and consequent death of the patient. The incidence and prevalence of CRF and ESRD have increased steadily such that nearly half a million patients were involved in ESRD treatment programs in the United States in 1998 compared with almost 200,000 in 1989 *(7)*. New approaches to the treatment of CRF are now being developed [reviewed by Gilbert et al. *(8)*], focusing on the treatment of diabetes and hypertension, which accounts for the vast majority of patients suffering CRF/ESRD *(9)*. These interventions include blockade of the renin-angiotensin system *(10,11)* and inhibition of protein kinase C (PKC) activity *(12,13)*.

Renal inflammation, both in its acute and chronic forms, plays an important role in the pathophysiology of both ARF and CRF *(14,15)*, and is particularly important in the aetiology of allograft rejection following renal transplantation *(16,17)*. Within the kidney, the inflammatory process involves a complex and interrelated sequence of events, resulting in injury to, and the eventual death of renal cells *(18,19)*. Furthermore, it appears that certain renal cells such as mesangial cells within the glomerulus, and proximal tubular (PT) cells, can themselves act as proinflammatory cells *(18,20)*. The inflammatory process is invariably characterized by a production and release of biologically active mediators including histamine, bradykinin, platelet-activating factor (PAF), and interleukin 1 (IL-1) from tissues and migrating cells. Generation of proinflammatory cytokines including tumor necrosis factor-α (TNF-α), IL-1, and IL-6 contributes to the extension of the inflammatory process. The contribution of inflammatory mediators to renal inflammation is reflected by the fact that their removal by dialysis can provide beneficial actions *(21,22)*. Several studies also support the conclusion that i) cell adhesion molecules such as intercellular cell adhesion molecule-1 (ICAM-1) and vascular cell adhesion molecule-1 (VCAM-1); and ii) vasoactive agents such as nitric oxide (NO$^\bullet$) derived from inducible nitric oxide synthase (iNOS); and iii) arachidonic acid metabolites such as prostaglandin E_2 (PGE_2) derived from cyclo-oxygenase-2 (COX-2), all play important roles in the pathogenesis of renal inflammation *(23–25)*. Furthermore, induction of proinflammatory proteins such as iNOS and COX-2 implicate the involvement of nuclear factor (NF)-κB activation in renal disease *(26)*.

There is a now a large amount of evidence that the production of reactive oxygen species (ROS) at the site of inflammation such as hydrogen peroxide (H_2O_2), superoxide ($O_2^{\bullet-}$) and hydroxyl radicals (OH$^\bullet$) and reactive nitrogen species (RNS) such as NO$^\bullet$ contribute to renal I/R injury *(27,28)* and subsequent ARF *(24,29)*. In addition to NO$^\bullet$, generation of peroxynitrite (ONOO$^-$), which is produced when equimolar amounts of NO$^\bullet$ reacts with $O_2^{\bullet-}$ *(30)*, has also been implicated in inflammation *(31)*. Overall, the roles of ROS and RNS in renal inflammation have been confirmed in studies involving reduction of the production of, or scavenging of ROS or RNS, in which renal inflammation is attenuated *(31–33)*.

This chapter will concentrate on renal ischemia/reperfusion (I/R) in the anesthetized rat. Renal I/R causes significant dysfunction and injury of the kidney *(27,32,34)* and is one of the major causes of ARF *(34)*. Significant renal ischemia commonly occurs during aortic surgery, renal transplantation, or subsequent to cardiovascular anesthesia, leading to renal dysfunction and injury *(35,36)*. This is complicated by the fact that reperfusion, although essential for the survival of ischemic renal tissue, causes additional cellular injury (reperfusion-injury) *(37)*, which is a major contributor to early allograft rejection and adversely affects long-term allograft survival subsequent to renal transplantation *(38)*.

Renal inflammation plays a significant role in the renal dysfunction and injury associated with I/R of the kidney, via infiltration of inflammatory mediators such as polymorphonuclear neutrophils (PMNs) and expression of iNOS and COX-2 *(32,39)*. Several models of renal I/R and oxidative stress, using different species have been used to investigate the role of renal inflammation and the contribution of ROS/RNS to the development of ARF. These range from in vivo models of renal I/R in the rat and mouse involving bilateral clamping of the renal artery or pedicles *(32,39–41)* to in vitro models using cultures of human or rat glomerular mesangial or PT cells exposed to oxidative or nitrosative stress *(18,32,41–43)*, in the form of H_2O_2 *(32,43)* or via cytokine-stimulated NO• production *(42)*, respectively.

The aim of this chapter is to introduce the reader to a reliable in vivo (nonrecovery) model of renal I/R in the anesthetised rat, which involves ischemia (produced by bilateral clamping of the renal pedicles for 45 min) followed by reperfusion for 6 h. The renal I/R protocol described results in significant and severe (but not fatal) renal dysfunction and injury, with particular injury to the PT, against which different interventions have shown beneficial effects *(32,39,41)*. A reperfusion period of between 6 and 24 h has been shown to produce a similar levels of renal I/R injury in the rat *(44)* and the use of a 6 h reperfusion period in the model described here allows it to be performed and completed in one day. Renal dysfunction and injury can be characterized by biochemical analysis of serum and urinary parameters and glomerular or tubular dysfunction, tubular injury and I/R injury can be distinguished (*see* **Figs. 1–4**). Additionally, sections of kidney can be used for histological analysis of renal injury *(32,39)*, immunohistochemical analysis of the expression of proinflammatory proteins including iNOS or COX-2 *(39)*, markers of inflammation such as nitrotyrosine (for ONOO⁻) or poly(ADP-ribose) (PAR, for activation of

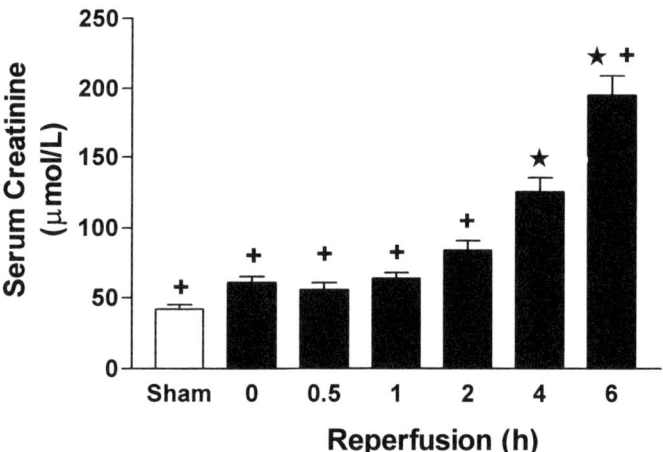

Fig. 1. Alterations in serum creatinine (sCr) concentrations during renal I/R; after increasing periods of reperfusion. ★$P < 0.05$ vs Sham-operated group (Sham), +$P < 0.05$ vs 4 h reperfusion group ($N = 8–12$).

poly(ADP-ribose) polymerase) *(32)* or for the measurement of biochemical markers of inflammation, e.g., myeloperoxidase (MPO) activity as a marker of PMN infiltration or malondialdehyde (MDA) levels as a marker of lipid peroxidation *(32,39)*. We have previously used this model to demonstrate how various interventions can significantly reduce renal dysfunction and injury mediated by I/R of the rat kidney *(29,39,41)*. Furthermore, we have shown how several of these interventions markedly reduce renal inflammation including the reduction of i) MPO activity (reduced PMN infiltration); ii) MDA levels (reduced lipid peroxidation); iii) iNOS protein expression (reduced NO• production); iv) COX-2 protein expression (reduced PG production); v) evidence of nitrotyrosine production (reduced ONOO• formation); and vi) reduced PAR formation (attenuated PARP activation) *(32,41)*.

2. Materials

1. Saline solution: 0.9% (w/v) saline (NaCl), sterile, nonpyrogenic (Baxter Healthcare Ltd., Thetford, Norfolk, UK).
2. Heparin-Saline 'Hepsal' solution: Add 1 mL Heparin (Multiparin™, stock solution 25,000 IU/mL, National Veterinary Supplies, Stoke on Trent, Staffordshire, UK) to 1 L 0.9% (w/v) saline to produce a 25 IU/mL working solution.
3. Anesthetic solution: Prepare a 3% (w/v) dosing solution of sodium thiopentone (Intraval™ Sodium, Merial Animal Health Care, Dublin, Republic of Ireland) in 0.9% (w/v) saline.

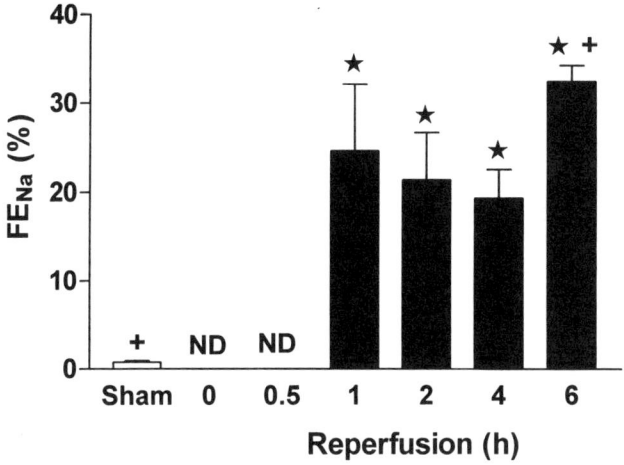

Fig. 2. Effect of renal I/R on fractional excretion of Na^+ (FE_{Na}); subsequent to increasing periods of reperfusion. ★$P < 0.05$ vs Sham-operated group (Sham), +$P < 0.05$ vs 4 h reperfusion group ($N = 8–12$).

4. 10% (w/v) formaldehyde in phosphate buffered saline (PBS):
   a. Dissolve 1 PBS tablet (Sigma Chemcial Co., Poole, Dorset, UK) in 200 mL distilled water to produce a 0.01 M phosphate buffer containing 0.0027 M potassium chloride and 0.137 M sodium chloride, pH 7.4 at 25°C.
   b. Carefully add 20 g paraformaldehyde (Sigma Chemical Co., store at 4°C. See Caution below) to 200 mL PBS and stir until dissloved. The solution will dissolve over several days if left at room temperature or faster if heated to 50–60°C in a water bath. Caution: Paraformaldehye is both toxic and highly flammable and appropriate precautions (lab coat, gloves, eye/face protection) must be taken when weighing out. The final solution must be labeled with the appropriate warning labels (e.g., toxic).
5. Heating mat (Harvard Apparatus Ltd., Kent, UK).
6. Silk braided suture (1.5, Pearsalls Sutures, Taunton, Somerset, UK).

3. Methods

Male Wistar rats (200–300 g) are used in this procedure although male Sprague-Dawley rats have also been used *(44)* (*see* **Note 1**). Rats are kept in normal night/day conditions and receive a standard diet consisting of rat chow and water *ad libitum*. The protocol described later has been approved and licensed by the UK Home Office and the care and use of animals described below is in accordance with the *Guidance in the Operation of the Animals (Scientific Procedures) Act 1986* (*see* **Note 2**).

1. After weighing, anesthetize the rat by administering an interperitoneal (ip) bolus of sodium thiopentone at 120 mg/kg (*see* **Note 3**).
2. Place the fully anesthetised rat on its back, with its head closest to you, on a thermostatically controlled heating mat and maintain body temperature at 37.5 ± 1°C by means of a rectal temperature probe attached to a homoeothermic blanket (*see* **Note 4**).
3. Make a 4 cm incision into the fur on the neck and separate the underlying layers of tissue using blunt-pointed surgical scissors to expose the trachea (*see* **Notes 5 and 6**). Using the scissors, separate the trachea from the surrounding tissue by separating it from the tissue below it, taking care not to damage it. Feed two small (approx 10 cm) lengths of silk-braided suture underneath the trachea, leaving the ends free on either side of the rat. Perform a tracheotomy by making a small incision into the top of the trachea and inserting a pointed polyethylene fine bore tube (1.67 mm bore, 0.375 mm wall, Scientific Laboratory Supplies Ltd., Nottingham, UK). Secure the trachea tube in place using the silk thread. Check airway patency (*see* **Note 7**).
4. Locate and isolate the carotid artery (CA) which is close to the trachea. Stretch the CA by placing a pair of open forceps underneath it (*see* **Note 8**). Feed two sections of silk thread under the exposed artery, leaving the ends free on either side of the rat. Tie off the CA using the silk thread closest to the head of the rat (i.e., furthest away from the heart) and secure the silk thread with a closed 15-cm clamp. Place the clamp such that the CA remains stretched and remove the forceps. Using a 3.5-cm "bulldog" artery clip (Dieffenbach's, Holborn Surgical and Medical Instruments Ltd., Margate, Kent, UK), occlude the CA at the point closest to the heart (i.e., furthest away from the head) (*see* **Note 9**). Using entomological scissors, make a small incision on the top of the CA. Carefully feed in a pointed polyethylene cannula (0.58 mm bore, 0.29 mm wall, Scientific Laboratory Supplies Ltd.) containing hepsal (*see* **Note 10**). Tie this firmly in place using the two silk threads (including the one already attached to the CA). Release the artery clip (*see* **Note 11**).
5. Locate and isolate the jugular vein (JV) from its surrounding tissue, close to the CA (*see* **Note 12**). Feed two 10-cm sections of silk thread under the exposed vein, leaving the ends free on either side of the rat. Tie off the JV using the silk thread closest to the head of the rat (i.e., furthest away from the heart). Using entomological scissors, make a small incision of the top of the JV (*see* **Note 13**). Carefully feed in a pointed polyethylene cannula (0.40 mm bore, 0.2 mm wall, Scientific Laboratory Supplies Ltd.) containing saline (*see* **Note 14**). Tie this firmly in place using the two silk threads (including the one already attached to the JV). Slowly administer 0.5 mL saline to clear the JV line and to replace any lost fluid.
6. Carefully turn the rat around, taking care not to dislodge the CA/JV lines, so that the rat's head is furthest away from you.
7. Using forceps, lift the fur on the abdomen and make an incision along the midline from the base of the abdomen up to the diaphragm, exposing the tissue below.

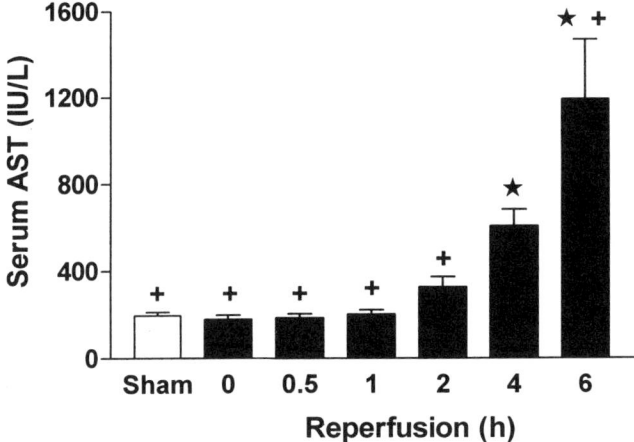

Fig. 3. Alterations in serum aspartate aminotransferase (AST) concentrations during renal I/R; after increasing periods of reperfusion. ★$P < 0.05$ vs Sham-operated group (Sham), +$P < 0.05$ vs 4 h reperfusion group ($N = 8$–12).

Lift the tissue at the base of the abdomen and make a small incision into the peritoneum. Use this space to carefully cut the tissue along the midline, stopping just short of the diaphragm (*see* **Note 15**). Attach clamps to the tissue on each side of the incision and position such that the peritoneum is exposed.

8. Locate and isolate the bladder at the lower end of the midline incision and attach a Dieffenbach's bulldog artery clip to the top of it. Loop a 10-cm section of silk thread around the bladder and, using the clip to hold the bladder upright, make a small incision at the top. After the bladder has emptied, insert the bulbed cannula (0.76 mm bore, 0.23 mm wall, Scientific Laboratory Supplies Ltd., *see* **Note 16**) into the bladder and secure in place by tightening the silk thread. Pull the cannula out of the bladder slightly so that the bulbed end catches at the top of the bladder where the silk thread has been tightened. Collect urine into a microcentrifuge tube. Remove the clamps used to expose the peritoneum and place a swab, kept moist with saline, over the midline incision.

9. Administer another 0.5 mL of saline to the rat via the JV line to replace lost fluid. Connect the JV cannula to an infuser and administer saline at a rate of 8 mL/kg/h (*see* **Note 17**). Allow the rat to stabilize for at least 10 min, or until MAP stabilizes, while monitoring cardiovascular parameters (*see* **Note 11**). After stabilization, a 1-mL blood sample can be taken via the CA line, and in combination with urine collected during the stabilisation period, can be used to measure baseline serum/plasma and urinary biochemical markers of renal function (*see* **Note 18**). The amount of blood taken should be replaced with an equivalent amount of saline administered slowly via the JV line.

10. Use a cotton bud to carefully move away the spleen and small intestine on the right-hand side of the rat, exposing the right kidney and pedicle (containing the

renal artery, vein, and nerve). Using a pair of forceps, carefully isolate the renal pedicle by separating it from the surrounding tissue, but keeping away from the ureter emerging from the kidney. Use a Differenbach's bulldog artery clip to clamp the isolated pedicle, thus occluding the blood supply to (and from) the kidney. However, ensure that the ureter, emerging nearby from the kidney, is *not* occluded. Move the spleen/small intestine to the other side of the rat to expose the left kidney and its pedicle, just below and behind the liver (*see* **Note 19**). As for the other kidney, isolate the renal pedicle and clamp.

11. Check to ensure that the kidneys are ischemic by monitoring their color. Occlusion is verified visually by a change in the color of the kidneys to a paler shade and then to a darker (cyanotic) color within minutes (prerenal azotaemia). Move the small intestine/mesentery back into the peritoneum and douse with saline (to replace fluid lost from the peritoneum). Cover with gauze moistened with saline and leave the pedicles clipped for 45 min.

12. To begin reperfusion, move the intestine/mesentery to expose the artery clips. Open and remove the clips using a pair of large forceps. Ensure that the kidneys reperfuse by visually observing a blush as the blood flow is reestablished (i.e., a change in color from dark (cyanotic) to a pink/brown color) (*see* **Note 20**). Replace the intestine/mesentery into the peritoneum and after adding saline to keep the internal organs moist, close up the peritoneum using a Differenbach's bulldog artery clip. At this point, saline infusion is reduced to 2 mL/kg/h.

13. During the reperfusion period: i) closely monitor the cardiovascular parameters of the rat (*see* **Note 11**); ii) ensure that the rat remains fully anesthetized (*see* **Note 21**); iii) the rat maintains the correct body temperature (*see* **Note 4**); and iv) the patency of the airway is maintained (*see* **Note 7**).

14. At the end of the experimental period, collect 1-mL blood samples via the CA cannula into labeled microcentrifuge tubes containing either serum gel or heparin (*see* **Note 22**). Centrifuge samples at 6000 rpm to separate serum/plasma, which are then transferred into new, labeled microcentrifuge tubes. Measure the volume of urine produced. Samples of serum/plasma and urine can then be used for biochemical analysis as required or frozen and stored at −80°C for later analysis (*see* **Notes 23** and **24**).

15. Kill the rat using an overdose of anesthesia (*see* **Notes 25** and **26**).

16. Remove the kidneys from the rat. Using a scalpel, gently cut along the top of the kidney and peel away and remove the renal capsule. Bisect and examine the kidney for gross histology. Kidneys can then be stored as required in 10% (w/v) PBS-buffered formaldehyde at room temperature or stored frozen after snap freezing in liquid N_2 (**Caution**: wear appropriate body/hand/eye/face protection because of risk of burns caused by extremely low temperatures).

4. Notes

1. We find that the use of rats below 200 g causes problems when the CA is isolated, as the vagus nerve, which runs alongside, is more susceptible to bruising, leading to breathing problems. The use of rats larger than 350 g causes problems

with administration and maintenance of anesthesia and in performing surgery due to the increased levels of body fat.
2. Published by Her Majesty's Stationery Office (H.M.S.O.), London, UK. All procedures undertaken that involve the use of animals in vivo *must* be approved and licensed by the UK Home Office or the equivalent national body.
3. Inject into the peritoneum of the rat using a brown (26-gauge, 0.45 × 10 mm) needle (Microlance 3, Beckton Dickinson UK Ltd., Oxford, UK). If the rat is held firmly and upright, the injection can be given quickly into the exposed abdomen without causing undue stress to the rat. We find that anesthetizing rats with sodium thiopentone at this concentration leads to a long-lasting surgical anesthesia.
4. It is important to maintain the right body temperature (37.5 ± 1°C). Body temperature within a clinically relevant range (i.e., 32–40°C) has a profound influence on the degree of renal I/R-mediated dysfunction/injury. For example, reduction in body temperature to 32°C (e.g., because of anesthesia or during abdominal surgery) can significantly reduce plasma creatinine levels in the rat subjected to 40 min bilateral renal ischemia followed by 24 h reperfusion *(45)*. Increased body temperature (40°C, e.g., as a result of pyrexia or overheating of the rat caused by lighting during surgery) subsequently results in significantly increased plasma creatinine levels in the same model *(45)*. Similar effects of temperature were observed in vitro in PT exposed to hypoxia *(46)*. If required, we use a surgical or table lamp for short periods to increase temperature if required or gauze soaked in saline and placed on the body of the rat to lower temperature to compliment the temperature regulation provided by the heating mat if required.
5. For surgery, ensure surgical equipment used is of the highest quality (e.g., stainless steel equipment from Holborn Surgical and Medical Instruments Ltd., Margate, Kent, UK). Also ensure good lighting for close surgical work using either a surgical lamp (which will not produce excessive heat) or a good table lamp (but take care not to increase the temperature of the rat).
6. To avoid excessive bleeding and tissue damage, use the ends of the blunt-pointed surgery scissors to separate the layers of tissue rather than cutting.
7. Maintain airway patency by using a small length of cannula (0.58 mm bore, 0.29 mm wall) attached to a blunted green (21-gauge, 0.8 × 40 mm) needle (blunt the needle by removing the sharp end using a pair of pliers) attached to an empty 10-mL syringe to clear the airway of any mucus. Withdraw air gently from the lungs to avoid damaging or collapsing the lungs. Take care not to make the length of the cannula not longer than approx 4 cm or there is a chance of damaging the lungs. Performing the tracheotomy first allows airway patency to be maintained throughout the remaining procedure and facilitates spontaneous respiration. However, if at any point, breathing should stop, the rat can be given artificial respiration using an animal ventilator (we use a small animal ventilator [Harvard Apparatus Ltd., Kent, UK] set at 8–10 mL/kg and 70 strokes/min) until spontaneous respiration is reestablished.
8. The CA can be located quite easily by looking for its pulsing. However, it can

often lie quite deep toward the back of the neck. Once located, isolate it by carefully stripping away the surrounding tissue and separate it carefully from the vagus nerve, which is white and runs alongside the CA. Take care not to snap or bruise the vagus nerve or respiration will slow down or stop. Once isolated, the CA is quite elastic and can be handled quite firmly, yet carefully.
9. When attaching the artery clip, ensure that the CA is totally occluded by checking its attachment to the CA and ensuring that none of the surrounding tissue has also been inadvertently clipped.
10. The cannula (0.58 mm bore, 0.29 mm wall) is connected to a 2-mL syringe containing hepsal via a blunted blue (23-gauge, 0.6×25 mm) needle. Trim the end of the cannula to a point to help insertion into the CA by "hooking" the edge of the incision, then push along carefully. Be careful not to push too close to the clip or you will risk tearing the CA and causing a hemorrhage when the clip is released.
11. When the artery clip is released, the residual blood in the cannula should pulse indicating a clear line. If not, gently push through some hepsal to clear the line. After occluding the cannula using a clamp (on which the teeth have been blunted using thick adhesive tape to avoid damaging to the cannula), it can be connected to a pressure transducer (Senso-Nor, Horten, Norway) allowing measurement of MAP and derivation of HR from the pulse waveform, using a data-acquisition system (MacLab 8e, AD Instruments, Hastings UK) installed on a personal computer.
12. The JV is located a short distance from the CA and can be spotted by looking for its dark color. Expose it (carefully, as it is not as robust as the CA) by stripping away surrounding tissue and isolate it.
13. On making this incision, there may be a small amount of bleeding from the JV. This can be stopped by gently stretching the JV by pulling upward on the silk thread already attached to the JV.
14. The cannula (0.40 mm bore, 0.2 mm wall) is connected to a 1-mL syringe containing saline via a blunted brown (26-gauge, 0.45×10 mm) needle. As with the CA cannula (*see* **Note 10**), trim the end to a point to allow easier insertion into the incision on the top of the JV. The cannula will have been inserted correctly when no resistance can be felt as it is pushed gently along the JV. However, be careful not to push it too deeply toward the heart. The JV line can be then be used for the iv infusion of saline or administration of drugs or supplementary anesthesia as required.
15. Cutting along the midline will avoid damaging surface blood vessels and excessive bleeding. As the incision gets closer to the diaphragm, take care not to damage the liver, which can often remain attached to the midline. Lift the tissue and check to ensure that the liver is not attached to the tissue. If it is, gently push it down and out of the way using a cotton bud.
16. The bladder cannula is "bulbed" by placing it briefly into a flame. However, ensure that the end does not become blocked. Bulbing the cannula prevents it from coming out of the bladder after being secured in place.
17. Administration of saline at this rate provides a saline infusion of 2 mL/h for a 250-g

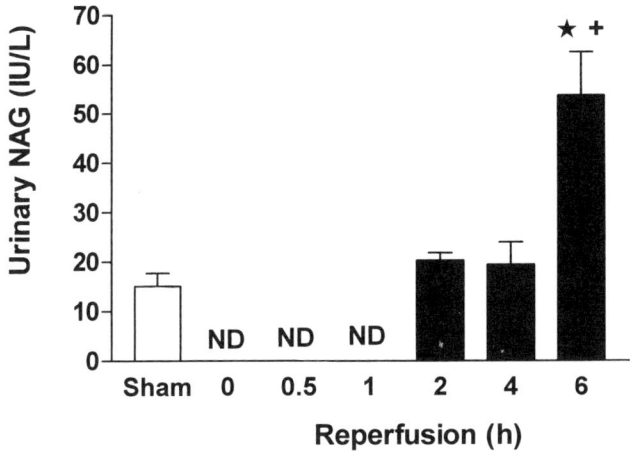

Fig. 4. Effect of renal I/R on urinary N-acetyl-β-D-glucosaminidase (NAG) levels during renal I/R; subsequent to increasing periods of reperfusion. ★$P < 0.05$ vs Sham-operated group (Sham), +$P < 0.05$ vs 4 h reperfusion group ($N = 8–12$).

rat, allowing fluid lost during surgery to be replaced and is sufficient to produce a urine output of at least 2 mL/kg/h, which provides enough urine for measurement of urinary parameters which, in conjunction with serum/plasma samples collected after stabilisation, can be used to determine baseline renal function.

18. We have previously taken a 1-mL plasma/serum sample from rats after the stabilization period and found that if replaced with an equal volume of saline administered iv via the JV line, no adverse effects are observed.

19. Aim to separate the pedicle from its surrounding tissue a short distance away from the kidney, avoiding the ureter emerging from the kidney close by. If the ureter is clipped by mistake, it can become stenosed and prevent urine leaving the kidney causing postrenal azotemia. Also take care when trying to isolate the pedicles to avoid bleeding from the renal vein, which is delicate. In most rats, the renal pedicle of the right kidney is much easier to locate than the left kidney. If the liver covers the left renal pedicle, carefully move it out of the way using a cotton bud. Finally, the length of the left renal pedicle is quite short so aim to separate it close to the junction of the renal artery/vein with the descending aorta/vena cava.

20. Clamping of the renal pedicles should not cause any lasting damage to the renal vein, artery or nerve, and reperfusion should commence without any problems. Occasionally, the kidney will not reperfuse. This can sometimes be alleviated by manipulating the renal pedicle using forceps, however, if the kidney does not reperfuse, the rat will have to be excluded from the study.

21. Regularly check that the rat remains fully anesthetised by looking for the standard indicators of anesthesia in the rat (e.g., no response to squeezing of the paw using a pair of forceps). Anesthesia is maintained by administration of supple-

mentary injections of sodium thiopentone (10 mg/kg, iv) to rats as required.
22. To obtain serum, serum one-third gel tubes are used (Vetlab Services, Sussex, UK). To obtain plasma, a small drop of heparin (25,000 IU/mL) is place into the microcentrifuge tubes before collection of blood.
23. Serum and urine samples are analyzed within 24 h after collection for measurement of serum/plasma and urinary parameters (Vetlab Services, Sussex, UK) for determination of renal function (see later).
24. Serum and urine samples are analysed for the following biochemical parameters of renal (glomerular and tubular) function, tubular injury and I/R injury.
Serum urea concentration: (sUr), increased levels indicate glomerular dysfunction and/or increased catabolism *(47,48)*. sUr is expressed in μmol/L.
Serum creatinine concentration: (sCr), increased levels indicate reduced creatinine clearance and glomerular filtration rate, and hence, renal failure *(47,48)*. sCr is expressed as mmol/L.
Creatinine clearance: (C_{CL}), an indicator of glomerular filtration rate and, hence, glomerular function. C_{CL} can be calculated using a standard formula involving the ratio of serum and urinary creatinine concentrations (sCr and uCr) and urine flow as shown:
C_{CL} (mL/min) = (uCr [mmol/L] × urine flow [mL/min] / sCr [mmol/L]).
Fractional excretion of Na^+: (FeNa), an indicator of tubular function. Fe_{Na} can be calculated using a standard formula incorporating the ratio of serum and urinary Na^+ concentrations (sNa and uNa), C_{CL} and urine flow as shown:
FE_{Na} (%) = (uNa [μmol/L] × urine flow [mL/min]) / (C_{CL} [mL/min] × sNa [μmol/L]) × 100
Urinary glutathione S-transferase: (uGST), an indicator of tubular injury *(49)*, expressed as IU/L
Urinary N-acetyl-β-D-glucosaminidase: (uNAG), a specific indicator of tubular damage *(50)*, expressed as IU/L
Serum aspartate aminotransferase level: (sAST), an indicator of renal I/R injury *(32,39)*, expressed as IU/L
Serum γ-glutamyl transferase levels: (sγGT), an indicator of renal I/R injury *(32,39)*, expressed as IU/L
25. We find that an administration of an iv bolus of up to 1 mL 3% (w/v) sodium thiopentone is adequate for producing rapid euthanasia.
26. Dispose of the rat carcass and related biological waste in an appropriate manner following local rules for the disposal of biological waste.

Acknowledgment

P. K. Chatterjee was funded by the National Kidney Research Fund (Grant R41/2/2000) and C. Thiemermann was supported by a Senior Research Fellowship (Grant FS/96/018) from the British Heart Foundation. We would like to thank Drs. Helder Mota-Filipe and Rui Pinto and the Clínica Médica e Diagnóstico Dr Joaquim Chaves, Lisbon, Portugal, for the urinary NAG measurements.

References

1. Thadhani, R., Pascual, M., and Bonventre, J. V. (1996) Acute renal failure. *N. Engl. J. Med.* **334,** 1448–1460.
2. Star, R. A. (1998) Treatment of acute renal failure. *Kidney Int.* **54,** 1817–1831.
3. McCarthy, J. T. (1996) Prognosis of patients with acute renal failure in the intensive care unit: a tail of two eras. *Mayo Clinic Proc.* **71,** 117–126.
4. Breen, D. and Bihari, D. (1998) Acute renal failure as a part of multiple organ failure: the slippery slope of critical illness. *Kidney Int.* **66,** S25–S33.
5. Maisonneuve, P., Agodoa, L., Gellert, R., Stewart, J. H., Buccianti, G., Lowenfels, A. B., et al. (2000) Distribution of primary renal diseases leading to end-stage renal failure in the United States, Europe, and Australia/New Zealand: results from an international comparative study. *Am. J. Kidney Dis.* **35,** 157–165.
6. Ritz, E., Rychlik, I., Locatelli, F., and Halimi, S. (1999) End-stage renal failure in type 2 diabetes: a medical catastrophe of worldwide dimensions. *Am. J. Kidney Dis.* **34,** 795–808.
7. U.S. Renal Data System (USRDS) at http://www.usrds.org
8. Gilbert, R. E., Kelly, D. J., and Atkins, R. C. (2001) Novel approaches to the treatment of progressive renal disease. *Curr. Opin. Pharmacol.* **1,** 183–189.
9. Bakris, G. L., Williams, M., Dworkin, L., Elliott, W. J., Epstein, M., Toto, R., et al. (2000) Preserving renal function in adults with hypertension and diabetes: a concensus approach. National Kidney Foundation Hypertension and Diabetes Executive Committees Working group. *Am. J. Kidney Dis.* **36,** 646–661.
10. Lewis E. J., Hunsicker L. G., Bain, R. P., and Rohde, R. D. (1993) The effect of angiotensin-converting enzyme inhibition on diabetic nephropathy. The collaborative study group. *N. Engl. J. Med.* **329,** 1456–1462.
11. The GISEN group (Gruppo Italiano di Studi Epidemiologici in Nephrologia). (1997) Randomized placebo-controlled trial of effect of ramipril on decline in glomerular filtration rate and risk of terminal renal failure in proteinuric, non-diabetic nephropathy. *Lancet* **349,** 1857–1863.
12. Goekjian, P. G. and Jirousek, M. R. (1999) Protein kinase C in the treatment of disease: signal transduction pathways, inhibitors, and agents in development. *Curr. Med. Chem.* **6,** 877–903.
13. Koya, D., Haneda, M., Nakagawa, H., Isshiki, K., Sato, H., Maeda, S., et al. (2000) Amelioration of accelerated diabetic mesangial expansion by treatment with a PKC β inhibitor in diabetic db/db mice, a rodent model for type 2 diabetes. *FASEB J.* **14,** 439–447.
14. Eckardt, K. U. (2000) Acute renal failure - more than kidney ischemia? *Wein. Klin. Wochenschr.* **112,** 145–148.
15. Kaysen, G. A. (2000) Inflammation and oxidative stress in end-stage renal disease. *Adv. Nephrol. Necker Hosp.* **30,** 201–214.
16. Vos, I. H., Rabelink, T. J., Dorland, B., Loos, R., Van Middelaar, B., Grone, H. J. et al. (2001) L-arginine supplementation improves function and reduces inflammation in renal allografts. *J. Am. Soc. Nephrol.* **12,** 361–367.
17. Albrecht, E. W., van Goor, H., Tiebosch, A. T., Moshage, H., Tegzess, A. M., and

Stegeman, C. A. (2000) Nitric oxide production and nitric oxide synthase expression in acute human renal allograft rejection. *Transplantation* **70,** 1610–1616.
18. Couser, W. G. (1998) Pathogenesis of glomerular damage in glomerulonephritis. *Nephrol. Dial. Transplant.* **13,** 10–15.
19. van Kooten, C., Langers, A. M., Bruijn, J. A., and Daha, M. R. (1999) Role of tubular cells in progressive renal disease. *Kidney Blood Press. Res.* **22,** 53–61.
20. Daha, M. R. and van Kooten, C. (2000) Is the proximal tubular cell a proinflammatory cell? *Nephrol. Dial. Transplant.* **15,** 41–43.
21. Inthorn, D. and Hoffman, J. N. (1996) Elimination of inflammatory mediators by hemofiltration. *Int. J. Artif. Organs* **19,** 124–126.
22. Montoliu, J. (1997) Clearance of inflammatory mediators through continuous renal replacement therapy. *Blood Purif.* **15,** 305–308.
23. Molitoris, B. A. and Marrs, J. (1999) The role of cell adhesion molecules in ischemic acute renal failure. *Am. J. Med.* **106,** 583–592.
24. Lieberthal, W. (1998) Biology of ischemic and toxic renal tubular cell injury: role of nitric oxide and the inflammatory response. *Curr. Opin. Nephrol. Hypertens.* **7,** 289–295.
25. Baud, L. and Ardaillou, R. (1986) Reactive oxygen species: production and role in the kidney. *Am. J. Physiol.* **251,** F765–F776.
26. Guijarro, C. and Egido, J. (2001) Transcription factor-κB (NF-κB) and renal disease. *Kidney Int.* **59,** 415–424.
27. Grace, P. A. (1994) Ischaemia-reperfusion injury. *Br. J. Surg.* **81,** 637–647.
28. Weight, S. C., Furness, P. N., and Nicholson, M. L. (1998) Nitric oxide generation is increased in experimental renal warm ischemia-reperfusion injury. *Br. J. Surg.* **85,** 1663–1668.
29. Nath K. A. and Norby, S. M. (2000) Reactive oxygen species and acute renal failure. *Am. J. Med.* **109,** 665–678.
30. Pryor, W. and Squadrito, G. (1995) The chemistry of peroxynitrite: a product from the reaction of nitric oxide with superoxide. *Am. J. Physiol.* **268,** L699–L772.
31. Wei, X. Q., Charles, I. G., Smith, A., Ure, J., Feng, G. J., Huang, F. P., et al. (1995) Altered immune responses in mice lacking inducible nitric oxide synthase. *Nature* **375,** 408–411.
32. Chatterjee P. K., Cuzzocrea, S., Brown, P. A., Zacharowski, K., Stewart, K. N., Mota-Filipe, H., et al. (2000) Tempol, a membrane-permeable radical scavenger, reduces oxidant stress-mediated renal dysfunction and injury in the rat. *Kidney Int.* **58,** 658–673.
33. Klahr, S. (2001) The role of nitric oxide in hypertension and renal disease progression. *Nephrol. Dial. Transplant.* **16,** 60–62.
34. Weight, S. C., Bell, P. R., and Nicholson, M. L. (1996) Renal ischemia-reperfusion injury. *Br. J. Surg.* **83,** 162–170.
35. Novis, B. K., Roizen, M. F., Aronson, S., and Thisted, R. A. (1994) Association of preoperative risk factors with postoperative acute renal failure. *Anesth. Analg.* **778,** 143–149.
36. Aronson, S. and Blumenthal, R. (1998) Perioperative renal dysfunction and car-

diovascular anesthesia: concerns and controversies. *J. Cardiothorac. Vasc. Anesth.* **17,** 117–130.
37. Paller, M. S. (1994) The cell biology of reperfusion injury in the kidney. *J. Investig. Med.* **42,** 632–639.
38. Shoskes, D. A. and Halloran, P. F. (1996) Delayed graft function in renal transplantation: etiology, management and long-term significance. *J. Urol.* **155,** 1837–1840.
39. Chatterjee, P. K., Brown, P. A. J., Cuzzocrea, S., Zacharowski, K., Stewart, K. N., Mota-Filipe, H., et al. (2001) Calpain inhibitor-1 reduces renal ischemia/reperfusion injury in the rat. *Kidney Int.* **59,** 2073–2083.
40. Singbartl, K., Green, S. A., and Ley, K. (2000) Blocking P-selectin protects from ischemia/reperfusion-induced acute renal failure. *FASEB J.* **14,** 48–54.
41. Chatterjee, P. K., Zacharowski, K., Cuzzocrea, S., Otto, M., and Thiemermann, C. (2000) Inhibitors of poly (ADP-ribose) synthetase reduce ischemia-reperfusion injury in the anesthetised rat in vivo. *FASEB J.* **14,** 641–651.
42. Chatterjee, P. K., Hawksworth, G. M., and McLay, J. S. (1999) Cytokine-stimulated nitric oxide production in human renal proximal tubule and its modulation by natriuretic peptides: a novel immunomodulatory mechanism? *Exp. Nephrol.* **7,** 438–448.
43. Chatterjee, P.K., Cuzzocrea, S., and Thiemermann, C. (1999) Inhibitors of poly (ADP-ribose) synthetase protect rat proximal tubular cells against oxidant stress. *Kidney Int.* **56,** 973–984.
44. Williams, P., Lopez, H., Britt, D., Chan, C., Ezrin, A., and Hottendorf, R. (1997) Characterisation of renal ischemia-reperfusion injury in rats. *J. Pharm. Toxicol. Meth.* **37,** 1–7.
45. Zager, R. A. and Altschuld, R. (1986) Body temperature: an important determinant of severity of ischemic renal injury. *Am. J. Physiol.* **251,** F87–F93.
46. Zager, R. A., Gmur, D. J., Bredl, C. R., and Eng, M. J. (1991) Temperature effects on ischemic and hypoxic renal proximal tubular injury. *Lab. Invest.* **64,** 766–776.
47. Baum, N., Dichoso, C. C., and Carlton, C. E. (1975) Blood urea nitrogen and serum creatinine: physiology and interpretations. *Urology* **5,** 583–588.
48. Stogdale, L. (1981) Correlation of changes in blood chemistry with pathological changes in the animal's body: II Electrolytes, kidney function tests, serum enzymes, and liver function tests. *J. South Afr. Vet. Assoc.* **52,** 155–164.
49. Harrison, D. J., Kharbanda, R., Scott-Cunningham, D., McLellan, L. I., and Hayes, J. D. (1989) Distribution of glutathione S-transferase isoenzymes in human kidney: basis for possible markers of renal injury. *J. Clin. Pathol.* **42,** 624–628.
50. Bosomworth, M. P., Aparicio, S. R. and Hay, A. W. M. (1999) Urine N-acetyl-β-D-glucosaminidase - a marker of tubular damage? *Nephrol. Dial. Transplant.* **14,** 620–626.

25

In Vivo Models of Inflammation

Immune Rejection and Skin Transplantation In Vivo

Isabelle Binet and Kathryn J. Wood

1. Introduction
1.1. Immune Rejection: What Is It?

One of the main functions of the immune system is the recognition and subsequent elimination of cells bearing foreign or "nonself" antigens. When cells bearing a foreign histocompatibility antigen are recognized, they become the target of the host immune response. Transplantation of an organ, tissue, or cells between genetically disparate individuals within the same species, allografts, or between species, xenografts, almost inevitably results in rejection of the graft if active steps are not taken to control the destructive immune response that is triggered immediately after transplantation.

The rejection process is complex. Many factors, including the nature of the tissue transplanted and the genetic disparity between the donor and recipient, the site of transplantation, as well as the immune status of the recipient, all contribute to determining the character of the rejection response.

In brief, the removal of the skin graft from the donor and transplantation into the recipient always triggers an inflammatory response. These "danger" signals are responsible for activating both the innate and adaptive immune systems that will act in concert to destroy the graft (*1*). For acute allograft rejection, activation of the adaptive immune system requires recognition of molecules that are mismatched or polymorphic, so-called histocompatibility molecules or antigens, between the donor and the recipient. The interaction between the triggering donor antigen and the recipient lymphocytes can take place in one or more of three sites, in the host lymphoid tissue, in the interstitial area of the graft, and on the endothelium of the graft. Host lymphoid tissues are involved in the triggering of the response *(2)*. Donor-derived passenger leukocytes in the skin, the Langerhans cells, migrate from the graft to the host lymphoid tissue that drains the graft site in response to "danger" signals triggered by the transplantation procedure *(3)*. As the donor-derived passenger leukocytes migrate to the host lymphoid tissue, they also undergo a process of maturation such that once they arrive at their destination they can present the donor antigens efficiently to host T cells. Antigen recognition in combination with additional, so-called costimulatory signals will lead to the activation of donor-reactive lymphocytes, both T cells and B cells. Clonal expansion, in other words proliferation of the donor-reactive lymphocytes, is triggered such that many more daughter cells with specificity for donor antigens are produced rapidly. The environment created by this lymphocyte activation will result in the differentiation of the activated donor-reactive lymphocytes into effector cells, including cytotoxic T cells and mature B cells or plasma cells that secrete antidonor antibodies. These antigen-specific effector cells in combination with activated components of the innate response, such as activated macrophages and natural killer (NK) cells, migrate to the graft site where, together, they orchestrate the destruction of the skin graft.

1.2. Which Actors are Involved in Immune Rejection?

The first actor responsible for initiating rejection, as aforementioned, is the inflammatory response triggered by the transplantation procedure itself. Chemokines, a family of cytokines whose main function is chemoattraction, are among the mediators produced and act as the primary regulators of lymphocyte trafficking *(4)*. Chemokines trigger both chemotaxis of donor-derived passenger leukocytes from the graft, thereby initiating the response and the recruitment of activated recipient leukocytes back to the graft to enable its destruction as the rejection response progresses.

Donor antigen-presenting cell (APC) triggered to migrate to the recipient lymphoid tissue can present donor alloantigens via the direct pathway of allorecogntion to recipient T cells. In this pathway, donor major histocompatibility complex (MHC) molecule-peptide complexes, expressed by the donor APC, are recognized by T-cell receptors (TCR) specific for one of the donor MHC-peptide complexes expressed by recipient T cells. Donor MHC class II molecules interact with $CD4^+$ T cells and MHC class I molecules with $CD8^+$ T cells.

In addition, recipient-derived APCs may also be involved in triggering the rejection response *(5)*. In this case, antigen recognition occurs via the indirect pathway where donor antigens are processed by a recipient APC, the peptides produced are then bound to recipient MHC molecules and presented at the cell surface to a recipient T cell. This pathway can also involve an interaction between recipient MHC class II molecules and CD4$^+$ T cells or recipient MHC class I molecules and CD8$^+$ T cells. Both the direct and indirect pathways of allorecognition can lead to graft rejection. Recognition of a MHC-peptide complex by TCR delivers the first signal to the responding T cell, so-called signal 1.

In order to activate the T-cell efficiently, APCs need to deliver not only "signal 1," but also other signals collectively referred to as "signal 2" or costimulation *(6)*. An increasing number of costimulatory pathways are being characterized, but two of these pathways appear to play a central role, the B7-CD28 and CD40-CD154 pathways *(7)*. CD80 and CD86 are two members of the B7 family of molecules expressed by mature APC. These two molecules can act as ligands for CD28 expressed by T cells. CD40 is also expressed by APC and binds to CD154 on the responding T cell. The signals delivered to the T cell through CD28 and CD154 integrate with those coming via the TCR to initiate T-cell proliferation and clonal expansion. These interactions need to be stabilized to ensure that the responding T cell receives all of the information required for activation. Adhesion molecules like LFA1 or ICAM ensure that this occurs by facilitating formation of the immunological synapse between the APC and the T cell *(8)*.

The third actor responsible for the development of the immune response is the recipient T lymphocyte. Intracellular signaling is initiated by the TCR–CD3 complex, enhanced by accessory and costimulatory molecules and involves a cascade of protein kinases and intracellular phosphorylation events in the T cell. The result is the activation of transcription factors (NFκB, NFAT, and AP-1) that bind to the promoters switching on the expression of new genes such as cytokines genes. This results in the production of, among other molecules, interleukin 2 (IL-2), the main cytokine responsible for lymphocyte proliferation and differentiation. IL-2 both initiates and sustains the clonal expansion of T lymphocytes through the production of IL-2, enhancing the inflammatory response through the release and upregulation of other cytokines and membrane receptors, thereby providing help for the differentiation of effector cells, including cytotoxic T lymphocytes (CTL), macrophages, and B cells *(9)*.

1.3. Which Effector Cells Damage the Transplanted Tissue?

CTL, B cells, macrophages, and NK cells represent four types of effector cells that can be involved in the destruction of the graft. In general, activated CD4$^+$ T cells will provide help for the activation of CD8$^+$ T cells, B cells, and monocytes. Once activated, T cells do not necessarily need any further costimulation to turn into effector cells when the specific allopeptide is encountered. However, the cytokine microenvironment in which these events take place will have a marked influence on the outcome of the response.

Cytotoxic T-cell activity mediated by the perforin—granzyme pathway and by the *Fas–Fas* ligand pathway induces antigen-specific lysis and apoptosis of target cells expressing donor alloantigens in the graft. B-cell differentiation leads to the production of alloantibodies, which cause tissue damage by activating the complement and by antigen-dependent cell-mediated cytotoxicity (ADCC). Macrophages and NK cells can also use the ADCC mechanism to lyse antibody-coated target cells by binding to the *Fc* portion of the antibody. In a sensitized host, preformed donor-specific antibodies will bind immediately to the graft endothelial cells, thus causing hyperacute rejection. This phenomenon plays a major role in the destruction of xenografts as a result of the presence of natural crossreactive preformed antibodies in the recipient.

In parallel with the activation of effector cells, a wide array of cytokines are released from APCs, activated T cells, and macrophages and play a central role as mediators of inflammation. Cytokines like TNFα and IFNγ can become directly cytotoxic when present at high concentrations, but their principal action is to amplify the process by which tissue injury promotes inflammation and cellular infiltration, increases immune recognition through upregulation of MHC expression, which makes graft cells even better targets for T-cell mediated killing, and thus further amplifies the inflammation.

In an attempt to distinguish functionally different types of lymphocytes, T cells have been classified as Th1 or Th2 on the basis of their cytokine production *(10)*. Th1 cells produce IL-2 and IFNγ, Th2 cells produce IL-4, IL-10, and IL-13. Th1 cells tend to favor cell-mediated immunity, whereas Th2 cells favor antibody-mediated immunity, and both patterns have a reciprocal inhibitory effect on each other. Graft infiltrating cells in rejection seem more frequently to be of a Th1 rather than a Th2 type, however, Th2 cells have also been shown to be capable of destroying allografts and the high degree of redundancy in the cytokine network does not allow such clear-cut distinction in vivo.

1.4. What Are the Histological Features of Rejection?

The acute rejection process is characterized by cellular infiltration, mostly T cells and macrophages, together with signs of acute inflammation and edema. Cellular infiltration occurs by perivascular infiltration, promoted by the upregulation of adhesion molecules on endothelial cells.

The hallmark of chronic rejection is the combination of interstitial fibrosis and graft vasculopathy. Graft vasculopathy is characterized by neointimal thickening secondary to smooth muscle cell proliferation and increased extracellular matrix leading to a narrowing of the vessel lumen. In certain circumstances, eosinophils are also observed and may play a causative role in the fibrosing process.

1.5. Skin Transplantation In Vivo

Skin transplantation is often referred to as a "strong" model of rejection as skin grafts are highly susceptible to destruction. The rapid rejection of skin grafts has been suggested to result from the high number of donor-derived passenger leukocytes, Langerhans cells, present in the graft. This may be part of the explanation but other factors are also involved. Indeed, recent work has shown that despite rejection, a skin graft is relatively inefficient at generating alloreactive T cells in the draining lymph node. The susceptibility of skin to rejection may reside in a capacity for amplification of the inflammatory response by particularily enhancing the expression of adhesion molecules and by recruiting keratinocytes as APCs. Keratinocytes are known to produce chemokines like IL-8 and MCP-1. Moreover, the microvasculature of the skin may be highly susceptible as a target for the effector mechanisms triggered after transplantation.

Rejection of allogenic skin transplants in mice is principally a T-cell-dependent process; depletion or blocking of B cells and NK cells does not prevent skin rejection, whereas T-cell-deficient hosts do not reject skin grafts. Allorecognition after skin transplant can occur through both the direct and the indirect pathway as a consequence of mismatching for the MHC or minor antigens including the male H-Y antigen.

Skin transplant in mice is a suitable model for investigating different aspects of the immune response and tolerance mechanisms in vivo such as:

- Effects of costimulatory blockade, donor-specific transfusions, and the role of new thymic emigrants on rejection vs prolonged skin graft survival.
- Role of regulatory T-cell subsets in the abrogation of skin allograft rejection.
- Impact of the induction of microchimerism in skin graft models under specific circumstances.
- Chemokines expression: MIP-1α, MIP-1β, and IP-10 are apparently expressed at equivalent levels in allografts and isografts in the early posttransplant period, then return to low levels. However, shortly before skin allograft rejection occurs, an increased expression of IP-10 in the epidermis and of Mig in the lower dermis can be observed.

The in vivo skin transplantation technique is detailed in **Subheading 2.** Full thickness tail skin transplantation has been adapted from the original skin graft technique established in 1951 by Billingham and Medawar *(11)*. The procedure described applies to rodents, particularly to mice, and can be applied to immunocompetent, as well as to immunodeficient strains.

2. Materials
2.1. Anesthesia

1. Hypnovel® (midazolam 10 mg/2 mL ampoule) solution with 2 ampoules in 36 mL NaCl 0.9%.
2. Hypnorm® (10 mL ampoule with fentanyl citrate 0.315 mg/mL and fluanisone 10 mg/mL) solution with 1.66 mL in 50 mL NaCl 0.9%.
   Both solutions can be kept sterile at 4°C for up to 1 mo. However, if crystallization or flocculation occurs, the solution should be discarded. The route of administration is subcutaneous.

2.2. Preparation of Donor Skin

1. 70% Alcohol to sterilize.
2. Petri dish covered with a swab and sterile 0.9% NaCl.
3. Scalpel blade and handle.
4. Curved and straight fine forceps (sterile).

2.3. Preparation of the Recipient

1. Shaver.
2. Q-tips and swabs.
3. 70% Alcohol.
4. Fine sharp scissors and fine straight forceps (sterile).

2.4. Skin Transplantation

1. Inadine(dressing (Providone Iodine nonadherent dressing).
2. Flexible collodion BP methylated (nitrocellulose solution). Collodion should be kept in a dark glass bottle, tightly closed, and in a fume cupboard.
3. Tape (type autoclave tape approx 1.5 cm large).

2.5. Unwrapping and Assessing the Transplant

1. Large round scissors and fine sharp scissors (sterile).
2. 0.9% NaCl in a syringe.
3. Ruler (in millimeters) (sterile).

3. Methods
3.1. Preparation of Donor Skin (Full Thickness Tail Skin)

1. The donor is sacrificed (see **Notes 1** and **2**) and the tail is sprayed with 70% alcohol
2. With the scalpel blade, an incision is made all around the base of the tail. A straight longitudinal incision is performed along the ventral part of the tail, from the base down to the tip.
3. The proximal corners are lifted with the forceps. The tail skin is held just under-

neath its base with the curved forceps so as to remove the whole length of the tail skin toward its tip.
4. The tail skin, with its inner side on a sterile swab, is immersed in sterile NaCl in a Petri dish and completely flattened (*see* **Note 3**).
5. Because it has been traumatized by the forceps during stripping, the proximal part of the tail is sectioned across with the razor blade and discarded (approx 3–4 mm). The skin is then divided into neat pieces, each piece representing one graft of approx 1–1.5 cm long (*see* **Note 4**).

3.2. Preparation of the Recipient

1. The recipients are anesthetised with 0.25–0.3 mL of each of the two anesthetics (*see* **Subheading 2.2.1.**) (*see* **Notes 5** and **6**).
2. According to the number of grafts per recipient, one or both sides of the trunk are shaved against the fur until the skin is apparent. The shaved fur is then removed from the skin using Q-tips soaked in 70% alcohol (*see* **Notes 7** and **8**).
3. The skin is stretched on the side of the trunk slightly and the graft bed is cut out with fine sharp scissors thus exposing the sc tissue; the size of the bed should match the size of the skin transplant (*see* **Note 9**). With alcohol-soaked Q-tips, the transplant bed is cleaned thoroughly.

3.3. Skin Transplant

1. The skin graft is held with the forceps by the hair and transferred to the graft bed. The graft is adjusted and completely flattened in its bed, then a wet Q-tip is rolled on the surface of the graft to remove any air bubbles underneath (*see* **Notes 10–12**).
2. The graft position is fixed using a Q-tip dipped in collodion and starting at each of the four corners. The edges of the graft are then sealed to the adjacent recipient skin with careful application of collodion sparing the centre of the graft. Collodion is left to air-dry.
3. Iodine gauze dressing is cut in rectangles slightly larger than the graft and approx 1 cm longer than the dorsal and ventral edges. When the collodion is completely dry the graft is covered with the iodine gauze.
4. To protect the skin transplant during engraftment and to maintain the gauze in place tape or sticking plaster is wrapped around the recipient trunk (*see* **Notes 13** and **14**).
5. When the procedure is completed, the recipients are placed in a heated recovery area and monitored (*see* **Note 15**).

3.4. Unbandaging and Monitoring

1. Seven days after grafting, the recipient is anesthetised with a balanced regimen of midazolam and hypnovel (0.2 mL of each, *see* **Subheading 2.1.**).
2. The bandage is loosened from the fur on the ventral side using round scissors, so that sharp scissors can then safely be used to cut across the bandage, without cutting the recipient ventral skin.

3. Tape and iodine gauze are cautiously removed (*see* **Note 16**). Desquamation of the graft epidermis is a normal phenomenon. The collodion will fall out spontaneously.
4. The length and width of graft are measured with a ruler and the appearance is observed daily for retraction, thickening, color, necrosis, hair growth, or hair loss (*see* **Note 17**).

3.5. Interpretation and Assessment of Full Thickness Skin Grafts

3.5.1. Macroscopy

1. When the graft is accepted, the skin appearance is similar to that of the recipient skin and hair growth is present (i.e., in syngenic graft). Hair growth progresses from a central line toward the edges of the graft.
2. When acute rejection develops, necrosis and retraction of the graft occur, progressing until it involves the whole transplant and the graft turns into a scab.
3. When chronic rejection develops, the graft appears thickened, hardened, and loss of new hair occurs.

3.5.2. Microscopy

1. Graft skin histology can be performed on tissue sections after OCT (Tissue Tech) embedding followed by snap freezing in liquid nitrogen.
2. Histology is particularly useful if chronic rejection is suspected or if the skin appearance is normal or subnormal. Thickening of the dermis because of cellular infiltration and/or collagen deposition (interstitial fibrosis), reduced number, and shrinking of the hair follicles and sebaceous glands, vascular intimal thickening (graft vasculopathy) can be observed.

3.6. Conclusion

Skin transplantation is a standardized procedure and an easily reproducible model in mice. It allows the investigation of both acute and chronic rejection mechanisms. The concomitant use of syngenic grafts as control in the recipient of an allogenic transplant helps to differentiate the effects as a result of nonspecific surgical injury from those secondary to the allogenic response. However, because of tissue-specific factors, intervention studies to prolong graft survival may show a different outcome to that achieved in other types of solid organ transplants.

4. Notes

1. One donor usually provides skin grafts for four recipients (three to five depending on strain and tail size).
2. Sex-matched or female donors and male recipients are always used to avoid immunization against male Y antigen.
3. Once removed from the tail, the skin has a tendency to roll and the curved forceps

can be used to flatten the skin on the swab; if the corners or the edges of the graft need to be lifted, pinching with the forceps tips should be avoided as this will damage the graft.
4. The narrow tail tip (less than approx 0.8 cm large) is best discarded as a reduced transplant surface may influence the graft survival time.
5. The number of recipients depends of the number of skin grafts obtained *per* donor.
6. Using both allogenic and syngenic skin transplants on the same recipient provides an internal control.
7. Animal hair is released during shaving, to decrease the risk of sensitization it is advisable to shave the recipients under an aspiration hood.
8. The shaved area should be approx 1 cm wider than the graft size.
9. For proper engraftment, graft and bed size have to be as closely matched as possible. The edges of the graft should not slip under the recipient skin, particularly at the corners, the edges of the graft should not lie on top of the recipient skin and any gap between donor and recipient skin should not be wider than 1 mm.
10. The graft orientation should be opposite to that of the recipient hair growth, to enable donor hair to be distinguishable from recipient hair.
11. Forceps must be used carefully while transferring and adjusting the graft in its bed so as not to traumatize the edges, the corners or the surface of the donor skin.
12. The recipient must have a relaxed muscle tone during the bandaging procedure. A small dose of the balanced anesthetic regimen mentioned under **Subheading 2.1.** can be used (0.1–0.15 mL sc of each anesthetic is usually enough at this stage).
13. Bandaging should be neither too tight (the recipient should not have any difficulty moving, breathing or eating normally) nor to loose (litter and food should not accumulate underneath, the bandaging should not slip down toward the hips and hinder walking, the graft should not become accessible to scratching). The bandage should be observed daily, and replaced if necessary.
14. If the whole procedure has taken more than 1 h, 0.5 to 1 mL NaCl 0.9% sc should be administered to avoid dehydration. Injection should be as far as possible from the transplant site to avoid swelling of the graft bed.
15. Approx half the recommended number of recipients per cage is advisable.
16. If gauze sticks to the graft, preliminary soaking with NaCl 0.9% will help loosen it. The graft should not become displaced while removing the bandage, as this will disrupt engraftment and cause necrosis, notably at the corners, and thus influence transplant outcome.
17. In naïve immunocompetent mice, the time-point of acute skin allograft rejection has to be determined for each strain combination but is usually expected around day 9. Increased surgical or external trauma to the graft may influence the outcome.

Acknowledgment

I. Binet was supported by the Else-Kröner-Fresenius Grant, the Fujisawa-ESOT Grant, the Novartis Research Grant, and the Roche Research Foundation.

Further Reading

- *Immunobiology. The Immune System in Health and Disease*. Janeway, C. A. and Travers, P., eds.) 3rd edition, 1997. Current Biology LTD and Garland.
- *The Handbook of Transplant Immunology*. (Wood, K. J., ed.) 1st edition, 1995. MedSci Publication.
- *Oxford Textbook of Medicine*.
- VanBuskirk AM, et al. Transplantation Immunology (1997) *JAMA* **278**: 1993–1999.
- Hancock WW, et al. (2000) Chemokines and their receptors in allograft rejection, *Current Opinion in Immunology* **12**: 511–516

References

1. Matzinger, P. (1994) Tolerance, danger and the extended family*Ann. Rev. Immunol.* **12,** 991–1045.
2. Lakkis, F., Arakelov, A., Konienczny B., and Inoue, Y. (2000) Immunologic 'ignorance' of vascularised organ transplants in the absence of secondary lymphoid tissue. *Nat. Med.* **6,** 686–688.
3. Larsen, C., Steinman, R., Witmer-Pack, M., Morris P., and Austyn, J. (1990) Migration and maturation of Langerhans cells in skin transplants and explants. *J. Exp. Med.* **172,** 1483–1493.
4. Cyster, J. (1999) Chemokines and cell migration in secondary lymphoid organs. *Science* **286,** 2098–2102.
5. Shoskes, D. and Wood, K. (1994) Indirect presentation of MHC antigens in transplantation. *Immunol. Today* **15,** 1–7.
6. Lechler, R., Ng, W., and Steinman, R. (2001) Dendritic cells in transplantation—friend or foe? *Immunity* **14,** 357–368.
7. Lenschow, D. J., Walunas, T. L., and Bluestone, J. A. (1996) CD28/B7 system of T cell costimulation. *Ann. Rev. Immunol.* **14,** 233–258.
8. Bromley, S., Burak, W., Johnson, K., Somersalo, K., Sims, T., Sumen, C. et al. (2001) The immunological synapse. *Ann. Rev. Immunol.* **19,** 375–396.
9. Dallman, M. J. and Morris, P. J. (1994) The immunology of rejection. In *Kidney Transplantation Principles and Practice*. (Morris, J., ed.) W. B. Sanders, Philadelphia, PA, pp. 8–25.
10. O'Garra, A. and Murphy, K. (1996) Role of cytokines in the development of Th1 and Th2 cells. *Chem. Immunol.* **63,** 1–13.
11. Billingham, R. E. and Medawar, P. B. (1951) Technique of free skin grafting in mammals. *J. Exp. Biol.* **28,** 385–391.

26

Wound Healing

A Model of Dermal Wound Repair

Annette Tomlinson and Mark W. J. Ferguson

1. Introduction

Wound healing in adult mammals proceeds by a series of overlapping, highly coordinated events. The sequence in dermal wound repair, which is principally analogous in other anatomical locations, starts with the arrest of hemorrhage, followed by an inflammatory response; reepithelialization of the wound; formation of granulation tissue within the wound space and finally the production of a scar *(1,2)*.

Initial deposition of a fibrin plug, prevents leakage from damaged blood vessels and the production of a provisional fibrin-containing matrix within the wound, facilitates the migration of inflammatory cells, directed by a variety of chemotactic factors.

Neutrophils initially predominate at the wound site in rodent dermal incisional wounds, peaking at 24 to 48 h. Therafter, macrophages accumulate, reaching maximum numbers at 3 to 5 d postwounding and returning to baseline levels by day 14. T lymphocytes in much smaller numbers than macrophages are first observed in murine wounds at day 3 postwounding. The largest numbers of CD4+ cells are observed at day 5 and decline by day 14. CD8+ cells are also present at the same time, but in much smaller numbers. Extremely small numbers of B cells are also present in adult murine incisional wounds, peaking at day 5 *(3)*.

Keratinocytes from dermal appendages and the wound margins, migrate laterally across the healing surface, effecting reepithelialization of the wound. Granulation tissue is formed in the wound space by the migration and proliferation of influxing fibroblasts, endothelial cells, and angioblasts, the latter two forming new blood vessels by angiogenic and vasculogenic processes. Synthesis and deposition of fibronectin, collagen, and other extracellular matrix molecules within the granulation tissue results in a neodermis. Fibroblasts differentiate into myofibroblasts and wound contraction occurs.

During the process of granulation tissue maturation, significant apoptosis of blood vessels, inflammatory cells, and myofibroblasts reduces wound cellularity and vascular density. Remodeling of the wound extracellular matrix over a period of many months results in the formation of a mature scar. All adult dermal injury results in visible and functional scarring to a greater or lesser extent, characterized by abnormal patterns of extracellular matrix organization by comparison to the surrounding normal dermis *(4)*.

Orchestration of the of the overlapping biological processes of wound repair is controlled by numerous chemokines, cytokines, growth factors, extracellular matrix molecules and their receptors, and proteases and their inhibitors *(2,5)*.

This sequence of healing is typical of acute injuries, terminating in mature scar formation, however, peturbation of this ordered response results in chronic nonhealing wounds, *(2,6)* or at the other extreme, excessive scarring, e.g., keloids or hypotrophic scars. Microvascular pathology and high blood-sugar levels are underlying factors in the development of diabetic ulcers and venous insufficiency in chronic venous ulcers, but alterations in the levels and activities of cytokines, growth factors, proteolytic enzymes and their inhibitors are implicit in preventing progress into a healing phase.

Surgical and medical procedures can interfere with normal wound healing causing fibrotic disorders. Abdominal surgery and radiation treatment can trigger fibrosis. In abberent wound healing such as keloids and hypertrophic scars, disorders of the fibroproliferative response result in altered cellularity, elevated collagen accumulation, and excessive scar formation.

In the majority of cases, the embryonic response to injury is fundamentally different to that of the adult, tissue is regenerated and healing occurs without scar formation *(7)*. There is a gradual transition to scarring with increasing fetal age. Young adults, in general, heal rapidly, but produce excessive scarring in comparison to the elderly. Slower rates of healing in the elderly are associated with alterations in inflammation, adhesion molecule expression, levels of proteases and their inhibitors, and cytokine and growth factors and their inhibitors, however, scar quality is improved *(8,9)*. In aged, healthy postmenopausal females, a reduced rate of cutaneous healing and improved scar quality was associated with reduced levels of transforming growth factor-beta 1 (TGF-β1). Estrogen reversed these age-related changes with an increase in TGF-β1 *(10)*. Manipulation of the ratios of TGF-β superfamily members, particularly the reduction of β1 and β2 or elevation of β3 is the most effective known way of reducing/preventing scarring and fibrosis *(11)*.

At the present time, there is no model of chronic wound healing in laboratory animals that accurately mimics the cellular and molecular alterations seen in biopsies of human chronic wounds *(12,13)*. Attempts to mimic other abberent healing states, including keloids and hypertrophic scar, have also had little success *(14)*. On the contrary, models of acute healing are excellent. There are a number of animal models of acute wound healing in various anatomical sites including stab injuries, surgical incisions/excisions, skin flaps, and burns. The most widely used models to evaluate healing therapies, or investigate wound healing mechanisms are incisional and excisional wounds on the dorsum of rodents. These wounds are termed full thickness and involve incising or excising the epidermis, the dermis, subcutaneous (sc) tissues, and the underlying muscular layer found in rodents, the panniculus carnosus (*see* **Fig. 1**). Excisional wounds involve a loss of tissue and, therefore, mimic such situations in humans except that the degree of contraction in rodents is greater than in humans. Pig wounds contract less and the skin has fewer hairs rendering human bandaging/dressing techniques feasible *(15)*. However, they are more expensive and often die under anesthesia. Rodent and porcine incisional wounds accurately mimic the situation in humans. Rodent models will be described in this chapter.

Dermal incisional and excisional wounds allow qualitative and quantitative evaluation of treatments at all stages of wound repair, including granulation tissue formation, resolution of the inflammatory response, rate of reepithelialization, measurement of wound strength, and assessment of scarring.

2. Materials

1. "Wella Contura" hair clippers (IMS, Industrial Medical Supplies, Congleton, Cheshire, UK). These are excellent for removing fine underhair on mice.
2. 70% alcohol and swabs.
3. No. 11 scalpel blades and holder. Use a new sterile scalpel blade per animal for incisional wounds.
4. Sterile biopsy punches from Stiefel (Wooburn Green, Bucks, UK). These are available in 2–8 cm diameter. Biopsy punches rarely last for more than 2–4 wounds before blunting.
5. 15-cm ruler.
6. Nontoxic and permanent marker pens. Secureline 2 marker pens (Raymond Lamb, Eastbourne, East Sussex, UK) will survive histological processing.

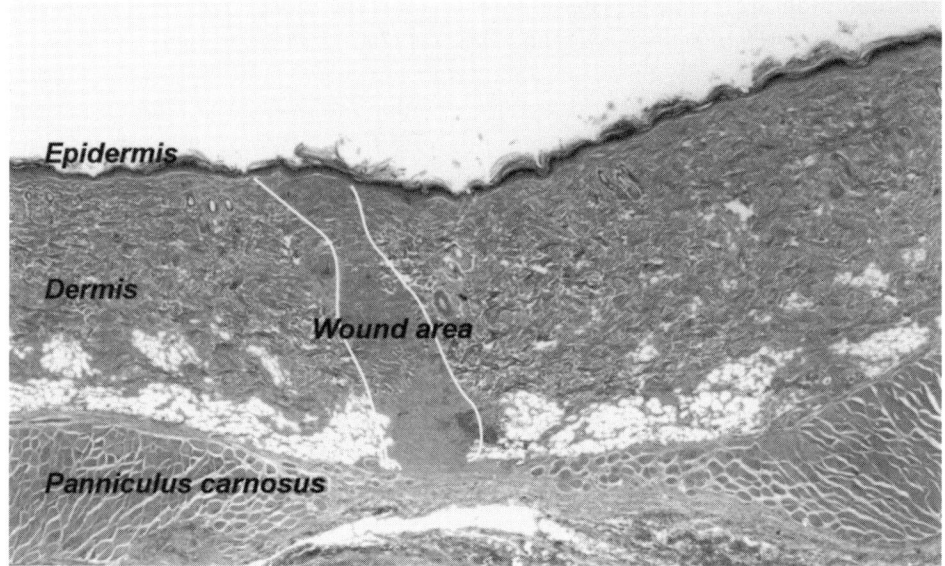

Fig. 1. Micrograph of a dermal full thickness incisional wound in rat 70 d postwounding.

3. Methods

The method of wounding described here is based on a 25–30 g mouse or 180–250 g rat. Modifications of placement of wounds may be necessary for smaller or larger animals. Male adult animals are used routinely, as hormonal status affects wound parameters in adult females. In order to prevent skin lesions from fighting males, which may interfere with the evaluation of wound repair, animals are housed singly for approx 1 wk prior to wounding.

The number and size of incisional and excisional wounds described in this protocol are routinely used in our laboratories, however, dependent on Home Office approval under the Animals (Scientific Procedures) Act 1986, a larger number, or longer wounds may be permitted.

The spatial positions of the wounds on the dorsum have been experimentally derived in our laboratories to minimize differences in wound gape and interference with the wound by the animal biting, scratching, or rubbing against the cage. Variability in wound gape may be attributable to the underlying skeleton, blood supply, or the position being accessible to biting or scratching.

A combination of incisional and excisional wounds can be applied in the same animal.

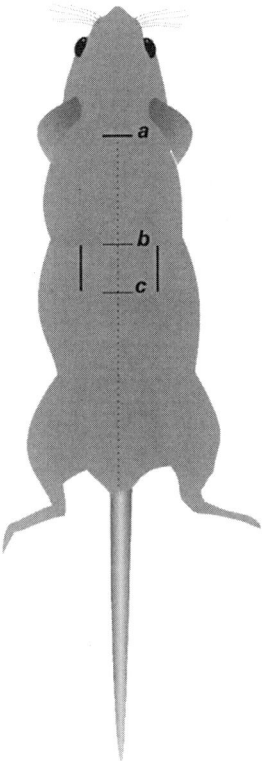

Fig. 2. Template for incisional wounds on the dorsum of a mouse. Distance **a–b** is 3 cm from the base of the skull along the midline (dotted line). Distance **a–c** is 4 cm. The two linear incisions (solid lines) are 1 cm in length and placed 1 cm to the side of the midline.

3.1. Incisional Wounds (see Notes 1–3)

1. The procedure is carried out under general anesthesia. Swab the dorsum with 70% alcohol and shave the entire area, removing the fine underhair.
2. In mice, from the base of the skull, measure and mark two points 3 and 4 cm along the midline using a nontoxic marker pen (*see* **Fig. 2**). Mark further points, 1 cm either side of the midline, two each at the 3- and 4-cm points. These delineate the position for two 1-cm incisions, running parallel to the midline.
3. In rats, measure and mark four points 5, 6, 8, and 9 cm from the base of the skull along the midline (*see* **Fig. 3**). Mark eight further points, 1 cm either side of the midline, two at each of the 5, 6, 8, and 9-cm points. These delineate the position of four 1-cm incisions, running parallel to the midline.

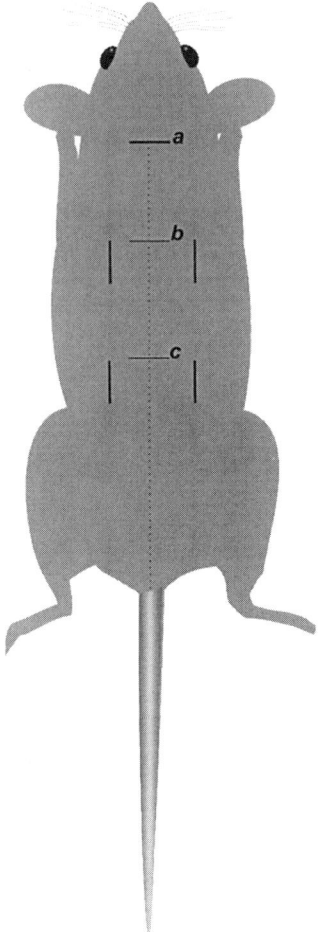

Fig. 3. Template for incisional wounds on the dorsum of a rat. Distance **a–b** is 5 cm from the base of the skull along the midline (dotted line). Distance **a–c** is 8 cm. The four l inear incisions (solid lines) are 1 cm in length and placed 1 cm to the side of the midline.

4. To make a 1-cm incisional wound, lift the skin of the animal between the finger and thumb of one hand, slightly above the cranial marked point. Insert the tip of the scalpel blade at the marked point, piercing the epidermis, dermis, and panniculus carnosus. Applying even pressure, pull the scalpel blade between the two marked points in a cranial/caudal direction, keeping the incision linear.
5. Lift the skin on either side of the wound and pull apart gently, checking that a full thickness incision has been made and that the underlying muscle is visible. Cut through any remaining connective tissue strands. There should be little or no bleeding from the wound.

Wound Healing 255

6. Repeat for the remaining wounds. Allow the animal to regain consciousness and house singly. The wounds are allowed to heal open to the atmosphere and no further procedures are required.

3.2. Excisional Wounds

1. Anesthetize and shave the animal as aforementioned.
2. In mice, from the base of the skull, measure and mark a point 3.5 cm along the midline. Mark two further points, 1 cm either side of this point. These delineate the centers of two excisional wounds.
3. In rats, measure and mark two points 5.5, and 8.5 cm from the base of the skull along the midline. Mark four further points, 1 cm either side of the midline, two at each of the marked points. These delineate the centers of four excisional wounds.
4. Align the biopsy punch vertically over the center of a mark and pierce the epidermis, dermis, and panniculus carnosus by applying pressure and twisting at the same time. Remove the skin plug (*see* **Note 4**).
5. Lift the skin to ensure a full thickness excisional wound has been made and that the underlying muscle is visible. Cut through any remaining connective tissue strands. There should be little or no bleeding from the wound.
6. Repeat for the remaining wounds. Allow the animal to regain consciousness and house singly. The wounds are allowed to heal without further procedures.

3.3. Harvesting and Processing of Wounds

The time of harvesting postwounding depends on the parameter to be evaluated, however, the method is the same.

Evaluation of the inflammatory response is carried out in wounds from 1 h to 14 d postwounding. A typical time-course would be 1, 6, 12, 24, and 48 h, and 3, 5, 7, 10, and 14 d. Measurement of reepithelialization can be carried out from immediately postwounding to about day 7. Assessment of vascularisation would cover approx 1 to 7 d. Appraisal of scar quality is carried out at least 70 d postwounding in mice and 80 d in rats. Measurement of wound breaking strength and image analysis of a variety of measurements can occur at any of the above times.

1. The animal is sacrificed by anesthetic overdose or carbon monoxide inhalation, the dorsum shaved, and top and bottom of each incisional wound marked. The orientation of excisional wounds with respect to the dorsum can be marked using a "Secureline 2" marker pen, which will survive subsequent processing for histology.
2. A photographic record of the wound or scar may be taken at this point using suitable apparatus such as a 35 mm or digital camera, with a 60 mm lens and flash.
3. Excise the wound leaving 3 to 4 mm of surrounding tissue, cutting through the body wall to give support to the excised part.

4. At this stage tissues can be fixed and processed for histology. Routinely used stains are hematoxylin and eosin for inflammatory infiltrates and Masson's and Mallory's trichromes and Picro Sirius Red to illustrate extracellular matrix deposition. Alternatively, wounds can be frozen for immunohistochemistry. A convenient method is to bisect the wound and freeze the block, cut surface down, in OCT in small foil boats.

3.4. Administration of Agents to Wounds (see Note 5)

The optimal method of delivering therapeutic agents to incisional and excisional wounds is by intradermal injection. The dosing regimen has to be experimentally derived, but there are a number of basic principles. If the animal is to be dosed prior to wounding, the agent can be injected intradermally into the skin where the incision or excision is to be made. The wound is then produced through the bleb.

By injecting different substances into each wound, a single animal can act as its own control and thereby highlight intra-animal variability. For example, two of the four incisional wounds in a rat can be injected with two doses of the therapeutic agent under investigation, the third is injected with the vehicle, and the fourth left unmanipulated. This pattern of injection can be distributed around the wound sites thus minimizing any effects of wound placement on the outcome.

3.5. Evaluation of Wound Parameters

3.5.1. Inflammation

Markers to antigens expressed on neutrophils, T and B lymphocytes, and macrophages can be used to quantify the temporal and spatial expression in untreated, control, and treated wounds. Cell numbers can be quantified in immunolabelled frozen or wax sections by image analysis. Antibodies are available that identify the state of maturation, activation, or subset marker of macrophages, either resident within the skin or newly elicited from the blood at different times during the healing process *(16)* (*see* **Note 6**).

3.5.2. Reepithelialization

Reepithelialization can be easily identified in stained sections by the proliferating epidermis at either side of the wound.

1. Using image analysis software, or manually on micrographs, measure the distance from the junction between normal and proliferating epidermis on one side of the wound, across the healing surface to the similar junction on the other wound margin.
2. Measure the length of proliferating epidermis on both sides and express this as a percentage of the total length. Measurement of the rate of reepithelialization can be compared at various times during postwounding.

3.5.3. Vascularization

The newly formed blood vessel component of granulation tissue can be measured by image analysis in immunolabeled sections at various time-points postwounding. Antibodies to CD31 can to used to evaluate the angiogenic response, development from existing blood vessels and CD 34 is a marker of vasculogenesis, from precursor cells.

3.5.4. Scarring

Dermal scarring is quantified on macroscopic and histological appearance (*see* **Fig. 4**). Evaluation of the macroscopic appearance involves allocating a score of 0 to 10 by placing a mark on a 10-cm line, 0 indicating normal skin and 10 indicating a severe scar. This is termed a visual analog scale and the data can be subjected to statistical analysis.

Compilation of a standard set of micrographs of the macroscopic and histological appearance of scars, selected to be representative of all severities of scar quality encountered, is used for training personnel and minimizing inter- and intra-observer variability. A second set of data slides generated from wounds, which are unmanipulated, will be representative of the normal distribution of macroscopic and histological appearance. Each set of macroscopic and histological data should be scored by a number of observers blind to the experimental intervention.

When the histological appearance of a scar is assessed, various parameters within the wound area can be scored individually on the visual analog scale. These include wound width at the epidermis, midwound, and panniculus carnosus; wound perimeter; orientation of collagen bundles; size of collagen fibers, and spacing between fibers. Alternatively, the observer can allocate an overall score, taking into account all the abovementioned parameters. For example, a narrow wound, with collagen deposited in a pattern similar to the normal surrounding dermis, i.e., in a basket weave pattern, with similar fibre size and spacing, would score at the lower end of the scale. A wide scar with densely packed linear collagen would conversely score high.

3.5.5. Analysis of Wound Strength

Traditional methods of measurement of wound strength involved subjecting excised tissues to disruption by tensiometry. The preferred method is now to assess breaking strength by applying stress to wounds in vivo. Briefly, multi-axial stress is applied to wounds in an anesthetized animal. A plastic ring is secured over the wound area using cyanoacrylate adhesive, two infrared reflective markers are positioned across the wound, a vacuum chamber is placed over the plastic ring and negative pressure applied. Displacement of the

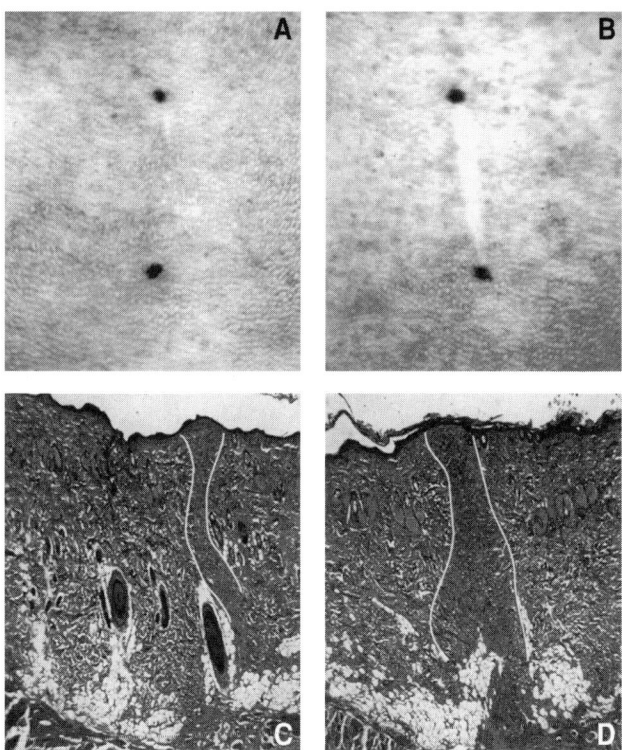

Fig. 4. Micrograph illustrating the macroscopic (**A,B**) and the histological (**C,D**) appearance of scars from a murine full thickness incisional wound, 70 d postwounding. (A) Example of a good scar scoring 0.5 on the visual analog scale, (B) scored 6, (C) is an example of a narrow wound with basket weave-like collagen (outlined in white), and (D) is a wide wound with parallel bundles of linear collagen.

infrared targets is videotaped when the wound is ruptured and the change in pressure and skin deformation analyzed to determine wound strength *(17,18)*.

4. Notes

1. Inhalation anesthetics such as halothane, delivered with O_2 and N_2O, are suitable and recovery is rapid. N_2O gives a level of analgesia. Isofluorane is a safer anesthetic, but is delivered only with O_2. With practice, wounding is a rapid procedure and anesthesia can be maintained using a facemask.
2. Incisional wounds should be linear and a small deviation from the line is acceptable, however, dogleg wounds are not.
3. Mini-pigs such as Gothenburg or Yucatan are used for wound healing experiments. They allow increased numbers of wounds and, therefore, greater variety in treatments. Their tethered skin structure is closer to that of humans than rodents.

4. If difficulties are experienced in producing clean excisions owing to blunting of the biopsy punch or movement of the untethered skin in rodents, an alternative procedure is to cut out a square of roughly the same proportions.
5. Animals have to be anesthetized to receive intradermal injections into wounds subsequent to initial wounding. Similarly, if agents are administered intraperitoneally or by any other route, it is impossible to scruff the animal as this would damage a healing wound.
6. A greater range of antibodies is available for mice than rats. BMA Biomedicals AG, Switzerland, Serotec, and Pharminogen are good sources.

References

1. Clark, R. A. F. (1996) Wound repair overview and general consideration, in *The Molecular and Cellular Biology of Wound Repair*, (Clark, R. A. F., ed.), Plenum, New York, pp. 3–35.
2. Ferguson, M. W. J. and Leigh, I. M. (1998) Wound Healing, in *Rook/Wilkinson/Ebling, Textbook of Dermatology 6th Edition* (Champion, R. H., Burton, J. L., Burns, D. A., and Breathnach, S. M., eds.), Blackwell Science, Oxford, U.K., pp. 337–356.
3. Cowin, A. J., Brosnan, M. P., Holmes, T. M., and Ferguson, M. W. J. (1998) Endogenous inflammatory response to dermal wound healing in the fetal and adult mouse. *Dev. Dyn.* **212,** 385–393.
4. Ferguson, M. W. J., Whitby, D. J., Shah, M. J., Siebert, J. W., and Longaker, M. T. (1996) Scar formation: the spectral nature of fetal and adult wound repair. *Plast. Reconst.Surg.* **97,** 854–860.
5. Cherry, G. W., Hughes, M. A., Leeper, D. J., and Ferguson, M. W. J. (2001) Wound Healing, in *Oxford Text Book of Surgery 2nd Edition* (Morris, P. J. and Wood, W. C., eds.) pp. 129–159
6. Agren, M. S., Eaglstein, W. H., Ferguson, M. W. J., Harding, K. G., Moore, K., Saarialho-Kere, U. K., et al. (2000) Causes and effects of the chronic inflammation in venous leg ulcers. *Acta. Derm. Venerol.* **210,** 3–17.
7. McCallion, R. L. and Ferguson, M. W. J. (1996) Fetal wound healing and the development of antiscarring therapies for adult wound healing, in *The Molecular and Cellular Biology of Wound Repair* (Clark, R. A. F., ed.), Plenum, New York, pp. 561–600.
8. Ashcroft, G. S., Horan, M. A., and Ferguson, M. W. J. (1997) The effects of ageing on wound healing: immunolocalisation of growth factors and their receptors in a murine incisional model. *J. Anat.* **190,** 351–365.
9. Ashcroft, G. S., Horan, M. A., and Ferguson, M. W. J. (1998) Aging alters the inflammatory and endothelial cell adhesion molecule profiles during human cutaneous wound healing. *Lab. Invest.* **1,** 47–58.
10. Ashcroft, G. S., Dodsworth, J., van Boxtel, E., Tarnuzzer, R. W., Horan, M. A., Schultz, G. S., et al. (1997) Estrogen accelerates cutaneous wound healing associated with an increase in TGF-β1 levels. *Nat. Med.* **3,** 1209–1215.
11. O'Kane, S. and Ferguson, M. W. J. (1997) Transforming growth factor betas and wound healing. *Int. J. Biochem. Cell. Biol.* **29,** 63–78.

12. Herrick, S. E., Sloan, P., McGurk, M., Freak, L., McCollum, C. N., and Ferguson, M. W. J. (1992) Sequential changes in histologic pattern and extracellular matrix deposition during the healing of chronic venous ulcers. *Am. J. Pathol.* **141,** 1085–1095.
13. Ferguson, M. W. J., Herrick, S. E., Spencer, M. J., Shaw, J. E., Boulton, A. J., and Sloan, P. (1996) The histology of diabetic foot ulcers. *Diabet. Med.* **13,** S30–S33.
14. Morris, D. E., Wu, L., Bolton, L., Roth, S. I., Ladin, D. A., Mustoe, T. A. (1997) Acute and chronic animal models for excessive dermal scarring: quantitative studies. *Plast. Reconstruct. Surg.* **100,** 674–681.
15. Sullivan, T. P., Eaglstein, W. H., Davis, S. C., and Mertz, P. (2001) The pig as a model for human wound healing. *Wound Rep. Regener.* **9,** 66–76.
16. Leenen, P. J. M., de Bruijn, M. F. T. R., Voerman, J. S. A., Campbell, P. A., and van Ewijk, W. (1994) Markers of mouse macrophage development detected by monoclonal antibodies. *J. Immunol. Methods* **174,** 5–19.
17. Charles, D., Williams, K., Perry, L. C., Fisher, J., and Rees, R. S. (1992) An improved method of in vivo wound disruption and measurement. *J. Surg. Res.* **52,** 214–218.
18. Clugston, P. A., Vistnes, M. D., Perry L. C., Maxwell, G. P., and Fisher, J. (1995) Evaluation of silicone-gel sheeting on early wound healing of linear incisions. *Ann. Plast. Surg.* **34,** 12–15.

III

PHARMACODYNAMIC ENDPOINTS IN EXPERIMENTAL MODELS AND IN CLINICAL STUDIES IN HUMANS

27

An Iconoclastic Approach to Pharmacodynamics in Model Systems: Their Relevance to Humans

Introduction to Part 3

David R. Blake and Gordon J. Taylor

> "History belongs to those who own the future."
> –George Orwell.

D. R. Laurence, in his seminal textbook *Clinical Pharmacology*, provides us with an essential text still relevant to all interested in drug development. It defines pharmacology, as he says "conveniently," into two branches.

1. **pharmacodynamics** (the study of the biology and therapeutic effects of drugs);
2. **pharamacokinetics** (the study of the absorption, metabolism, and excretion of drugs).

His definition certainly has the advantage of brevity. It disguises, however, a problem that continues to confound, as it implies simplicity in a system that Laurence knew well was inordinately complex. The problem to be tackled was summarized by Laurence—"little can be profitably written here on the mode of action of drugs for though much is known of drug effects, the way in which they occur is often complicated and obscure."

This complexity can be dissected by an analysis of what makes a **complex** structure or problem.

Let us consider one drug with which rheumatologists and the pharmaceutical industry are very familiar. A drug whose basic action appears to have been dissected, and a drug on which multiple copies have been developed—cyclo-oxygenase inhibitors [nonsteroidal anti-inflammatory drugs (NSAIDs)]. The credit for generating the "obscure" hypothesis which underlies NSAID development is attributed to Paracelsus, honored as the father of modern medicinal chemistry. Paracelsus had already defined the concept of the "Therapeutic Index," a concept that underlines much of pharmacokinetics. He then turned his attention to more difficult matters and found apparent simplicity, stating, though I paraphrase, "that where a disease is found the treatment will lie nearby." He thereby formulated a proposal that now underpins homeopathy and the search for pharmaceutical agents that are founded in nature.

Many considered (including Laurence) that his initial hypothesis was ill-founded, but observation makes this unlikely. Plant life has little ability to escape noxious insults in its immediate environment and is, to some extent, compelled to manufacture chemical species that will deal with proximate insults. Many primitive insults were consequent upon redox stresses, generated by evolutionary centred climatic change, which led to the transition from a reductive to an oxidizing environment. The defense mechanisms generated here are essentially antioxidants (see below—vitamin C and citrus fruits). Later in evolution, insect predators posed a major threat, and by similar and fairly rapid adaptive mechanisms, plants have produced a wide range of insect repellent systems now utilized by primitive human societies as natural remedies and by the pharmaceutical industry in a more standardized and convenient form. At one level Paracelsus's hypothesis, now known as the "Doctrine of Signatures" has served us well.

Overinterpretation and ignorance of the basic premise then generated some surprising and apparently serendipitous drug discoveries, resulting eventually in Sir John Vane's discovery of the mode of action of aspirin. It was the Reverend Stone, utilizing what we would now consider to be De Bono theory—a knight's move in thought—who made this "inventive step."

The Reverend Stone argued on the basis of the Doctrine of Signatures, that rheumatic symptoms appeared most prevalent in damp and wet environments. He deduced simply that this environment should produce a species capable of healing rheumatic pains. Reference to preexisting literature suggested that bark was a fruitful place to look as malaria had already been suppressed by cinchona bark. Perhaps no one was more surprised when the taking of this cocktail by the first patients proved successful. We can now understand why rheumatic diseases are more symptomatic in environments where humidity changes—diseased joints function as barometers and we can now accept the elementary theories behind the original hypothesis. There is, however, a major step missing in the argument.

The advent of molecular biology, nevertheless, has allowed all subsequent steps to appear rational and comprehensible and to some extent, therefore, predictable and facile (and therefore fundable). I use the word facile with care. Many model systems that we utilize in pharmacological practice are based on a facile system. It is known that the injection of carageenan, among other substances, will act quickly to activate the cyclo-oxygenase pathway. It, therefore, follows that if this were the primary enzyme target for a NSAID, it should suppress the system, and of course such compounds do. However, if one takes a more complex system such as Freund's adjuvant arthritis, which is considered by many (though not this author) to generate a T-cell dependent disease, one finds that an almost identical dose of an identical inhibitor will suppress this much more complex process. Adjuvant arthritis is characterized by bone destruction, a cardinal feature of rheumatoid arthritis and a major primary end point for human-based pharmacodynamic studies. It is clear that in clinical practice, nonsteroidals do not influence rheumatoid-based erosions. Herein lies the problem. Cyclo-oxygenase inhibitors do suppress adjuvant bone disease. The model clearly has no validity as a pharmaceutical tool for screening drugs. We are not able to conclude that this or any agent, because it acted in this model on the erosive process, will then suppress rheumatoid disease. This mistake is made continuously, and to some extent purposefully, by the pharmaceutical industry. It has, in their defense, nevertheless spawned many drugs that have with "Stone-like serendipity" proved partially effective in rheumatoid disease. No doubt many more agents that failed in the model could have been successfully and logically developed if we could understand the basis for the apparently anomalous situation that I present.

There is a glimmer of light here that would allow us to explain the problem and does point to a new way of designing model systems. A facile model I define as a simple system where the influence of the initiating factor relates to the proposed mechanisms of action of the drug, and relates to aspects of the outcome in a near-linear fashion. Such a model will never be achieved in a pure state but carageenan edema would appear to approximate to a linear sequence. This we know is not true of the Freund's-based system as all pharmacokinetic and pharamacodynamic studies illustrate this is a nonlinear system with multiple iterating loops. Understanding the basics of linear and nonlinear systems is the province of mathematicians and, to some extent, beyond the scope of this essay, but reference to any textbook of "chaos theory" provides us with simple answers and possible solutions.

If you perturb a nonlinear system in any direction you will create change. Change and the direction of change will be unpredictable. If, however, you can only measure change in one direction, perhaps because you have chosen to drive the system very hard, then it follows that change can only be measured in the opposite direction and this, in a pharmacological setting, is improvement. Almost any agent that can perturb the system will, therefore, appear effective and providing the system is perturbed reasonably close to the point of insult, then the changes downstream will be self-similar. Chaos theory thereby provides a rudimentary understanding of why so many drugs acting apparently on totally different pathways all end up giving self-similar clinical results. There is no "head" of the cascade when one is dealing with complex iterating systems generated by a small number of deterministic values where the conditions are set such that their activation generates a chaotic pathway.

This might appear a prophecy of doom, but where there is death there is hope. Death is a very easily measurable end point. Death has rarely proved to be an outcome that we can use in rheumatological studies unless of course we concern ourselves with drug toxicity. Death, however, did prove an end point that was utilized by one young investigator prior to undertaking a medical career in Edinburgh. In the 16th century, "three ships left England with crews of 961 men. Only one returned laden with booty and 626 men had died." Scurvy, arguably the first rheumatic disease that was cured on the basis of a pharmacodynamic study, has as one of its initial manifestations, joint pains. Hemorrhagic periostitis and death follow shortly after. Joint pains, as our investigator knew, were not suitable end points for the proposed pharmacodynamic study having far too much variability inherent in the system. James Lind (1716–1794) achieved fame by demonstrating both the preventative and curative effects of the antioxidant and redox cycling citrus fruit. His story is outlined succinctly by Laurence, but is worthy of further dissection as we can now see the major pharmacoeconomic consequences of his studies, and are able to analyze the government's reaction to a major therapeutic advance. This has resonance today and will no doubt continue to do so in the future.

James Lind in 1747 took "12 patients with the scurvy, on board *The Salisbury* at sea. Their cases were as similar as I could have them. They all in general had putrid gums, the spots and lassitude, with weakness of their knees. They lay together in one place... and had one diet common to all."

James Lind has clearly provided the basic structure to permit a randomized, controled clinical trial. We would perhaps consider it underpowered were not death the final outcome measure... "Two of these were ordered each a quart of cider a-day, two others took 25-gutts of *elixir vitriol* three times a day upon an empty stomach...two others took two spoonfuls of vinegar three times a day, upon an empty stomach. Two of the worst patients, with the tendons in the ham rigid... were put under a course of sea water. Two others had each two oranges and one lemon given them every day. The two remaining patients took the bigness of nutmeg three times a day, of an electuary recommended by a hospital surgeon...The consequence was that the most sudden and visible good effects were perceived from the use of the oranges and lemons."

Modern statistical analysis shows that using the Fisher's exact test on the data to test for association between improvement in the condition and the treatment that was taken, i.e., oranges and lemons: the exact P value is 0.01 and, therefore, is statistically significant.

The cured, being now fit for duty we presume, buried their colleagues at sea and James Lind's novel treatise was published in 1753. An almost identical anecdotal observation had been made somewhat earlier but was unpublished! As to the medico-economic consequences, they were subtle. Sailors were paid when they returned from their voyages and were often held just out of port for a suitable time, designated a "quarantine period" to allow the sick to die in the comfort of their own homes. Failure to pay the sick and dying provided the Naval Board with an opportunity that was hard to resist. Indeed Lind's discoveries challenged health boards for a further 40 yr, and it was only an argument centred upon manpower difficulties that led to a change in attitude. The introduction of citrus fruits (predominantly limes) to all ships doubled the strength of our Navy (the limeys) during the Napoleonic Wars, and led to the beginning of the end of the Napoleonic Empire. An impressive outcome for a pharmacodynamic study.

The identification of vitamin C and the understanding of the redox reactions it controls awaited the discoveries of Albert Szent-Gyorgi. His work laid the foundation for Hans Krebs' elucidation of the conversion of carbohydrate breakdown products to carbon dioxide, water, and other substances necessary for the production of usable energy by the cell. This was a classic example of a chaotic system with positive and negative feedback loops which generates apparent order.

I end by quoting from Szent-Gyorgi, "in studying life, you keep diving from higher levels to lower ones until somewhere along the way life fades out, leaving you empty handed. Molecules and electrons have no life." Chaos theory predicts otherwise—nature repeats itself at progressively lower levels with self-similar patterns. As all pharmacology students are aware, no rodent-based model would have assisted James Lind with his studies, nor would they assist in optimising the pharmacokinetics. Rodents prevalent on *The Salisbury* did not and could not suffer from the scurvy. They could, however, harbor the insect vector for the Plague.

Acknowledgment

This essay is dedicated to my friend and colleague, Professor D. Willoughby, who taught me much that is unprintable and a little more beside. This essay is based on a lecture first presented to the Royal College of Physicians, Edinburgh, (2001) "Inflammation and pain in arthritis—new concepts, new treatments." Professor D. Blake et al. are supported as an integrated clinical arthritis center by the Arthritis Research Campaign. I am grateful to Alison MacKenzie for all the help given with the historical research underpinning this essay.

Additional Reading

1. Pharmacology, (1973) *Clinical Pharmacology*, D. R. Laurence, Churchill Livingstone, Edinburgh and London, 4th ed., ISBN 0 443 01004 8
2. From Paracelsus to Aspirin, (1992) *Encyclopaedia Britannica*: vol. 9 p. 135, Paracelsus, ISBN 0-85229-553-7
3. Concerning James Lind, (2001) Fellows of Edinburgh's College of Physicians during the Scottish Enlightenment Reginald Passmore, Royal College of Physicians of Edinburgh, ISBN 0-854405057-4
4. Beyond Molecular Biology, (1960) *Encyclopaedia Britannica*: vol. 11, p. 475, Szent-Gyorgy, Al., Introduction to a Submolecular Biology, ISBN 0-85229-553-7.

28

A Reply to "An Iconoclastic Approach to Pharmacodynamics in Model Systems: Their Relevance to Humans"

Derek A. Willoughby

As I lift up my pen to undertake this reply to the outstanding essay by David R. Blake, this being requested by himself and my co-editor Professor Paul Winyard, I feel myself becoming overcome by trepidation and fear. Frankly, I cannot write in the elegant style of David! Furthermore, I have always been convinced that David Blake is a direct descendant of William Blake (1757–1827), the artist, poet, and philosopher who was always wildly controversial, but outstanding in his perception of life and death.

If William Blake had been Professor of Rheumatology at Bath, he would undoubtedly have seized upon obscure hypotheses and quoted Paracelsus to explain the development of the therapy of nonsteroidal antiinflammatory drugs (NSAIDs). He too would have extensively quoted chaos theory to support his views. One does not need DNA analysis to appreciate the similarities between these two outstanding men and their contributions to their chosen subjects. Bearing in mind this familial background, much of what David has written becomes easier to understand. It is necessary to express novel concepts and write them into a script such that they appear controversial despite, perhaps, the tacit agreement of many!

None would disagree that an extract of seaweed (carrageenan) injected into a rat's paw fails to simulate all aspects of rheumatic disease in man—even among English Channel swimmers! However, it does provoke inflammation, i.e., heat, redness, swelling, and pain, the classical signs described by Celsus (30BC-38AD), one of the few observations in inflammation that has truly withstood the test of time. Not surprisingly, reversing these cardinal signs has proved the basis for the development of many of the NSAIDs. However, it is ever-increasingly realized that the NSAIDs, already renowned for their gastrointestinal side effects, will also accelerate cartilage breakdown, the very process at the heart of the pathology of diseases such as rheumatoid and osteoarthritis (*see* **Chapter 18**). Many of these drugs, despite the risk of these side effects, improve the "quality of life" of the rheumatoid patient and are thus widely prescribed, even if not improving the underlying pathology.

In defense of the basic biologists working on the inflammatory response, I also would refer extensively to Hans Selye who divided research into instinct and intellect. His view is that the general biologist, naturalist, or clinician's exploration of life is aided much more by keen observation, and an instinctive feeling for nature, rather than by complex instruments and elaborate planning. He bemoans the loss of this type of scientist. For him, the "Problem Finders" are phenomenologists, interested in new configurational wholes rather then structural details. In his second group are the "Problem Solvers," who start with something already known and try to take it apart to understand its composition and mechanism. He goes on to describe the original work of Mendel, planting and cross-fertilizing his garden peas. His simple observations were the foundation of modern genetics. A further example quoted by Selye is the discovery of penicillin by Sir Alexander Flemming. Certainly, once again, not a planned discovery but, thanks to his peripheral vision, he made an important discovery. Perhaps many of us working on models of inflammation are still using a combination of gut instinct, serendipity, and "obscure" hypothesis (*see* **Chapter 27**), even while focusing on small subunits like a cytokine or an enzyme in these models, and suggesting new therapeutic agents. On the other hand, once the target becomes very small—one of these subunits—is this guaranteed to enjoy more success? As David writes, Szent-Gyorgi makes the point that "in studying life, you keep diving from higher levels to lower ones until somewhere along the way, life fades out, leaving you empty handed. Molecules and electrons have no life."

I would respectfully point out to my friend David that what has retarded the advance of basic technology in the search for antirheumatic drugs is largely the responsibility of his clinical colleagues. The basic scientist has a rough, and rather ignorant, view of rheumatoid arthritis. It would seem from the response of different patients to the same therapy that there must be different forms of rheumatoid arthritis which require, in turn, different therapies. If we consider hypertension, this started as simply Bright's Disease and was slowly subclassified into many different forms of hypertension. We are aware that a common therapy cannot be applied, indeed once one includes phaeochromocytomas, some treatments could be fatal! I was briefly on a European League Against Rheumatism committee and invoked a meeting of clinical rheumatologists.

Sadly, to investigate responders and nonresponders to common NSAIDs, the committee wanted a huge quantity of blood to carry out the appropriate investigations! I decided at the end of the meeting the patients would be exsanguinated!! Presumably, this would have represented the ultimate cure, halting any disease process, and would be consistent with the observations of David and William Blake.

Please David, provide us with separate subclassifications of rheumatoid arthritis, which will perhaps suggest differing therapeutic targets, and help us struggling scientists. A "facile" model (*see* **Chapter 27**) is useful to develop new therapies providing it reflects the mechanisms important in a disease process; the trick is to identify the disease process in the patient! It is true, however, regarding to novel therapies and side effects, if a "facile" model is used and the new drug specifically inhibits the inflammatory response by inhibiting a specific mediator of inflammation, one must pose the question, "What is the physiological role of the new therapeutic target?" This may be important, but is oft ignored until the clinic. Recently, for example, new drugs are being designed and introduced clinically to abolish key cytokines. Do these cytokines have a physiological role, as well as their pathological one? If so, one can predict any potential side effects.

Even with our woefully inadequate models of rheumatoid arthritis and so on, I would, respectfully, point out that it is impossible to produce inflammation in a test tube. The inflammatory milieu changes every second, this really cannot be reproduced in vitro despite the high-powered technology that can be brought to bear in this situation. It is a sad reflection that when one discusses inflammation with some of the most erudite molecular biologists, they often fail to recognize that, in vivo, we are effectively dealing with a constantly changing tissue. For example, at the outset of inflammation there are many polymorphonuclear leukocytes that subsequently undergo apoptosis and are replaced by macrophages derived from monocytes. The changing cell populations secrete or release different factors into the exudate. Even the local tissue at the site of the inflammatory response is changing and may act as a source of inflammatory signals and generate an endogenous antigen perpetuating the inflammation. Hence, the impossibility of the task to reproduce these events in vitro.

I repeat once more, if the rheumatologists gave better indicators of what is taking place in humans, we would hopefully have greater opportunities to get closer to mimicking human rheumatoid arthritis. David, you place the responsibility for inadequate models on us; I would return the responsibility to you and your clinical colleagues.

To address a specific point raised in your essay, you appear distressed that the facile test, carrageenan paw edema, responds to the same drugs as the more complex adjuvant arthritis. This merely points out that inflammation as described by Celsus is the endpoint of a complicated and chaotic series of steps. A huge variety of stimuli or insults provoke these ultimate signs. I do agree that certain agents may act earlier on the chain of events and these need to be identified. Lapsing into optimism, I find that certain groups who are now focusing on the naturally occurring endogenous host factors that switch off inflammation may ultimately lead to a safer and, indeed, more effective therapy for inflammatory disease. Using the Doctrine of Signatures it does appear more logical to use man's own built-in systems for switching off inflammation and attempting to enhance these responses. If we suppress the inflammation successfully with little consideration as to whether this is by perturbing a linear or nonlinear system this will be a success—analysis of chaos can follow later! A little bit of serendipity may also not go amiss—more than a few Nobel Prizes have been gained from the exploitation of Lady Luck!!

Having reached the end of this limited reply, I am reminded that William Blake, David's forebear, was advised to reform to ensure tenure in his afterlife in heaven. Blake's reply was most of the "good people" seemed dull and boring—he would prefer hell, with the more lively adjudged "wicked people," whom he thought would be more entertaining. David, wherever I go, please come and join me—even if it may be a trifle warm! Thank you for your essay. I, too, would have liked to quote more of Hans Selye and Szent-Gyorgi—unfortunately David, you have borrowed my book by Selye and preempted many of the appropriate quotes. In the meanwhile, please follow your own advice and absorb bountiful amounts of citrus fruits—I hear polyphenols in grapes may represent a new breakthrough in the fight against inflammation by inhibiting a few key enzymes...!! Perhaps all is not lost.

29

Quantifying Inflammation In Vivo Using Radiolabeled Antibodies and Leukocytes

Diane Marshall and Dorian O. Haskard

1. Introduction

Although histological techniques are frequently used to study inflammation, precise quantification allowing an analysis of the dynamics of the inflammatory response is often hard to achieve. This chapter describes the application of intravenously injected radiolabeled antibodies and leukocytes for investigating endothelial activation, adhesion molecule expression, and leukocyte recruitment.

Adhesion molecules expressed on vascular endothelial cells are essential for regulating the migration of leukocytes to sites of inflammation. The endothelial selectins, E- and P-selectin, which mediate the initial rolling of leukocytes along the vessel wall, are expressed at low-absent levels in the absence of inflammation, but are upregulated in response to inflammatory stimuli. The adhesion molecules ICAM-1 and VCAM-1 are also expressed on endothelial cells at increased levels in response to inflammatory mediators and are critical for the subsequent firm adhesion of leukocytes to endothelial cells prior to their migration through the endothelial barrier *(1,2)*. Using radiolabeled monoclonal antibodies directed against these regulated adhesion molecules, we have been able to investigate changes in the endothelial activation and the capacity of endothelial cells to recruit leukocytes during experimental inflammatory responses *(3–7)*.

Our established protocol involves the simultaneous injection of two anti-adhesion molecule antibodies, together with a negative control antibody, each labeled differentially with ^{125}I, ^{111}In, or ^{99m}Tc to permit their separate detection in tissues. Because each animal is injected with negative control antibody, it is possible to distinguish specific binding to antigen from nonspecific antibody localization. Intravenously injected antibodies are allowed to circulate for 5 min, during which time they can bind to their respective antigens. Each animal is then sacrificed, tissues of interest collected, and the amount of antibody present, as measured by the level of radioactivity for each radioisotope, counted in a gamma counter.

Quantification of inflammation with antibodies to endothelial adhesion molecules can be complemented by assessment of leukocyte traffic into inflamed tissue *(8–10)*. Isolated leukocytes [polymorphonuclear cells (PMN) or mononuclear cells (MNC)] are differentially radiolabeled with ^{99m}Tc or ^{111}In and injected simultaneously into the animal to be studied. One hour later, the animal is exanguinated and the inflammatory sites collected and counted in a gamma counter. The uptake of the leukocyte populations into sites of inflammation, as measured by radioactivity counts, is then quantified as a percentage of the injected dose per gram of tissue. Thus, studying animals over the course of an inflammatory response can reveal the precise dynamics of PMN and MNC infiltration. In fact, simultaneous injection of radiolabeled anti-adhesion molecule antibodies with radiolabeled leukocytes can reveal the relationship between endothelial adhesion molecule expression and the recruitment of specific leukocyte populations.

2. Materials
2.1. Radiolabeling of Antibodies
2.1.1. With Iodine

1. Phosphate-buffered saline (PBS, approx pH 7.3).
2. Antibody in PBS (preferably at a concentration of 1 mg/mL or above).
3. 1.5 mL polypropylene tube coated with Iodogen (1,3,4,6-tetrachloro-3α, 6α-diphenylglycouracil) (Pierce & Warriner, Chester, UK), prepared by the addition of 40 μL of iodogen at 0.4 mg/mL in dichloromethane. This is followed by evaporation at room temperature in a fume hood for 2 h (*see* **Note 1**).
4. Prepacked PD10 Sephadex G25 gel filtration column (Amersham Pharmacia Biotech, Uppsala, Sweden) that has had nonspecific binding sites blocked (*see* **Note 2**).
5. Na^{125}I (carrier-free) in NaOH (IMS30, Nycomed Amersham, Little Chalfont, UK).
6. Instant thin layer chromatography (ITLC) silica gel impregnated glass fiber sheets (Gelman Sciences, Ann Arbor, MI).

2.1.2. With Technetium

1. PBS, approx pH 7.3.
2. 1.5 mL polypropylene tube containing frozen reduced antibody. The antibody is reduced by the addition of 2-mercaptoethanol (0.5 μL/mg antibody) for 30 min at room temperature, followed by gel filtration on a prepacked PD10 Sephadex G25 gel filtration column that has nonspecific binding sites blocked (*see* **Note 2**). The

protein concentration of the eluted fractions (1 mL) is measured using a spectrophotometer (A_{280nm}) and aliquots of reduced antibody frozen **immediately** in 1.5 mL polypropylene tubes on dry ice and then stored at –70°C (*see* **Note 3**).
3. Vial of Amerscan Medronate II Agent (Nycomed Amersham) reconstituted with 2 mL saline (this reagent can be stored at 4°C for up to 1 wk after reconstitution).
4. Prepacked PD10 Sephadex G25 gel filtration column that has nonspecific binding sites blocked (*see* **Note 2**).
5. $Na^{99m}TcO_4$- (product of fission ^{99}Mo).
6. ITLC silica gel impregnated glass fiber sheets (Gelman Sciences).

2.1.3. With Indium

1. PBS, approx pH 7.3.
2. Diethylenetriaminepentaacetic acid (DTPA)-coupled antibody in 0.1 M sodium acetate, pH 6.0. DTPA coupling of the antibody is carried out by incubation with a 20-fold excess of DTPA anhydride in 0.1 M sodium bicarbonate buffer, pH 8.2 for 30 min. Excess DTPA is then removed by gel filtration over Sephadex G50 equilibrated with 0.1 M sodium acetate, pH 6.0, and fractions containing the antibody are then pooled [detected by measurement of protein using a spectrophotometer (A_{280nm})] and stored at –20°C or 4°C (*see* **Note 4**).
3. 3.8% sodium citrate.
4. Prepacked PD10 Sephadex G25 gel filtration column that has nonspecific binding sites blocked (*see* **Note 2**).
5. ^{111}In chloride (Nycomed Amersham).
6. ITLC silica gel impregnated glass fiber sheets (Gelman Sciences).

2.2. Radiolabeling Leukocytes

2.2.1. With Technetium

1. Freshly isolated leukocytes in 1 mL autologous plasma.
2. ^{99m}Tc-hexamethyl-propyleneamine oxime (^{99m}Tc-HMPAO, Ceretec™, Nycomed Amersham).
3. Autologous plasma.

2.2.2. With Indium

1. Freshly isolated leukocytes in 1 mL autologous plasma.
2. 4.4 mM tropolone (Fluka, Sigma-Aldrich, Dorset, UK) in HEPES-saline buffer (pH 7.6).
3. ^{111}In chloride (Nycomed Amersham).
4. Autologous plasma.

2.3. In Vivo Targeting with Radiolabeled Antibodies

1. Targeting and negative control radiolabeled antibodies mixed in equal volumes and made up to the appropriate concentration and volume for intravenous (iv) injection (*see* **Note 5**). Fill numbered syringes with the appropriate volume for injection and then weigh—use one syringe per animal. The syringe will also be

weighed at the end of the procedure, allowing the exact volume of radiolabelled antibody given to each animal to be calculated.
2. A measured aliquot of the above antibody mixture to count alongside the tissue samples (e.g., 500 μL of a 1:500 dilution)—this is the antibody standard and will be used to assess the injected dose of radiolabelled antibodies for each animal.
3. A measured aliquot of each of the individual radiolabeled antibodies—these will be used to assess any spillover of radioactivity counts between the channels of the gamma counter during sample counting.
4. PBS containing 10 U/mL heparin.
5. Preweighed tubes labeled appropriately with animal number and the tissue to be collected.
6. Gamma counter.

2.4. In Vivo Targeting with Radiolabeled Leukocytes

1. Numbered syringes filled with the appropriate volume of radiolabeled leukocytes (*see* **Note 6**) for injection—one syringe per animal, each weighed after filling. The syringe will also be weighed at the end of the procedure and therefore the exact quantity of radiolabelled leukocytes injected into each animal can be calculated.
2. A measured aliquot of the aforementioned radiolabeled leukocyte mixture to count alongside the tissue samples (e.g., 500 μL of a 1:500 dilution)—this is the standard and will be used to assess the injected dose of radiolabeled leukocytes for each animal.
3. A measured aliquot of each of the individual radiolabeled leukocyte preparations—these will be used to assess any spillover of radioactivity counts between the channels of the gamma counter during sample counting.
4. Preweighed tubes labeled appropriately with animal number and tissue to be collected.
5. Gamma counter.

2.5. Data Handling

1. Data handling program, e.g., Microsoft Excel.

3. Methods

3.1. Radiolabeling of Antibodies

3.1.1. With Iodine

1. Add 0.1–0.5 mg antibody to the iodogen tube.
2. Add 10 MBq Na^{125}I to the antibody and incubate for 15 min at room temperature, mixing gently by tapping the tube every 5 min.
3. To remove the excess "free" radioisotope from the radiolabeled protein, load the antibody mixture onto the equilibrated PD10 column and allow to enter the gel bed. Add 0.5 mL PBS to the column and collect the subsequently eluted fractions. Continue to elute 0.5 mL fractions from the column until 12 fractions have

been collected. Measure the level of radioactivity in each fraction to find the "hottest" fractions that contain the radiolabeled antibody (the majority of the antibody is usually eluted around fractions 6–8) and pool the 2 "hottest" fractions, (*see* **Note 7**).

4. Assess the radiolabeling efficiency by ITLC. Apply 2 µL of the pooled radiolabeled antibody approx 0.5 cm from the base to a 1-cm-wide strip of ITLC sheet and place in a bijou containing 0.5 mL PBS as the mobile phase. When the solvent front has almost reached the top of the strip, bisect the strip and measure the radioactivity levels in the top half of the strip compared to the bottom. Only "free" radioisotope will be carried with the solvent front to the top of the strip, whereas the radiolabeled protein remains at the origin. The proportion of radioactivity that is associated with protein can, therefore, be assessed and will ideally be above 95%.

3.1.2. With Technetium

1. Keep aliquot of reduced antibody frozen until ready to use.
2. Add 35 µL of Medronate to the thawed reduced antibody (0.1–0.5 mg).
3. Add approx 10 MBq ^{99m}Tc to the antibody, mix well, and leave at room temperature for 5 min.
4. Remove the excess "free" radioisotope from the radiolabeled protein, as in **Subheading 3.1.1.**, **step 3**. (*see* **Note 8**).
5. Assess the radiolabeling efficiency by ITLC as in **Subheading 3.1.1.**, **step 4**.

3.1.3. With Indium

1. Mix the required volume of ^{111}In chloride that is equivalent to 10 MBq of radioactivity with 1.5 times this volume of sodium citrate (3.8%).
2. Add the ^{111}In/citrate mixture to the aliquot of DTPA-coupled antibody (0.1–0.5 mg), mix, and incubate at room temperature for 15 min, mixing gently by tapping the tube every 5 min.
3. Remove the excess "free" radioisotope from the radiolabeled protein, as in **Subheading 3.1.1.**, **step 3** (*see* **Note 4**).
4. Assess the radiolabeling efficiency by ITLC as in **Subheading 3.1.1.**, **step 4**.

3.2. Radiolabeling Leukocytes

3.2.1. With Technetium

1. Add ^{99m}Tc-HMPAO to the leukocyte suspension (approx 10 MBq ^{99m}Tc to $1-3 \times 10^8$ cells).
2. After 10 min incubation at room temperature, add 5 mL autologous plasma and centrifuge at 1000g for 5 min to remove unbound radioactivity.
3. Remove supernatant and wash the cell pellet with a further 5 mL autologous plasma followed by centrifugation at 1000g for 5 min.
4. Resuspend cells in an appropriate volume of autologous plasma for injection.

3.2.2. With Indium

1. Add 100 µL tropolone to the leukocyte suspension, followed by ^{111}In chloride (approx 5 MBq ^{111}In to $1-3 \times 10^8$ cells).
2. After 5 min incubation at room temperature, add 5 mL autologous plasma and centrifuge at $1000g$ for 5 min to remove unbound radioactivity.
3. Remove supernatant and wash the cell pellet with a further 5 mL autologous plasma followed by centrifugation at $1000g$ for 5 min.
4. Resuspend cells in an appropriate volume of plasma for injection.

3.3. In Vivo Targeting with Radiolabeled Antibodies

1. Inject the animal intravenously with the appropriate amount/volume of radiolabeled antibody mixture.
2. After allowing time for the targeting antibody to bind to the appropriate antigen (5 min), inject the animal with a lethal dose of anesthetic.
3. Perfuse with PBS/heparin to minimize the level of unbound radiolabeled antibody present in the circulation (*see* **Note 9**).
4. Dissect out the tissues of interest, and place in the appropriate preweighed tubes.
5. Weigh the empty syringes used for injection of radiolabeled antibodies. Weigh tubes containing tissue samples.
6. Count all the tissue sample tubes together with the standard aliquot of the injected antibodies and the aliquots of the individual radiolabeled antibodies in a gamma counter.

3.4. In Vivo Targeting with Radiolabeled Leukocytes

1. Inject the animal intravenously with the appropriate amount/volume of radiolabeled leukocytes.
2. After allowing time for the cells to infiltrate the sites of inflammation (usually 1 h, but can be less), inject the animal with a lethal dose of anesthetic.
3. Dissect out the tissues of interest, place into the appropriate preweighed tubes.
4. Weigh the empty syringes used for injection of the radiolabeled leukocytes. Weigh tubes containing tissue samples.
5. Count all the tissue sample tubes together with the radiolabeled leukocyte standard and the aliquots of the individual radiolabeled leukocytes in a gamma counter.

3.5. Data Handling (see Notes 10 and 11)

3.5.1. With Radiolabeled Antibodies

1. Knowing the weight of each tissue sample, the counts per minute (cpm) for each isotope within the sample, and the total cpm of the injected antibodies (i.e., the injected dose), calculate the percentage of the injected dose of radiolabeled antibodies that has localized per gram of tissue (%ID/g). Subtract the %ID/g tissue of the nonspecific negative control antibody from the specific antigen-binding antibody. This value is the amount of antibody specifically bound to the tissue and hence reflects the amount of antigen on endothelium available for antibody binding.

3.5.2. With Radiolabeled Leukocytes

1. Knowing the weight of each tissue sample, the cpm for each isotope within the sample, and the cpm of the injected dose of leukocytes, calculate the percentage of the injected dose of radiolabeled leukocytes that has localized per gram of tissue (%ID/g).

3.5.3. Correcting for Differences in Body Weight

1. Plasma volume (and, therefore, volume of distribution of injected antibodies and/or leukocytes) is proportional to body weight. When experiments involve comparisons between animals of different weight, specific uptake of radiolabeled antibodies or leukocytes can be further normalized by multiplying by the weight of the animal in grams.

3.5.4. Correcting for Differences in Vascularity

1. To compare the relative density of antigen expression on the endothelium between different tissues, the data is corrected for vascularity and endothelial cell surface area. In mouse studies, 100 µg anti-CD31 (PECAM-1) antibody and 100 µg control antibody (each differentially labeled) are injected iv and the distribution of anti-CD31 antibody used for normalization of inducible adhesion molecule expression relative to endothelial cell surface area (*see* **Note 12**). The relative vascularity (RV) of each tissue is calculated by dividing the anti-CD31 uptake by the anti-CD31 uptake for the tissue with the lowest anti-CD31 uptake. The uptake of each antiadhesion molecule antibody is then divided by the RV for each tissue to give the relative density of the antigen with respect to endothelial cell surface area.

4. Notes

1. Iodogen coated tubes can be made in advance and stored desiccated at $-70°C$ for several months.
2. Nonspecific binding sites are blocked by addition of 500 µL 4.5% human serum albumin followed by equilibration with 25 mL PBS.
3. It is important to prevent reoxidation of the antibody during and after gel filtration. Therefore, use N_2 saturated PBS and measure the eluted fractions in the spectrophotometer rapidly. Freeze aliquots of reduced antibody *immediately* upon preparation and ensure the aliquots are never allowed to thaw before use.
4. Indium labeling is achieved by chelation via DTPA. To ensure maximum labeling efficiency, contact with other metal ions must be avoided. Therefore, avoid the use of metal (e.g., spatulas), remove metal tip ejectors from pipets and keep contact with glass to a minimum.
5. Successful in vivo quantification can usually be achieved with tracer doses of radiolabeled antibodies. The absolute amount of antibody required varies with the plasma volume and the amount of constitutively expressed antigen that is accessible for binding. The protocol we describe is similar to that developed by D. N. Granger et al. for studies of rodents, whose quantification technique

employs doses of antibodies which are receptor saturating *(11–13)*. We have found it best to establish the optimal quantity of antibody for a particular investigation by performing preliminary experiments. Targeting the endothelial selectins, E- and P-selectin, in the mouse requires only 2 µg antibody per mouse *(7,14)*. In contrast, ICAM-1 is highly expressed in mouse lungs and therefore 30 µg antibody per mouse is required to target ICAM-1 expressed at sites of inflammation *(5,6)*. ICAM-1 and VCAM-1 can be successfully quantified in the rat with 25 µg antibody per animal *(15,16)*, and VCAM-1 and E-selectin can be successfully quantified in the pig with 100 µg antibody per animal *(4)*.

6. Quantification of cell infiltration into sites of inflammation has been successfully achieved in the pig using approx $1-2 \times 10^8$ PMN and 3×10^8 MNC.
7. If very little of the applied radioactivity is eluted from the column in 12 fractions, then wash the column with a further 3 mL PBS and measure whether the radioactivity is present in this wash or is still bound to the PD10 column. If the radioactivity can be washed from the column as "free" isotope, then the iodogen procedure was unsuccessful. Steps to trouble-shoot unsuccessful radioiodination include: i) checking the buffer is at neutral pH; ii) checking antibody concentration, and, if necessary, concentrating antibody to ≥ 1 mg/mL; and iii) preparing fresh desiccated Iodogen tubes, as Iodogen reagent may have perished. If the radioactivity remains on the column, the antibody has bound nonspecifically to the column. This should have been prevented by the application of human serum albumin to block the column and may indicate the presence of damaged/aggregated antibody. Check the antibody is monomeric before labeling. If the damage appears to occur during the radiolabeling procedure, try reducing the concentration of Iodogen reagent used to coat the tube or reduce the incubation time.
8. Reoxidation of the antibody will prevent successful radiolabeling with ^{99m}Tc. Therefore, remove the aliquot of antibody from –70°C just before the radiolabeling is about to start and add the Medronate and ^{99m}Tc immediately upon thawing (while a few crystals of ice remain).
9. For our studies with rodents, we have found that perfusion with heparinized PBS reduces the background levels of radioactivity as a result of unbound antibody that remains in the circulation and hence improves the specificity of the targeting. The method of perfusion varies with the animal studied. For mice, immobilize the animal on a dissecting board and open the chest cavity to expose the heart. Insert a 25-gauge butterfly needle through the wall of left ventricle and cut a small incision in the right atrium. Connect a 20 mL syringe containing PBS/heparin to the butterfly needle and slowly depress the plunger to perfuse the animal, allowing blood/buffer to wash down the board and into a waste tray. Be sure the insertion of the butterfly needle is very shallow and, therefore, just pierces the wall of left ventricle. Hold the needle very steadily to minimize the possibility of also piercing the right ventricle. This part of the procedure greatly benefits from two pairs of hands: one person to hold the needle steady and make the incision in the right atrium and an assistant to fill, connect, and plunge the syringe. For rats, the perfusion is carried out with 50 mL of buffer via a cannula to the

abdominal aorta. For targeting pig skin, the animal is exanguinated and perfusion is not required. Be aware of handling radioactive needles, tissues, carcasses, and perfusate—use appropriate shielding and disposal of radioactive waste.

10. To ensure correct calculation of %ID/g tissue, be sure to count an aliquot of the injected material (to calculate the injected dose) and also an aliquot of each of the individual radiolabeled antibodies/leukocytes (to determine any crossover of radioactivity counts between the gamma counter channels used to count the different isotopes) at the same time as the tissue samples. ^{99m}Tc has only a 6-h half-life and, therefore, will decay during the period of counting the radioactive samples. Therefore, ensure each sample is corrected for radioactive decay by normalizing each sample to time zero (when the first sample was counted).

11. Quantification of endothelial antigen expression using radiolabeled antibodies (%ID/g tissue) does not provide an absolute value for the antigen of interest, but offers a relative value that can be compared with the same antigen under different conditions, i.e., over the time-course of an inflammatory response. To compare the relative density of antigen expression on the endothelium between different tissues, the data needs to be corrected for vascularity and endothelial cell surface area (*see* **Subheading 3.5.3.** and **Note 12**). As relative, not absolute, values for adhesion molecule expression are obtained, comparisons should not be used to define the relative quantity of one antigen vs another.

12. CD31 (PECAM-1) is constitutively present on endothelial cells and appears to show little variation in expression in inflammation *(13)*. The distribution of anti-CD31 antibody can, therefore, be employed to normalize the data to endothelial cell surface area.

References

1. Butcher, E. C. (1991) Leukocyte-endothelial cell recognition: Three (or more) steps to specificity and diversity. *Cell* **67,** 1033.
2. Springer, T. A. (1994) Traffic signals for lymphocyte recirculation and leukocyte emigration: the multistep paradigm. *Cell* **76,** 301.
3. Keelan, E. T. M., Licence, S. T., Peters, A. M., Binns, R. M., and Haskard, D. O. (1994) Characterization of E-selectin expression in vivo using a radiolabelled monoclonal antibody. *Am. J. Physiol.* **266,** H279.
4. Harrison, A. A., Stocker, C. J., Chapman, P. T., Tsang, Y. T., Huehns, T. Y., Gundel, R.H., et al. (1997) Expression of VCAM-1 by vascular endothelial cells in immune- and non-immune inflammatory reactions in the skin. *J. Immunol.* **159,** 4546.
5. McHale, J., Harari, O. A., Marshall, D., and Haskard, D. O. (1999) Vascular endothelial cell expression of ICAM-1 and VCAM-1 at the onset of eliciting contact hypersensitivity response in mice: evidence for a dominant role of TNFa. *J. Immunol.* **162,** 1648.
6. McHale, J. F., Harari, O. A., Marshall, D., and Haskard, D. O. (1999) TNFalpha and IL-1 sequentially induce endothelial ICAM-1 and VCAM-1 expression in MRL/lpr lupus-prone mice. *J. Immunol.* **163,** 3993.

7. Harari, O., McHale, J., Marshall, D., Ahmed, S., Brown, D., Askenase, P. W., et al. (1999) Endothelial cell E- and P-selectin up-regulation in murine contact sensitivity is prolonged by distinct mechanisms occurring in sequence. *J. Immunol.* **163,** 6860.
8. Binns, R. M., Whyte, A., Licence, S. T., Harrison, A. A., Tsang, Y., Haskard, D. O., et al. (1996) The role of E-selectin in lymphocyte and polymorphonuclear cell recruitment into cutaneous delayed hypersensitivity reactions in sensitized pigs. *J. Immunol.* **157,** 4094.
9. Binns, R. M., Licence, S. T., Harrison, A. A., Keelan, E. T. D., Robinson, M. K., and Haskard, D. O. (1996) In vivo E-selectin upregulation correlates with early infiltration of PMN, later with PBL-entry: mAbs block both. *Am. J. Physiol.* **270,** H183.
10. Chapman, P. T., Jamar, F., Harrison, A. A., Schofield, J. B., Peters, A. M., Binns, R. M., et al. (1996) Characterization of E-selectin expression, leukocyte traffic and clinical sequelae in urate crystal-induced inflammation: an insight into gout. *Br. J. Rheumatol.* **35,** 323.
11. Panes, J., Perry, M. A., Anderson, D. C., Manning, A., Leone, B., Cepinskas, G., et al. (1995) Regional differences in constitutive and induced ICAM-1 expression in vivo. *Am. J. Physiol.* **38,** H1955.
12. Eppihimer, M. J., Wolitzky, B. A., Anderson, D. C., Labow, M. A., and Granger, D. N. (1996) Heterogeneity of expression of E- and P-selectins in vivo. *Circ. Res.* **79,** 560.
13. Henninger, D. D., Panes, J., Eppihimer, M., Russell, J., Gerritsen, M., Anderson, D. C., et al. (1997) Cytokine-induced VCAM-1 and ICAM-1 expression in different organs in the mouse. *J. Immunol.* **158,** 1825.
14. Harari, O., Marshall, D., McHale, J., Ahmed, S., and Haskard, D. O. (2001) Limited endothelial E- and P-selectin expression in MRL/lpr lupus-prone mice. *Rheumatology* **40,** 889.
15. Allen, A. R., McHale, J., Smith, J., Cook, H. T., Karkar, A., Haskard, D. O., et al. (1999) Endothelial expression of VCAM-1 in experimental crescentic nephritis and effects of antibodies to VLA-4 or VCAM-1 on glomerular injury. *J. Immunol.* **162,** 5519.
16. Larbi, K. Y., Allen, A. R., Tam, F. W. K., Haskard, D. O., Lobb, R. R., Silva, P. M. R., and Nourshargh, S. (2000) VCAM-1 has a tissue-specific role in mediating interleukin-4-induced eosinophil accumulation in rat models:evidence for a dissociation between endothelial-cell VCAM-1 expression and a functional role in eosinophil migration. *Blood* **96,** 3601.

30

Immunoperoxidase Histochemistry for the Detection of Cellular Adhesion Molecule, Cytokine, and Chemokine Expression in the Arthritic Synovium

Zoltan Szekanecz and Alisa E. Koch

1. Introduction

The invasion of leukocytes into the synovial tissue (ST) eventually resulting in tissue damage is a crucial process in the pathogenesis of rheumatoid arthritis (RA) *(1–4)*. Augmented adhesion of inflammatory cells to the ST endothelia and to other ST components is mediated by a number of cell adhesion molecules (CAMs), whose expression may also be upregulated in RA, as well as in other inflammatory diseases *(1–3)*. Some cytokines, such as interleukin-1β (IL-1β) and tumor necrosis factor-α (TNF-α), as well as other pro- and antiinflammatory cytokines are also present in the RA ST. These soluble mediators have an effect on leukocyte activation, upregulation of cell adhesion receptors on lining cells and endothelial cells, tissue destruction, angiogenesis, and other important inflammatory processes *(2,4,5)*. Chemotactic cytokines termed chemokines drive inflammatory leukocytes into the synovium. The production of a number of chemokines is regulated by proinflammatory cytokines, such as TNF-α. In addition, chemokines act in concert with CAMs on the endothelial surface during leukocyte extravasation *(3,5,6)*. In summary, there is an existing regulatory network of cytokines, chemokines, and CAMs, which play an important role in the pathogenesis of synovitis underlying RA.

To determine which of these soluble or cell surface bound factors may play a role in RA, studies of the *in situ* distribution of cytokines, chemokines, and CAMs in the arthritic synovium are needed (**Fig. 1**). This should be the very first step, followed by more detailed functional analysis. Blocking studies using specific antibodies to soluble mediators or CAMs may also give relevant information on the relative role of these factors, as these antibodies may decrease the synovial expression of the targeted molecule. Thus, human studies using the anti-TNF-α monoclonal antibody Infliximab revealed that the synovial production of certain chemokines and CAMs, as well as other cytokines, was also attenuated *(7)*. In this chapter, we describe the use of immunohistochemistry in the detection of *in situ* synovial cytokine, chemokine, and CAM expression. We also discuss hematoxylin eosin staining, as this is used to analyze tissue morphology before immunohistochemistry. Additional procedures needed for immunohistochemistry, such as tissue processing and sectioning are also described.

2. Materials

2.1. Patients

1. Patients with RA, osteoarthritis, or other types of arthritis.
2. Patients are undergoing arthroplasty or arthroscopy, when ST is obtained.

2.2. Synovial Tissue Processing

1. 15-mL tubes, 5-mL vial, sealable plastic bags, sterile forceps, and scissors.
2. Liquid nitrogen (for snap-freezing).
3. OCT compound (Miles, Elkhart, IN), stored at room temperature.

2.3. Slide Coating with Vectabond

1. Clean glass slides, metal/plastic slide racks, glass staining dishes.
2. Vectabond reagent (Vector Laboratories, Burlingame, CA), stored at room temperature.
3. Acetone (Fisher), stored at 4°C; distilled water, stored at room temperature.

2.4. Synovial Tissue Sectioning

1. Gloves (must be worn when human samples are used !!!).
2. Sample synovial tissue, stored at –70°C.
3. OCT compound (Miles), stored at room temperature.
4. Cryostat chuck.
5. Vectabond-coated slides (*see* **Subheading 2.3.**), stored at room temperature.
6. Brushes, Kimwipes.

2.5. Hematoxylin-Eosin Staining

1. Slides to be stained, stored at room temperature; cover slips (22 × 22 mm), mounting medium.
2. 70% Ethanol, 95% ethanol, 100% ethanol (all from Fisher), stored at 4°C.
3. Alcoholic formalin: 10 mL 37% formaldehyde, 90.6 mL 95% ethanol (all from Fisher), stored covered at room temperature.

Immunoperoxidase Histochemistry

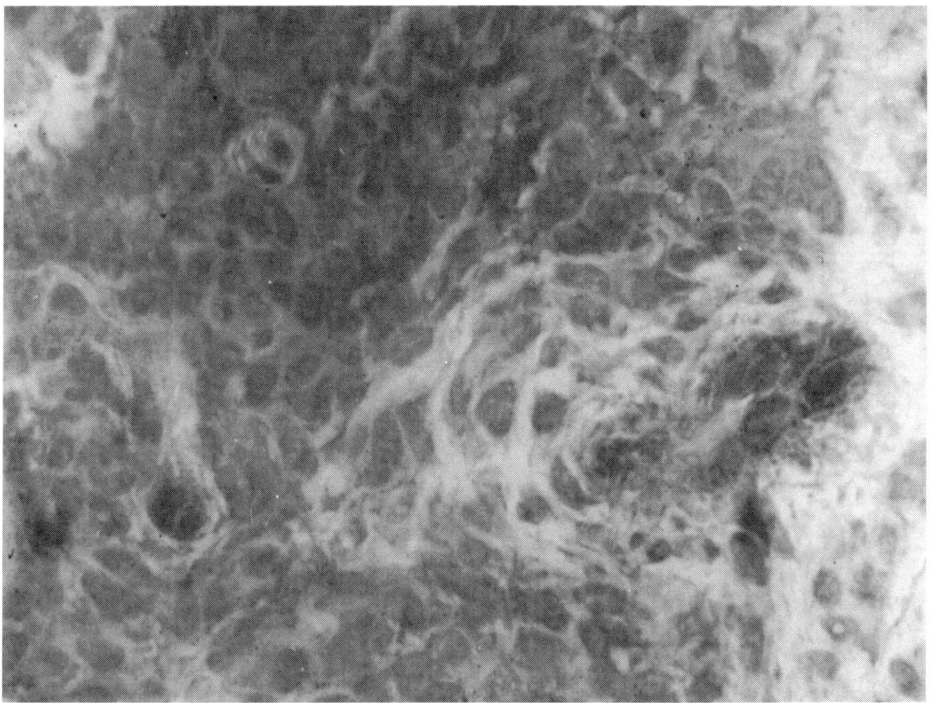

Fig. 1. Indirect immunoperoxidase staining of frozen ST, showing intercellular adhesion molecule (ICAM)-1 expression on synovial lymphocytes and endothelial cells. The massive lymphocytic infiltrate causes compression of the synovial venule (magnification: ×696).

4. Harris' hematoxylin (Sigma), stored at room temperature, filter before use.
5. Acid alcohol: 1 mL concentrated HCl, 100 mL 70% ethanol (Fisher), stored covered at room temperature.
6. Saturated lithium chloride: 10 g LiCl powder (Sigma), 500 mL distilled water, stored at room temperature.
7. Eosin stock solution: 2 g Eosin-y (Sigma), 40 mL distilled water, 160 mL 95% ethanol (Fisher), stored at room temperature.
8. Eosin working solution: 1 mL glacial acetic acid (Fisher). 100 mL stock eosin (from above), 100 mL 95% ethanol (Fisher), freshly prepared before use (to enhance eosin staining, add 1 to 2 mL extra glacial acetic acid).
9. Isopropyl alcohol (Fisher), stored at 4°C.

2.6. Immunoperoxidase Histochemistry

1. Tissue sections on Vectabond-coated slides (see above).
2. PAP pen or diamond pen (Dakopatts).

3. Centrifuge and microcentrifuge tubes, gloves, Kimwipes, cover slips, pipets, pipetors, 10–20 cm^3 syringes, needles, mounting medium, stick-on slide labels, incubator.
4. Vector ABC Elite immunoperoxidase staining kit (Vector Laboratories, Burlingame, CA); A, B, and C solutions freshly made before use, stored at 4°C (*see* **Note 1**).
5. Acetone (Fisher), stored at 4°C.
6. Gill's hematoxylin (Sigma), stored at room temperature (discard after 2 mo).
7. Saturated Li_2CO_3 (Sigma, 2% in distilled water), stored at room temperature.
8. 95% ethanol, 100% ethanol, methanol, isopropyl alcohol (all Fisher), stored at 4°C.
9. 1x PBS in 500-mL bottles, stored at room temperature.
10. 0.1 *M* Tris-HCl pH 7.6; 1 m*M* Tris-HCl pH 7.6; 0.1 m*M* Tris pH 7.6 (from 1 m*M* stock, Sigma), stored at room temperature.
11. Diaminobenzidine chromogen (Kirkegaard & Perry, Gaithersburg, MD), stored at –20°C.
12. 30% H_2O_2 (Sigma), stored at –20°C.
13. Distilled water stored at room temperature.
14. Avidin Non-Specific Binding (if needed): biotin blocking kit (Vector Laboratories).

3. Methods
3.1. Synovial Tissue Processing and Freezing

1. Under the hood, with sterile forceps and scissors, divide the tissue in small, embeddable pieces to be frozen in OCT compound.
2. Label sealable small plastic bags with information on the source of the tissue (initials or name of the patient, date, diagnosis, surgical procedure, and so on).
3. Layer OCT compound on the top of a cryostat chuck at room temperature, then dip the chuck with the OCT into liquid nitrogen using forceps until the solidification of the embedding compound (snap freezing).
4. Place the tissue piece on the top of the solid OCT layer.
5. Place another layer of OCT compound on top as described in **step 3**. To prepare a "sandwich." Again, snap freeze the embedded tissue in liquid nitrogen.
6. Remove the tissue embedded in OCT from the chuck by using a razor blade.
7. Place the embedded synovial tissue into the sealable bag, seal, and store in freezer at –80°C.

3.2. Vectabond Coating of Slides

1. Place clean glass slides in slide racks. Use either precleaned slides or wash slides thoroughly in detergent and rinse in water.
2. Immerse slides in acetone for 5 min.
3. Prepare Vectabond reagent treatment solution by adding the entire contents of the bottle (7 mL) to 350 mL of acetone and stirring well (*see* **Note 2**).

4. Remove slides from acetone, tapping rack several times to drain and place in Vectabond reagent solution for 5 min.
5. Remove slides and drain.
6. Eliminate excess reagents by gently dipping them several times for 30 s in deionized or distilled water (do not create bubbles), changing the water after every five racks. Remove rack of slides for drying. (Gentle agitation or tapping of the rack before allowing to dry will decrease water droplets and their resulting spots.)
7. Air-dry slides thoroughly at room temperature or at 37°C.

3.3. Synovial Tissue Sectioning

1. Always put on latex gloves when handling human tissue.
2. Layer OCT compound onto the chuck, place embedded tissue on top, and place the chuck on the cooling bar inside the cryostat.
3. While the sample is cooling, label your slides. Allow 10 min.
4. Mount the chuck into the microtome (inside the cryostat).
5. Advance microtome slowly (10–20 µm) until the tissue is exposed then change the section thickness to 6–8 µm and cut your specimen.
6. Use the brush to gently pull the section out as it is being cut.
7. When you have a good section, invert a Vectabond-coated slide and touch it to the section; thus the section will attach to the slide.
8. When you have enough sections cut, put one into alcoholic formalin (for hematoxylin-eosin staining), let the remainder of the slides air-dry for 2–16 h, put them in a slide box, wrap the box in aluminum foil to prevent evaporation, label box, and place slides into –80°C freezer.
9. When finished cutting, remove the chuck from microtome and place it on the freezer bar. Add a drop of OCT to cover tissue, and place heat extractor on the top of tissue.
10. Gently remove the embedded tissue from the chuck using a razor blade, place it in the plastic bag, seal the bag, and return the uncut tissue to the freezer.

3.4. Hematoxylin Eosin Staining

1. Fix slides in alcoholic formalin for at least 1 min.
2. Rinse in tap water for about 1 min or 15–20 dips.
3. Stain with hematoxylin for at least 1 min.
4. Rinse in tap water for about 1 min or 15–20 dips.
5. Quickly dip in acid alcohol for 0.2 s.
6. Rinse in tap water for about 1 min or 15–20 dips.
7. Place in lithium chloride for at least 1 min.
8. Stain in eosin working solution for 10 s.
9. Dehydrate in 95% ethanol for at least twice 1 min.
10. Dehydrate in 100% ethanol for at least twice 1 min.
11. Remove excess ethanol in isopropyl alcohol at least twice for 1 min.
12. Mount with medium and cover slip.

3.5. Immunoperoxidase Histochemistry

1. Remove slides from freezer and allow them to come to room temperature for about 5–10 min.
2. Circle sample with diamond/PAP pen and label slides with pencil.
3. Put slides into slide racks.
4. Fix slides in acetone at 4°C for 20 min. (Blood cell cytopreps are fixed in 95% ethanol at 25°C for 10 min).
5. To 2.5 mL PBS, add 37.5 µL of serum from Vector ABC kit.
6. Take slide rack from acetone and put it into PBS.
7. Block avidin nonspecific binding, if needed: add blocking solution (see **Subheading 2.**), incubate for 15 min at room temperature, then rinse with PBS.
8. Remove a slide, wipe off excess PBS, and apply 1 drop of serum solution from **step 5** to sample.
9. Incubate for 15 min, at 37°C in humidified CO_2 incubator, do not allow slides to dry out.
10. Allow the primary anti-CAM, anticytokine, or antichemokine antibody suitable for tissue staining to come to room temperature.
11. Remove excess moisture from slide with a Kimwipe and apply 20–50 µL of primary antibody on each tissue section.
12. Incubate for 30 min at 37°C in the incubator. Place rack in water bath, and check slides regularly for drying out.
13. Wash slides in two changes of PBS.
14. Label two glass tubes as #1 and #2.
15. Put 2.5 mL PBS into each tube.
16. Add 37.5 µL blocking solution from the yellow bottle in kit and 12.5 µL from the blue bottle in kit into tube labeled #1.
17. Add one drop of solution A and one drop of solution B into tube labeled #2 (see **Note 3**).
18. Remove a slide, wipe off excess moisture and apply 1 drop of solution #1 to the sample.
19. Incubate for 15 min at 37°C in incubator. Check slides for drying out.
20. Wash slides in two changes of PBS.
21. Block endogenous peroxidase, if needed (e.g., neutrophils are stained): make fresh solution of 3% H_2O_2 in methanol, incubate slides in this blocking solution for 30 min at room temperature, then wash slides in three changes of PBS (see **Note 4**).
22. Remove a slide, wipe off excess moisture, and apply 1 drop of solution #2 to sample.
23. Incubate for 15 min at 37°C in incubator. Check slides for drying out.
24. Wash slides in two changes of PBS.
25. Make diaminobenzidine (DAB) solution freshly, right before use: add 17 µL H_2O_2 in 1 mL distilled water to a microcentrifuge tube. Also add 100 µL of DAB in 5 mL 0.1 M Tris-HCl (pH 7.6) to a 15-mL centrifuge tube and vortex briefly. Add 100 µL of H_2O_2 solution to the DAB solution and vortex briefly. Draw this solution into a syringe with 0.2 µm microfilter, and filter solution into another 15-mL centrifuge tube.

26. Remove a slide, wipe off excess moisture, and add 20–50 μL of DAB solution prepared as in step 25.
27. After 5 min of incubation, put slides back in slide-rack standing in tap water.
28. Wait an additional 2 min, dispose of DAB waste into properly marked containers (*see* **Note 5**).
29. Put slide rack into Gill's hematoxylin, incubate for 1 min.
30. Rinse slides in tap water. Dip slides into Li_2CO_3 for one minute, then again rinse slides in tap water.
31. Run slides through ethanol sequence, for 1 min (or 15 dips) at each step as follows: two changes of 95% ethanol, three changes of 100% ethanol, then two changes of isopropyl alcohol. Leave slides in last isopropyl alcohol container until cover slipping.
32. Wipe off excess isopropyl alcohol, add one drop of mounting medium and cover slip. Remove bubbles by pressing down the coverslip for a few seconds.
33. Label slides.

3.6. Semiquantitative Microscopic Analysis

1. Identification of synovial cell types: Gill's hematoxylin counterstaining enables the observer to detect the following synovial cell types: synovial lining cells, sublining (interstitial) macrophages, vascular endothelial cells, interstitial fibroblasts, lymphocytes. Power light microscopy using x400 magnification is recommended (*see* **Note 6**).
2. The frequency of immunostaining is evaluated by counting a certain number (100–400) of cells and determining the percentage of immunoreactive cells. Thus immunostaining of ST components can be graded by frequency on a scale of 0–100%, where 0% indicates no staining and 100% indicates that all cells are immunoreactive. We usually examine five ×400 fields per section.

4. Notes

1. The type of Vector kit must be selected according to the species in which the secondary antibody was raised.
2. Vectabond reagent solution should be prepared just prior to use. The 357 mL of solution fills a standard size horizontal staining dish and is sufficient to process at least 500 slides. Slides can be used immediately after drying, or be stored at room temperature.
3. At this point return kit into refrigerator. Do not leave the kit on room temperature for a long time.
4. Never allow the slides to dry out at room temperature; use sufficient amount of solutions.
5. DAB may be carcinogenic. Do not drain DAB down the sink or dispose into trash cans.
6. For exact identification, specific primary antibodies detecting certain cell types may be used. We recommend antifactor VIII for endothelial cells, anti-CD68 for macrophage-type cells, anti-CD3 for T cells, anti-CD19 for B cells.

Acknowledgment

This work was supported by the National Institutes of Health Grants AR-30692 and AI-40987 (A.E.K.); funds from the Veterans' Administration Research Service (A.E.K.); the Gallagher Professorship for Arthritis Research (A.E.K.); grants from the Hungarian National Scientific Research Fund No. F 025813 (Z.S.), and an Educational Research and Development Grant (Z.S.)

References

1. Jalkanen, S. (1989) Leukocyte-endothelial cell interaction and the control of leukocyte migration into inflamed synovium. *Springer Semin. Immunopathol.* **11,** 187–198.
2. Haynes, B. F., Hale, L. P., Denning, S. M., Le, P. T., and Singer, K. H. (1989) The role of leukocyte adhesion molecules in cellular interactions: implications for the pathogenesis of inflammatory synovitis. *Springer Semin. Immunopathol.* **11,** 163–185.
3. Szekanecz, Z., Haines, G.K., Lin, T.R., Harlow, L.A., Goerdt, S., Rayan, G., et al. (1994) Differential distribution of intercellular adhesion molecules (ICAM-1, ICAM-2 and ICAM-3), and the MS-1 antigen in normal and diseased human synovia. *Arthritis Rheum.* **37,** 221–231.
4. Szekanecz, Z., Szegedi, G., and Koch, A.E. (1996) Cellular adhesion molecules in rheumatoid arthritis. Regulation by cytokines and possible clinical importance. *J. Invest. Med.* **44,** 124–135.
5. Szekanecz, Z., Strieter, R.M., and Koch, A.E. (1998) Cytokines in rheumatoid arthritis: potential targets for pharmacological intervention. *Drugs Aging* **12,** 377–390.
6. Szekanecz, Z., Kunkel, S.L., Strieter, R.M., and Koch, A.E. (1998) Chemokines in rheumatoid arthritis. *Springer Semin. Immunopathol.* **20,** 115–132.
7. Feldmann, M., Charles, P., Taylor, P., and Maini, R.N. (1998) Biological insights from clinical trials with anti-TNF therapy. *Springer Semin. Immunopathol.* **20,** 211–228.

31

Roles of Nitric Oxide and Superoxide in Inflammation

Daniela Salvemini, Harry Ischiropoulos, and Salvatore Cuzzocrea

1. Introduction

Nitric oxide (NO), superoxide, and the product of their reaction peroxynitrite play fundamental roles in inflammation (*see* **Fig. 1**). An understanding of the relative contribution of these species to the overall inflammatory response has been achieved by the ability to detect their presence and to block their effects.

NO is synthesized from the guanidino group of L-arginine by a family of enzymes known as nitric oxide synthases (NOS). Three isoforms have been described and cloned: endothelial cell NOS (ecNOS or type 3), brain NOS (bNOS, nNOS, or type 1), and inducible macrophage type NOS (iNOS or type 2). The production of NO by the two constitutive forms of NOS (cNOS) is calcium-dependent, whereas the production of NO by iNOS does not require increases in intracellular Ca^{2+} concentration. The inducible form of NOS is induced by proinflammatory agents such as endotoxin (bacterial lipopolysaccharide, LPS), interleukin 1β (IL-1β), tumor necrosis factor α (TNF-α), and interferon-γ in vivo and in vitro *(1–3)*. It is now well accepted that enhanced formation of NO following the induction of iNOS is implicated in the pathogenesis of inflammation *(1–4)*.

Another important radical that is involved in numerous inflammatory responses is superoxide anion (produced by the one electron reduction of molecular oxygen). This is formed via a large number of pathways, inflammatory cells, as well as in the metabolism of arachidonic acid *(5)*. In acute and chronic inflammation, the production of superoxide anion is increased at a rate that overwhelms the capacity of the endogenous superoxide dismutase (SOD) enzyme defense system to remove it. The consequence of this imbalance results

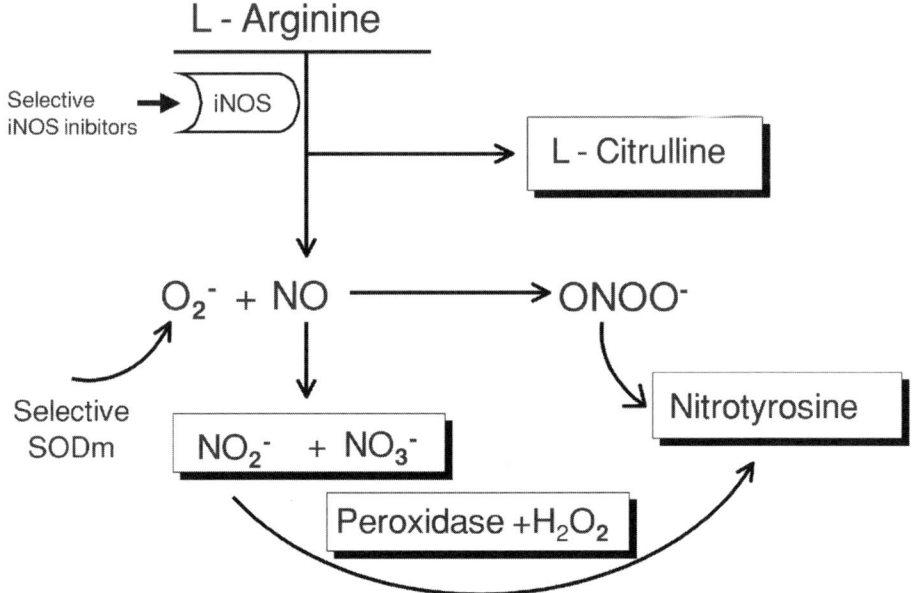

Fig. 1. Scheme of Nitric oxide (NO), superoxide and the product of their reaction peroxynitrite formation.

in superoxide anion mediated damage *(5)*. Some important proinflammatory roles for superoxide anion include: endothelial cell damage and increased microvascular permeability *(6–8)*, formation of chemotactic factors such as leukotriene B_4 *(9,10)*, recruitment of neutrophils at sites of inflammation *(11–13)*, autocatalytic destruction of neurotransmitters and hormones such as norepinephrine and epinephrine *(14)*, respectively, and the generation of the cytotoxic and proinflammatory peroxynitrite *(15,16)*. The detection of superoxide anion in vivo, in inflammatory settings, has been, and still is, a major challenge. This stems from the fact that this radical is short lived and reactive, making its detection problematic *(5)*. Techniques such as electron paramagnetic resonance are available, but the technology and equipment is not available in many laboratories. To date, the majority of evidence on the role of superoxide in inflammation has come from studies using pharmacological tools; use of the native SOD enzyme *(17)*, or by recently developed synthetic enzymes of SOD, which are selective for superoxide *(18–20)*.

Superoxide reacts with nitric oxide at a rate approaching the diffusion limit to form peroxynitrite a highly reactive oxidant *(21)*. Peroxynitrite is cytotoxic and is involved in numerous inflammatory responses *(16,22)*. Peroxynitrite also nitrates and deactivates the MnSOD *(23)* perpetuating the inflammatory response.

Experimental data gathered over the last decade strongly supports NO, superoxide anions, and peroxynitrite as key players in acute and chronic inflammation of various etiologies. Thus, a number of molecular, biochemical, and pharmacological tools have been developed and are available to assess their presence and contribution in inflammatory settings.

2. Materials
2.1. ^{3}H-Arginine/Citrulline Assay

1. Stop buffer: 20 mM HEPES pH 5.5, 1 mM EGTA, 1 mM ethylene diamine tetraacetic acid (EDTA).
2. Homogenation buffer: 50 mM Tris-HCl pH 7.4 (6.06 mg/mL), 0.1 mM EDTA (0.037 mg/mL), 2 μM leupeptin (100 μL/100 mL), 1 μM pepstatin, 12 mM 2-mercaptoethanol (84 μL/100 mL), 0.1 μM PMSF (added fresh).
3. Dowex 5OW: To generate Dowex 5OW, place 500 g Dowex 5OW into 2 L 1 N NaOH on stirrer for 6 h, decant NaOH, and replace with fresh 1N NaOH, stir overnight. The next day, wash the resin 6–8 times with 2 L distilled H$_2$0 then 6–8 times with 1 L Stop Buffer until pH 5.5 to 5.8.
4. ^{3}H-Arginine: To make clean ^{3}H-arginine, add 20 μL ^{3}H-arginine (10 μCi/mL) to 1.0 mL L-arginine (100 μM), vortex then place over 1.0 mL column of AG 1X8 anion exchange resin (100–200 mesh). Elute off the ^{3}H-arginine with 1.0 mL distilled H$_2$O. (This removes the free protons from the mixture.)
5. Agents: NADPH 10 mM.
6. Calmodulin 3000 U/mL (CAM).
7. Tetrahydrobiopterin 50 μM (BH4).
8. 100 μM L-Arginine HCl.
9. W Valine 5 mM (Val).
10. 20 mM CaC1$_2$.
11. 10 mM EGTA.
12. 100 mM phenyl methyl sulfonyl fluoride (PMSF) in dimethyl sulfoxide (DMSO).

2.2. Fluorometric Measurement of Nitrite in Biological Samples Using the 2,3-Diaminonaphthalene (DAN) Assay

1. 96-well plates for fluorometric measurements.
2. 0.62 N HCl.
3. 2.8 N NaOH.
4. 100 μM NaNO$_2$ in H$_2$O.
5. DAN; 2,3-diaminonaphthalene (Sigma).
6. Microcentrifuge filters (10 K NMWL cutoff filter unit) (Sigma).
7. Nitrate Reductase (from *Aspergillus niger*, Sigma) 1.38 U/mL in 500 mM Tris-HCl, pH 7.5.
8. 100 μM NADPH in 50 mM Tris-HCl pH 7.5 (0.833 mg/mL).

2.3. Immunohistochemical Localization of Nitrotyrosine

1. Buffer: 0.1 M phosphate-buffered saline (PBS), pH 7.2.
2. Blocking buffer: 0.1% Fraction V, fatty acid ultrafree BSA is added to PBS. This solution should be made fresh daily.
3. Sodium hydrosulfite and sodium borohydride solutions (Aldrich-Sigma).
4. Humidified chamber: A flat surface rectangular box 7" × 5" or larger lined with wet paper towels can be used for this purpose. All incubations are done in a humidified chamber.

2.4. Immunoprecipitation of Nitrotyrosine and Detection by Western Blotting

1. Gel electrophoresis and transfer apparatus.
2. Protein G Sepharose beads, Amersham Pharmacia Biotech AB (Arlington Heights, IL).
3. PROTRAN pure nitrocellulose membranes 0.2 μm, Schleicher & Schuell (Keene, NH).
4. ECL Western blotting detection reagent, Amersham Pharmacia Biotech AB.
5. Bio-Rad goat antimouse or antirabbit IgG (H+L)-HRP conjugate (Hercules, CA).
6. Kodak BioMax Autoradiography Cassette and Kodak X-Omat AR Film (Rochester, NY).
7. Homogenization Buffer: 25 mM Tris-HCl, 100 mM NaCl, 100 μM Detpac, 40 μM PMSF, 0.5 μg/mL aprotinin from Sigma (St. Louis, MO), 20 μM lactacystin from Calbiochem (La Jolla, CA).
8. Lysis Buffer: 20 mM Tris-HCl base, 150 mM NaCl, 10% glycerol, 1% Triton X-100, 4 mM EGTA, 1 mM PMSF, 10 μg/mL aprotinin, 20 μM lactacystin, pH 7.4.
9. TBS-T: TBS with 0.05% Tween-20 (Sigma, Bio-Rad, and so on).
10. Nonfat dry milk.
11. ECL antibody detection system (Amersham) or equivalent.

3. Methods

Use methods described in **Subheading 3.1.–2.** to detect and evaluate the roles of NO from inducible form of the enzyme. L-arginine (the precursor for NO) is converted to L-citrulline and NO by the iNOS enzyme (calcium independent). In biological fluids, NO decomposes to nitrite; and nitrite is subsequently converted to nitrates by hemoglobin. The presence of the iNOS enzyme can be detected in inflammatory settings by measuring the presence of the message of the enzyme in most tissues by Western blots. The activity of the enzyme can be measured by monitoring the conversion of L-arginine to L-citrulline, the formation of nitric oxide from the enzyme can be measured either by detecting NO directly by chemiluminescence (not discussed here) or by indirect methods by measuring the formation of its metabolites, nitrites, and nitrate (NOx) by fluorometric assays *(24)*. Finally, the pharmacological activity of the enzyme and the consequences of its induction in the overall inflammatory response can be assessed by the use of selective inhibitors of the enzyme such as aminoguanidine *(25,26)*.

3.1. ^{3}H-Arginine/Citrulline Assay

1. If you are using tissues as samples (i.e., lung, brain and so on), weigh your sample then add 5.0 mL Homogenation Buffer for every 1.0 g tissue and homogenize on ice. If you are using cells, for every T- 175 cm^2 flask use 1.0 mL Homogenation Buffer and homogenize on ice.
2. To test for total enzyme, inhibitable enzyme and iNOS for each sample you will need nine Eppendorf microfuge tubes. All tubes have 10 µL each of NADPH, CAM, Val, BH$_4$. Tubes 1–6 have 20 µL each CaCl$_2$, tubes 7–9 have 30 µL each EGTA. Tubes 4–6 also have 10 µL each 30 mM L-NMMA.
3. To each tube, 30 µL of Tissue/Cell Homogenate is added.
4. 20 µL ^{3}H-Arginine (10 µCi/mL) is added to each tube, tubes are capped, then vortexed and the reaction is allowed to proceed at room temperature for 30 min.
5. After 30 min, add 0.5 mL Stop Buffer to each tube. Place each reaction mixture over a separate 1.0 mL column of Dowex 50W. Elute with 0.5 mL Stop Buffer. Column eluates can be collected directly into 7.0 mL scintillation vials. To each vial add 5.3 mL Optiphase scintillation fluid and count each vial for 2 min in Beta scintillation counter, tritium spectrum. Two blank samples (no Tissue) should be include over Dowex 5OW for background.
6. After scintillation counts are secured, subtract background from all samples. The data can be platted as corrected CPM or as a percentage of control.

3.2. Fluorometric Measurement of Nitrite and Nitrate in Plasma Samples Taken from Endotoxin-Challenged Rats Using the DAN Assay

The assay can be used to detect 10 nM nitrite, making it 50–100 times more sensitive than the well-known Griess assay *(24)*. In blood, all of the nitrite is converted to nitrate by hemoglobin. Thus, nitrate reductase has to be used to convert the nitrate back to the nitrite. The same technique can be applied in other biological fluids.

NB: If measurements are to be done in cell culture media (for example, if one is interested to measure NOx release from endotoxin-stimulated macrophages in culture, then omit nitrate reductase.

1. Inject endotoxin (4 mg/kg, serotype 0111:B4) intravenously in anesthetized rats and collect blood an urine from 0 to 5 h postendotoxin as described in *(12)*. Endotoxin elicits a time-dependent increase in NOx formation that can be measured in plasma and urine; release of NOx from iNOS occurs within 2–3 h postendotoxin and as expected is blocked by aminoguanidine an iNOS inhibitor (*see* **Fig. 2**).

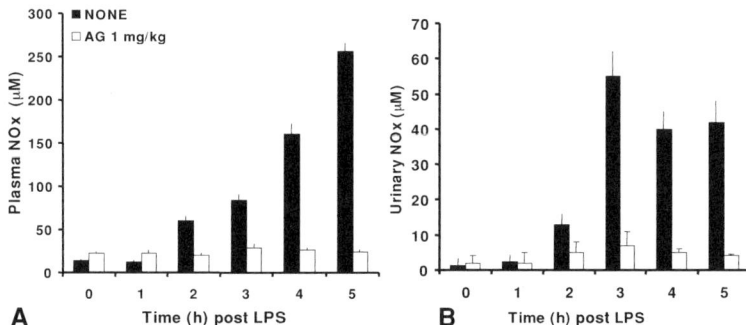

Fig. 2. The increase in plasma and urinary levels of nitrite/nitrate seen at different time point post LPS administration is attenuated in Aminoguanidine treatment (AG, 1 mg/kg infused from 0–5 h).

2. To obtain plasma, red blood cells are first removed by centrifugation (in the presence of heparin or EDTA) or by clot formation.
3. Remove plasma and filter through a 10,000 M_r cutoff filter such as a Centricon 10 (10,000 rpm for 15 min) to remove the hemoglobin resulting from cell lysis. Use the same filtration for urine sample (filter 100 µL of urine). The filter should contain mostly nitrate (recovery greater than 90%) because of the reaction of NO with the iron-heme center of the protein. Nitrate will be converted back to nitrite by the addition of nitrate reductase.
4. Allow microplate reader to warm up for at least 30 min prior use.
5. Prepare DAN; 0.05 mg/1 mL in 0.62 M HCl sonicate for 5 min, *keep in the dark until used*.
6. Prepare the following standard concentrations: 10, 5, 2.5, 1, 0.5, 0.25, 0.1, and 0.0 µM, and aliquot in triplicate 100 µL per standard concentration per well for 1000, 500, 250, 100, 50, 25, 10, and 0 pmol/100 µL.
7. Add 100 µL/well of sample diluted 1:10 to 1:100 .
8. Add 10 µL nitrate reductase and 10 µL NADPH and incubate 5 min prior to the addition of DAN (Skip this step if not assaying with nitrate reductase).
9. Add 10 µL/well DAN and mix gently.
10. Incubate for 10 min at room temperature.
11. Stop reaction with 5 µL of 2.8 N NaOH.
12. Read plate on fluorescence plate reader at 365 nM excitation and 450 nM emission, gain set to 50–75.
13. Express results as plasma or urinary levels of NOx in µM (*see* **Fig. 2**).

3.3. Nitrotyrosine Detection

Protein tyrosine nitration can be derived by the formation of reactive nitrogen intermediates, which includes peroxynitrite, the reaction product of nitric oxide and superoxide *(27)*. If the formation of peroxynitrite is inhibited by removal of superoxide (pharmacologically by using SOD enzyme or SOD mimetics) then its measurement can be used as an indirect measure of superoxide *(18)*. The production of peroxynitrite can be evidenced in part by evaluating the nitrotyrosine formation by immunohistochemistry and Western blot techniques using appropriate inhibitors (SOD enzyme or SOD mimetics, NOS, and peroxidase inhibitors).

3.3.1. Immunohistochemical Localization of Nitrotyrosine (see **Note 1**)

A number of polyclonal and monoclonal antibodies that specifically recognize tyrosine nitrated proteins have been developed and are available from commercial sources. The protocols described later utilize specific antibodies against protein 3-nitrotyrosine described by Giasson et al. *(28)* and by Viera et al. *(29)* but not for commercially available antibodies. The antibodies can be used for immunohistochemistry, which provides tissue and cellular distribution of nitrated proteins. Two protocols using chromogenic, 3,3'-diaminobenzidine tetrahydrochloride dihydrate (DAB), and fluorescence detection methods are described. A general rule for immunohistochemistry and other methodologies using antibodies is the use of appropriate controls. Fortunately, with nitrotyrosine a number of negative controls (described later) are available, thus ensuring both selectivity and specificity of detection. The use of antibodies for Western blotting have been hindered by a number of experimental difficulties mostly arising from the observation that the antibodies appear to preferentially recognize nitrotyrosine in specific protein conformations, which is disrupted by boiling in SDS. However, the antibodies tested appear to have high avidity and specificity and can detect as little as 0.01% of a given nitrated protein in a protein mixture. A protocol for immunoprecipitation of nitrated proteins has been developed for human plasma proteins, and it can be applied to tissue extracts and other biological fluids (*see* **Fig. 3**). However, not all nitrated proteins can be immunoprecipitated and conversely antibodies against specific proteins do not always immunoprecipitate-nitrated protein. Therefore, to optimize the use of the antinitrotyrosine antibodies for Western blot and immunoprecipitation some trial-and-error is required.

1. Paraffin-embedded slides are deparaffinized by placing the slides at 60°C for 15 min followed by two 10-min successive incubations in Xylene, two 5-min successive incubations in 100% ethanol, 95% ethanol, and 70% ethanol. Finally, rinses slides in PBS briefly and then wash them in PBS for 10 min.
2. *Blocking endogenous peroxidases*: Using an ImmEdge pen, make a circle around the tissue. Incubate slides with 5% H_2O_2 (30%) in methanol/ at room temperature for 20 min. Wash slides twice with PBS for 10 min.
3. *Positive control*: Apply peroxynitrite solution directly on the tissue, add equal volume of PBS (otherwise peroxynitrite will not react with tissue because pH is approx 11.0) incubating at room temperature for 5 min.

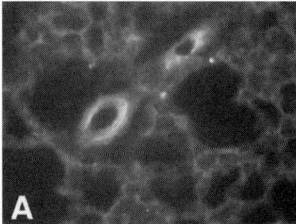 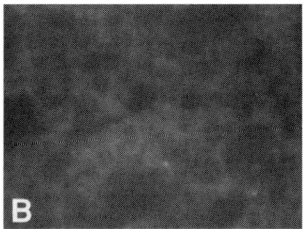 

Fig. 3. Immunohistochemical localization of 3-nitrotyrosine in rat lung following 1 h of ischemia and 1-h of reperfusion. (**A**) Ischemia/Reperfusion stained with polyclonal anti-3-nitrotyrosine antibody. (**B**) Ischemia/Reperfusion stained with Antigen Competed anti-3-nitrotyrosine antibody. (**C**) Perfusion Control stained with polyclonal anti-3-nitrotyrosine antibody.

4. *Negative control*: 3-Nitrotyrosine can be reduced to 3-aminotyrosine by sodium hydrosulfite (dithionite). Prepare fresh a 0.5 M dithionite solution by dissolving dithionite powder in nitrogen purged 0.01 N NaOH solution. Incubate the slides three times successively in fresh solutions of 0.5 M dithionite for 5 min each time.
5. *Negative control*: Preabsorb the antinitrotyrosine antibody with 10-fold excess (w/w) 3-nitrotyrosine. The antibody dissolved in PBS, pH 7.2 is incubated overnight a 4°C with 3-nitrotyrosine. The antibody complex with 3-nitrotyrosine is diluted in antibody buffer prior to use.
6. *Blocking*: Incubate slides at 37°C for 30 min with blocking solution, which contains 10 drops of goat serum in 10 mL of PBS-BSA buffer. Both primary and secondary antibodies should be diluted in the blocking solution.
7. *Primary Antibody*: Remove blocking solution by flinging the solution off or blotting off with absorbent paper. Do not rinse the sections. Apply antibody solution at the desired dilution in blocking buffer (suggested starting dilution is 1:100 or 1:200). Incubate at 37°C for 90 min. At the end of incubation, rinse slides briefly with PBS-BSA buffer, and then wash slides in PBS-BSA buffer for 5 min twice.
8. *Secondary Antibody*: Make up secondary antibody in blocking buffer at the dilution of 1:200. Apply the antibody solution to blotted tissue and incubate at 37°C for 40 min. Rinse slides with PBS-BSA buffer, and then wash slides in PBS-BSA buffer for 5 min, wash another 5 min in second dish.
9. *Color Development*: For 3,3'-Diaminobenzidine tetrahydrochloride dihydrate development the ABC-kit (Vector) is used. Make ABC solution 20 min before use by mixing 1 drop of solution A and 1 drop of solution B in 2.5 mL of PBS-BSA buffer. Blot excess PBS from slides and apply ABC reagent to sections. Incubate at 37 oC for 30 min. Wash slides twice in PBS-BSA buffer 5 min each. Make up DAB solution by adding 5 mg DAB solid to 10 mL PBS-BSA. Filter the DAB solution using a 45-µm syringe filter. Add 10 µL of 30% H_2O_2 solution right before use. Apply DAB solution to the tissue section and incubate until desired color is attained. Stop reaction by rinsing the slide with PBS and then rinse 2 min under running tap water. Handling DAB with great caution. All the

contaminated materials should be discarded into biohazard containers. If desired, counterstaining can be performed based on standard protocol.

10. *Use of fluorescence-labeled secondary antibody*: For fluorescence staining, it is important to reduce the background staining as much as possible. The background staining varies in different tissues and is strongly influenced by the fixation protocol. To reduce autofluorescence, incubate the slides six times for 5 min each in 1 mg/mL sodium borohydride. Sodium borohydride will not reduce 3-nitrotyrosine to 3-aminotyrosine, but will significantly reduce tissue autofluorescence. Examine the slides for autofluorescence at the end of the incubation. If needed repeat the borohydride treatment.

11. *Blocking*: Incubated slides for 30 min in blocking solution, made up of 0.3% Triton X-100, 5% fatty acid free-bovine serum albumin (BSA), and 10% normal goat serum in 0.05 M PBS (pH = 7.2). Incubate with anti3-nitrotyrosine antibodies as aforementioned. At the end of incubation, rinse slides with PBS-0.3% Triton X-100 buffer, and then wash slides in PBS buffer for 5 min twice.

12. *Secondary antibody*: Incubate slides tissues for 1 h with antirabbit goat secondary antibody labeled with fluorescence dye (diluted at 1:200 concentration in blocking solution). Wash with 0.05 M PBS three times for 5 min each time. Allow slides to air-dry and cover slip.

3.3.2. Immunoprecipitation of Nitrotyrosine and Detection By Western Blotting (see **Note 1**)

1. *Sample Preparation and Immunoprecipitation*: Homogenize sample in homogenization buffer. Usually 100 µg of homogenate is diluted in with (500 µL total volume) with lysis buffer. 5–20 µL antinitrotyrosine antibody is added and the solution is incubated on an orbital shaker at 4°C overnight. Protein G Sepharose beads, 30 µL, are added and incubated for 1 h at 4°C. Centrifuge the slurry for 2 min at 10,000 rpm to precipitate beads. Remove and discard supernatant, add 500 µL lysis buffer, and vortex gently to mix. Precipitate beads by centrifugation and repeat three times. Resuspend washed beads in 20–40 µL loading dye solution, boil 8–10 min, and centrifuge for 2 min at 10,000 rpm to precipitate beads. Transfer supernatant to a fresh tube and repeat centrifugation to fully remove beads. Sample can be run on gel or stored at –20°C.

2. *Western Blot Procedure* (*see* **Notes 2** and **3**): All steps below are performed at room temperature with gentle shaking. Following blotting to nitrocellulose, block nonspecific antibody binding with 5% nonfat dry milk in TBS-T (to avoid high background prepare TBS and TBS-T solution fresh and filter) for 2 h. Wash 3 times for 5 min each time in TBS-T. Dilute anti-3-nitrotyrosine antibody in TBS-T with 1% dry milk. Dilutions of 1:5000 or 1:10000 of the primary antibody is a good starting point. Incubate blot with primary antibody for 2 h. Rinse blot twice with TBS-T, followed by one 15-min wash and 4 x 5-min washes with TBS-T. Dilute secondary antibody 1/5000 to 1/10000 in TBS-T and incubate with blot for 1 h. Rinse and wash as in **step 4**, except perform last two 5-min washes with TBS (no Tween-20). Detect antibody binding by standard methods recommended by the manufacturers. We routinely use the ECL method (Amersham), (*see* **Figs. 4** and **5**).

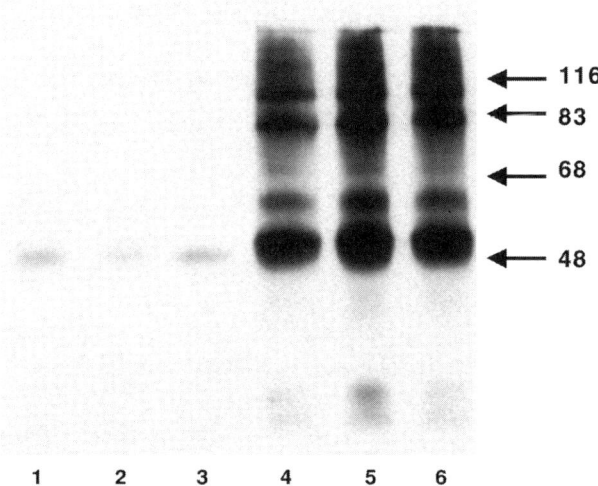

Fig. 4. Immunoprecipitation of nitrated human plasma proteins 1–3 is unreacted plasma 4–6 is plasma reacted with 1 mM SIN-1 for 1 hour at 37°C. The proteins were immunoprecipitated with polyclonal anti-3-nitrotyrosine antibody and the western blot was developed using monoclonal anti-3-nitrotyrosine antibody.

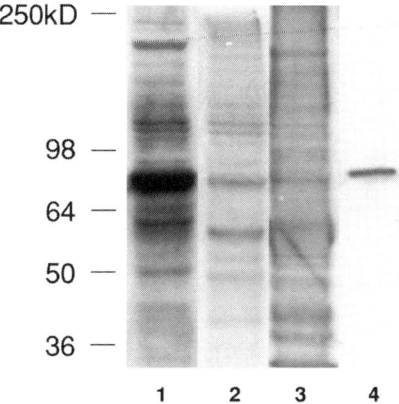

Fig. 5. Western blotting with anti-3-nitrotyrosine antibodies. Composite blot showing rat lung (1), spleen (2), and brain (3) homogenates nitrated by exposure to peroxynitrite. Nitrated bovine serum albumin (4) included as positive control.

4. Notes

1. The efficiency of precipitation can vary between proteins, and, thus, the antibody concentration can be varied to increase efficiency. A variation of immunoprecipitation and Western blotting protocol has been developed *(30)*. The dilution of

both the primary and secondary antibodies is determined partially by the sensitivity of the detection system employed, the properties of the antibodies themselves, as well as by the type and amount of immunoreactive material on the blot. It is advisable to determine the optimal dilution of the antibodies by serial dilution. Incubation times and temperature may vary as well. Preconjugation of the primary and secondary antibody as aforementioned may also help reduce background and increase sensitivity.
2. Do not allow the nitrocellulose membrane to dry at any time following protein transfer. Handle the membrane with gloved hands or clean forceps. Good general references for Western blotting are available from Bio-Rad, as well as from Current Protocols in Molecular Biology (Wiley).
3. Include a positive control on the blot. We commonly load one lane of the gel with 25 ng of BSA nitrated by standard methods with peroxynitrite. Negative controls (samples reduced with dithionite, preabsorbed primary antibody) can be performed as aforementioned.

References

1. Moncada, S., Palmer, R. M. J., and Higgs, E. A. (1991) Nitric oxide: Physiology, Pathophysiology and Pharmacology. *Pharmacol Rev.* **43,** 109–142
2. Nathan, C. (1996) Nitric oxide as a secretory product of mammalian cells. *FASEB J.* **6,** 3051–3064.
3. Alderton, W. K., Cooper, C. E., and Knowels, R. G. (2001) Nitric oxide synthases: structure, function and inhibition. *Biochem. J.* **357,** 593–615.
4. Knowels, R. G. and Moncada, S. (1994) Nitric Oxide syntases in mammals, *Biochem. J.* **298,** 249–258.
5. Fridovich, I. (1997) Superoxide anion radical (O2-.), superoxide dismutases, and related matters. *J. Biol. Chem.* **272,** 18,515–18,517.
6. Droy-Lefaix, M. T., Drouet Y., Geraud G., Hosfod D., and Braquet P. (1991) Superoxide dimutase (SOD) and the PAF-antagonist (BN 52021) reduce small intestinal damage induced by ischemia-reperfusion. *Free Rad. Res. Commun.* **13,** 725–735.
7. Haglind, E., Xia G., and Rylander R. (1994) Effects of antioxidants and PAF receptor antagonist in intestinal shock in the rat. *Circ. Shock* **42,** 83–91.
8. Xia, Z. F., Hollyoak M., Barrow R. E., He F., Muller M. J., and Herndon D. N. (1995) Superoxide dismutase and leupeptin prevent delayed reperfusion injury in the rat small intestine during burn shock. *J. Burn Care and Rehabilitation* **16,** 111–117.
9. Fantone, J. C. and Ward P. A. (1982) A review: role of oxygen-derived free radicals and metabolites in leukocyte-dependent inflammatory reactions. *Am. J. Pathol.* **107,** 395–418.
10. Deitch, E. A., Bridges, W., Berg, R., Specian, R. D., and Granger, N. (1990) Hernorrhagic Shock-induced Bacterial Translocation: The role of neutrophils and hydroxyl radicals. *J. Trauma* **30,** 942–951.

11. Boughton-Smith, N. K., Evans, S. M., Laszlo, F., Whittle, B. J., and Moncada, S. (1993) The induction of nitric oxide synthase and intestinal vascular permeability by endotoxin in the rat. *Br. J. Pharmacol.* **110,** 1189–1195.
12. Salvemini, D., Settle, S. L., Seibert, K., Masferrer, J. L., Currie, M. G., and Needleman, P. (1995) Regulation of prostaglandin production by nitric oxide; an in vivo analysis. *Br. J. Pharmacol.* **114,** 1171–1178.
13. Salvemini, D., Mazzon, E., Dugo, L., Riley, D. P., Serraino, I., Caputi, A. P., et al. (2001) Pharmacological manipulation of the inflammatory cascade by a selective superoxide dismutase mimetic, M40403. *Br. J. Pharmacol.* **132,** 815–827.
14. Macarthur, H., Westfall, T. C., Riley D. P., Misko, T. P. and Salvemini D. (2000) Inactivation of catecholamines by superoxide gives new insights on the pathogenesis of septic shock. *Proc Natl Acad Sci USA* **97,** 9753–9758.
15. Beckman, J. S. and Crow, L. P. (1993) Pathological implications of nitric oxide, superoxide and peroxynitrite formation. *Biochem. Soc. Trans.* **21,** 330–334.
16. Salvemini, D., Jensen, M. P., Riley, D. P., and Misko, T. P. (1998) Therapeutic manipulations of peroxynitrite. *Drug News and Perspect.* **11,** 204–214.
17. Flohe, L. (1988) Superoxide dismutase for therapeutic use: clinical experience, dead ends and hopes. *Mol. Cell Biochem.* **84,** 123–131.
18. Salvemini, D., Wang, Z., Q., Zweier, J. L., Samouilov, A., Macarthur, H., Misko, T. P., et al. (1999) Synzymes: potent non-peptidic agents against superoxide-driven tissue injury. *Science* **286,** 304–306.
19. Salvemini, D. and Riley, D. P. (2000) Nonpeptidyl mimetics of superoxide dismutase in clinical therapies for diseases. *Cell Mol. Life Sci.* **57,** 1489–1492.
20. Salvemini, D. and Riley, D. P (2000) M40403, drug of the future. *Drug News and Perspect.* **25,** 1027–1033.
21. Huie, R. E. and Padmaja, S. (1993) The reaction of nitric oxide with superoxide. *Free Radical Res. Commun.* **18,** 195–199.
22. Szabo, C. (1996) The pathophysiological role of peroxynitrite in shock, inflammation, and ischemia-reperfusion injury. *Shock* **6,** 79–88.
23. Yamakura, F., Taka, H., Fujimura, T., and Murayama, K. (1998) Inactivation of human manganese-superoxide dismutase by peroxynitrite is caused by exclusive nitration of tyrosine 34 to 3-nitrotyrosine. *J. Biol. Chem.* **273,** 14,085–14,089.
24. Misko, T. P., Schilling, R. J., Salvemini, D., Moore, W. M., and Currie, M. G. (1993) A fluorometric assay for the measurement of nitrite in biological samples. *Anal. Biochem.* **214,** 11–16.
25. Cuzzocrea, S., Zingarelli, B., Gilard, E., Hake, P., Salzman A. L., and Szabó, C. (1998) Anti-inflammatory effects of mercaptoethylguanidine, a combined inhibitor of nitric oxide synthase and peroxynitrite scavenger, in carrageenan-induced models of inflammation. *Free Rad. Biol. Med.* **24,** 450–459.
26. Salvemini, D., Wang, Z. Q., Wyatt, P., Bourdon, D. M., Marino, M. H., Manning, P. T., et al. (1996) Nitric oxide: a key mediator in the early and late phase of carrageenan-induced rat paw inflammation. *Br. J. Pharmacol.* **118,** 829–838.

27. Beckman, J. S., Beckman, T. W., Chen, J., Marshalland, P. A., and Freeman, B. A. (1990) Apparent hydroxyl radical production by peroxynitrite: implication for endothelial injury from nitric oxide and superoxide. *Proc. Natl. Acad. Sci. USA* **87,** 1620–1624.
28. Giasson, B. I., Duda, J. E., Murray, I., Chen, Q., Souza, J. M., Hurting, H. I., et al. (2000) Oxidative damage linked to neurodegeneration by selective a-synuclein nitration in synucleiopathy lesions. *Science* **290,** 985–989.
29. Viera, L., Zu, Y., Eztevez, A. G., and Beckman J. S. (1999) Immunohistochemical methods to detect nitrotyrosine. *Meth. Enzymol.* **301,** 373–381.
30. MacMillan, L. A. and Thompson, J.A. (1999) Immunoprecipitation of nitrotyrosine containing proteins. *Meth. Enzymol.* **301,** 135–145.

32

Analysis of Nitrite and Nitrate in the Study of Inflammation

Claire A. Davies, Sophie A. Rocks, Meg C. O'Shaughnessy, David Perrett, and Paul G. Winyard

1. Introduction

An acute inflammatory response is mounted in response to a stimulus such as tissue damage or the presence of an invading pathogen *(1)*. If this stimulus cannot be removed, then chronic inflammation will develop as classically shown in rheumatoid arthritis (RA). Along with the array of cytokines and chemokines released during inflammation infiltrating macrophages and neutrophils release nitric oxide (NO•), which is involved in killing the offending organism *(2,3)*. Additionally, NO• is known to mediate the inflammatory response by inhibiting or inducing inflammation via a variety of different pathways *(4–8)*. For example, NO• has been shown to activate and inhibit the transcription factor, nuclear factor-kappa B (NF-κB) (9). When NO• activates NF-κB it induces the generation of proinflammatory cytokines such as tumor necrosis factor alpha (TNFα), which are thought to drive the chronic inflammatory response *(10)*. However, NO• can also cause the inhibition of NF-κB by upregulating the production of its inhibitor IκB *(11,12)*. In a similar way, NO• has been shown to inhibit neutrophil adhesion, preventing white blood cells (WBC) from infiltrating the site of inflammation *(13)*. NO• also increases the vascular permeability of the vessel wall so that WBCs can reach the affected tissue *(14)*. The level of NO• produced is thought to determine whether NO• acts as a proinflammatory or antiinflammatory mediator. In many cases, the formation of peroxynitrite, from NO• and superoxide, is thought to be responsible for some of the proinflammatory actions of NO• *(15)*. For instance, NO• has been shown to inactivate tissue inhibitor of metalloproteinases-1 (TIMP-1) via the formation of peroxynitrite *(4)*.

From: *Methods in Molecular Biology, vol. 225: Inflammation Protocols*
Edited by: P. G. Winyard and D. A. Willoughby © Humana Press Inc., Totowa, NJ

A family of enzymes called the nitric oxide synthases (NOS) convert L-arginine into L-citrulline and NO• *(16)* (*see also* **Chapter 31**). Constitutive isoforms (eNOS and nNOS) are known to generate small amounts of NO• that are utilized in normal physiological processes such as neurotransmission and the vasodilatation of blood vessels *(17,18)*. However, during the inflammatory response, inducible NOS (iNOS) expressed in activated cells, such as macrophages, produce large amounts of NO•. The expression of iNOS is induced by proinflammatory cytokines, such as interleukin 1 (IL-1) and TNF, endotoxins, and lipopolysaccharide (LPS). More recently, NO• has also been shown to be produced via NOS-independent pathways. For instance, Zhang et al. *(19)* and Millar et al. *(20)* demonstrated that xanthine oxidase could generate NO• from nitrite or nitrate because of its nitrite and nitrate reductase activity. In this reaction, xanthine oxidase converts nitrite or nitrate to NO• by accepting an electron from nicotinamide adenine dinucleotide, reduced form (NADH), which is then converted to nicotinamide adenine dinucleotide (NAD$^+$).

Studying the level of NO• in biological fluids is particularly difficult because of its short half-life. Instead, the metabolites, nitrite and nitrate, are measured as markers of NO• production. Nitrite (NO_2^-) and nitrate (NO_3^-) are formed by the oxidation of NO•. Equation (1) demonstrates how NO• is oxidized in an aqueous solution *(21)*.

$$4NO^• + O_2 + 2H_2O \rightleftharpoons 4H^+ + 4NO_2^- \qquad \text{[Eq. 1]}$$

In whole blood, hemoglobin (Hb) can oxidize either NO• or nitrite to form nitrate (NO_3^-) as shown in Equations (2) and (3) *(21)*. Alternatively, nitrate can be formed by the decomposition of peroxynitrite.

$$4HbO_2 + NO^• \rightleftharpoons MetHb + NO_3^- \qquad \text{[Eq. 2]}$$

$$4NO_2^- + 4HbO_2 + 4H^+ \rightleftharpoons 4Hb^+ + O_2 + 2H_2O + 4NO_3^- \qquad \text{[Eq. 3]}$$

Plasma nitrite and nitrate concentrations have been shown to be elevated in patients with a variety of inflammatory diseases *(22–25)*. For example, Ueki et al. *(23)* detected higher serum nitrite levels in RA patients when compared to healthy control subjects. The nitrite concentrations detected in these RA patients were also shown to significantly correlate with serum TNF and interleukin 6 (IL-6) levels, thus suggesting that increased endogenous NO• synthesis reflects abnormalities of immunoregulation in the joints.

Nitrite and nitrate have previously been measured by the Griess reaction *(26)*, high-performance liquid chromatography (HPLC) *(27)*, gas chromatography-mass spectrometry *(28)*, electron paramagnetic resonance (EPR) spectrometry *(22)*, and chemiluminescence *(29)* (*see also* **Chapter 31**). The Griess reaction,

EPR spectrometry, and chemiluminescence methods often lack specificity as other nitrogen oxides or nitrosothiols present in the sample may be degraded to the compounds measured indirectly in these methods. The gas chromatography-mass spectrometry and HPLC methods are relatively sensitive (high picomolar to low nanomolar range). However, the samples often require extensive sample preparation, which is both time consuming and tedious. Capillary electrophoresis provides a sensitive technique for the direct measurement of nitrite and nitrate simultaneously. The sample volumes required are small and the amount of sample preparation necessary is minimal. Hence, the total analysis time is significantly reduced when compared to other techniques such as HPLC. The next section briefly explains the technique of capillary electrophoresis before going on to describe the method developed for the measurement of nitrite and nitrate concentrations in biological samples and two systems used in the study of inflammation.

1.1. Capillary Electrophoresis

This technique involves the application of an electrical field to a capillary filled with electrolyte solution. A sample is introduced onto the capillary by pressure or voltage injection. The components of the sample are separated on the basis of charge and mass, as illustrated in **Fig. 1**. The molecules are detected as they pass through a detector window in the capillary. The detector (usually UV) measures the absorbance of the components and plots the detector response versus time to give an electopherogram.

The capillary electrophoresis assay described later provides a simple and specific method for the measurement of nitrite and nitrate in biological samples. The simultaneous measurement of NADH and NAD^+ *(30)* is also described.

2. Materials

1. Buffer A stock solution: 150 mM sodium chloride, 5 mM Tris-HCl, pH 7.4. For 500 mL, dissolve 4.388 g of sodium chloride and 389 mg of Tris-HCl in deionized water. Adjust the pH to 7.4 with sodium hydroxide.
2. SAX solid phase extraction (SPE) cartridges (Merck Limited, Dorset, UK) preconditioned with 1 mL of deionized water. To precondition, add 1 mL water to each cartridge then centrifuge at 1000g for 5 min.
3. Tetradecyltrimethylammonium bromide (TTAB) stock solution: 20 mM in deionized water. For 10 mL, dissolve 67.28 mg in 10 mL of deionized water. Place 1 mL of the TTAB stock solution into two of the preconditioned SPE cartridges then centrifuge at 1000g for 5 min. Combine the filtrate obtained from the two SPE cartridges (*see* **Notes 1–3**).
4. Capillary electrophoresis buffer solution: For 10 mL, add 1 mL of the TTAB solution prepared in **step 3** to 9 mL of buffer A solution prepared in **step 1**. Pass this solution through a 0.45 µm syringe filter.

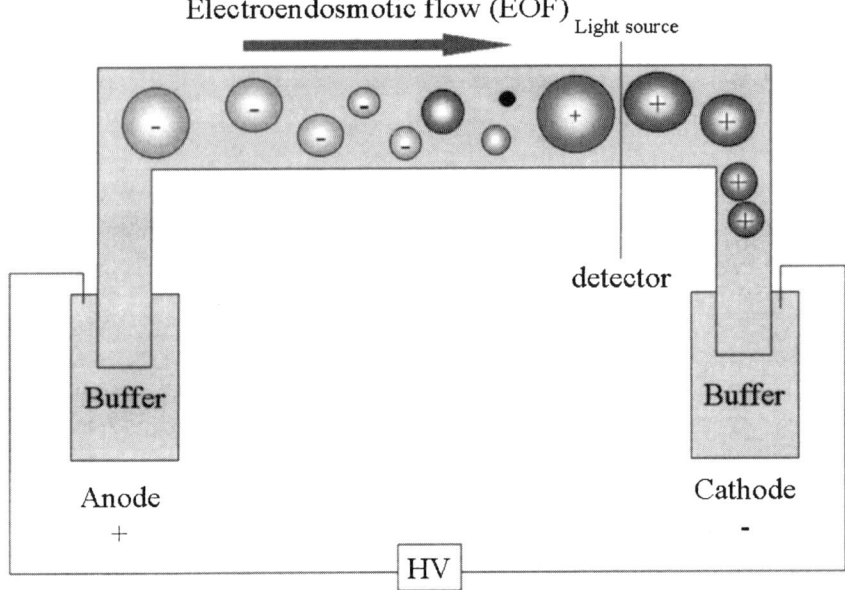

Fig. 1. Diagrammatic representation of capillary electrophoresis (CE) technique showing the migration of cations (+) toward the cathode (−) driven by electrophoretic migration. The initial migration of the anions (−) to the anode (+) is overwhelmed by the electroendosmotic flow (EOF). HV represents the presence of an electric current across the system.

5. Nitrite standard stock solution: 100 mM prepared in deionized water. Remake fresh every 1–2 d (*see* **Notes 4** and **5**).
6. Nitrate standard stock solution: 100 mM prepared in deionized water. Remake fresh every 1–2 d (*see* **Notes 4** and **5**).
7. Sodium hydroxide rinsing solution: Prepare a 0.1 M sodium hydroxide solution by dissolving 4 g sodium hydroxide in 100 mL (*see* **Note 6**).
8. Heat inactivated fetal calf serum (FCS): Heat FCS at 56°C for 30 min, aliquot into 50-mL vials and store at −20°C. For 10% FCS, add 50 mL to 450 mL Dulbecco's modified Eagle's medium (DMEM). For 0.1% FCS, add 0.5 mL FCS to 499.5 mL DMEM.
9. L-glutamine stock solution: 200 mM in normal saline. For 10 mL, dissolve 293 mg in 10 mL of sterile normal saline and filter sterilize through a 0.2-μm pore filter. Aliquot into 5-mL vials and store at −20°C until use.
10. Stock solution 10,000 U penicillin/mL and 10,000 μg streptomycin/mL in sterile normal saline. For 10 mL, dissolve 100,000 U penicillin/mL and 100,000 μg streptomycin/mL in 10-mL sterile normal saline and filter sterilize through a 0.2-μm pore filter. Aliquot into 5-mL vials and store at −20°C until use.
11. TNF-α stock solution: 25 μg/mL in sterile water. For 1 mL, dissolve 25 μg and

filter sterilize through a 0.2-μm pore filter. Store at –70°C. Make up 25 ng/mL–10 ng/mL solution immediately before use.
12. PBS solution: prepare a 0.01 M PBS solution by dissolving one PBS tablet in 200 mL of deionized water (*see* **Note 7**). If necessary, adjust to pH 7.4 using dilute phosphoric acid.
13. NADH stock solution: 1 mM NADH in 0.01 M PBS solution. For 100 mL, dissolve 70.9 mg NADH in 100 mL of 0.01 M PBS solution. Remake this solution on a daily basis.
14. NAD$^+$ stock solution: 1 mM NAD$^+$ in 0.01 M PBS solution. For 100 mL, dissolve 63.3mg NADH in 100 mL of 0.01M PBS solution. Remake this solution on a daily basis.
15. Xanthine oxidase stock solution: 1 U/mL in 0.01 M PBS. Dilute 75 μL xanthine oxidase (13.3 mg protein/mL Grade III from buttermilk) in 1 mL PBS solution.
16. Capillary electrophoresis system consisting of an automatic injector and an ultraviolet (UV) or diode array detector (*see* **Note 8**).
17. Capillary: 50 μm × 47 cm (40 cm to the detector) fused silica capillary (*see* **Note 9**).
18. Glass vials (4 mL) with rubber tops for use with the CE system. Microvials and microvial springs for holding small sample volumes (10–50 μL; Beckman Instruments, Beaconsfield, UK).
19. Microfuge capable of 9000g.
20. Centrifuge capable of 3000g.

3. Methods
3.1. Capillary Electrophoresis

1. Reverse the polarity of the electrodes so that the positive electrode is connected to the inlet side of the capillary and the negative electrode is connected to the outlet side (*see* **Note 1**).
2. Fill two glass vials with the capillary electrophoresis buffer solution (*see* **Subheading 2.4.**) and place one of the vials in the inlet tray and the other vial in the outlet tray of the autosampler.
3. Place an empty vial in outlet position. Rinse the capillary with the capillary electrophoresis buffer solution for 30 min.
4. Prerinse the capillary with 0.1 M sodium hydroxide for 1 min, then with the capillary electrophoresis buffer with 2 min.
5. Set the detector to a wavelength of 214 nm. If you are using a diode array detector, set the bandwidth to 4 nm (*see* **Note 8**).
6. Dilute the nitrite and nitrate stock solutions in buffer A to give two solutions, one containing 1 mM nitrite and the other containing 1 mM nitrate. A further solution containing both 1 mM nitrite and nitrate should also be prepared in buffer A (*see* **Note 10**). Place the standards in microvials and place them in the inlet tray of the autosampler.
7. Inject the solutions prepared in **step 6** onto the capillary by hydrodynamic injection using a pressure injection of 0.5 psi for 15 s.

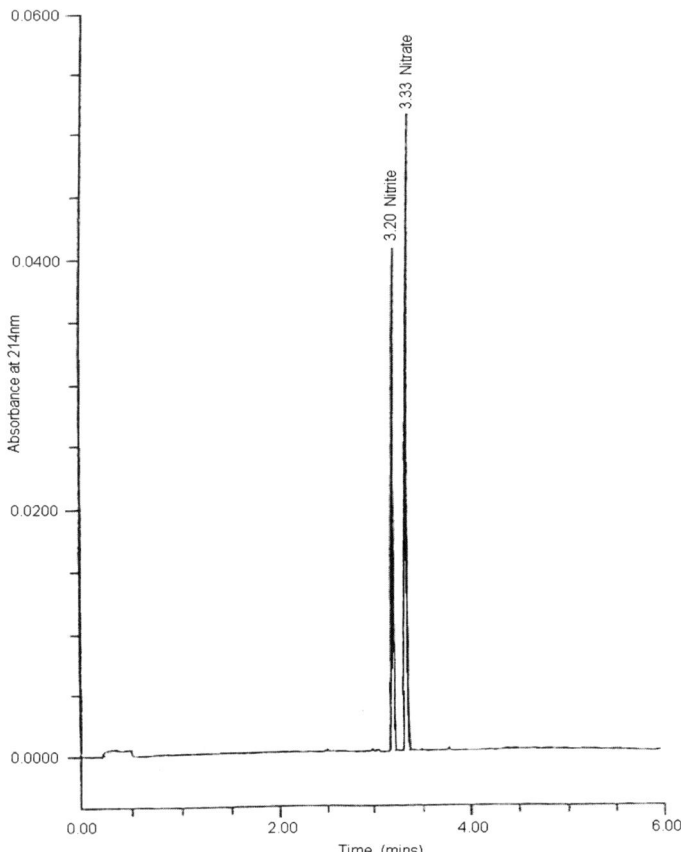

Fig. 2. Typical electropherogram of 1000 µM nitrite and 1000 µM nitrate standard solution prepared in deionized water. Migration times for nitrite and nitrate were 3.20 and 3.33 min, respectively. Reproduced from *(30)* with permission.

8. Separate the components in the standards/samples using a –10 kV voltage separation. **Figure 2** shows a typical electropherogram of a standard solution containing 1 mM nitrite and nitrate (*see* **Note 11**).

3.2. Calibration Curve

1. Calibration curve: dilute the 100 mM nitrite and nitrate standards in buffer A to give six standard solutions containing 0, 2, 4, 6, 8, and 10 µM nitrite and 0, 10, 20, 30, 40 and 50 µM nitrate, respectively, (*see* **Note 10**).
2. Analyze these standard solutions using the conditions described in **Subheading 3.1., steps 7 and 8**. Inject the standards in order of increasing concentration.

3. Use the peak area of the nitrite and nitrate peaks to construct a calibration curve for nitrite and nitrate. Plot the peak area against the concentration of the analyte present in the standard solution. Then calculate the line of best fit using linear regression.
4. Use this line of best fit to calculate the concentration of nitrite and nitrate in the samples from the peak area obtained from each electropherogram.

3.3. Biological Samples

Nitrite and nitrate are often measured to reflect the amount of NO· produced in a particular human disease state, or in animal models of inflammation. The combined measurement of both nitrite and nitrate provides a good marker of NO· production. However, care must be taken if measuring nitrite or nitrate alone in man. It is well known that the dietary intake of nitrate can influence the nitrate levels detected *(21)*. In a similar way, the measurement of nitrite alone should be avoided, as the amount of nitrite present in the sample is dependent on the hemoglobin concentration and/or the length of time it takes to process the sample (*see* **Note 12**; *30,31*).

1. Blood samples: collect whole blood into heparinized vacutainers for plasma and plain tubes for serum (*see* **Note 12**). Centrifuge for 10 min at 1000*g*.
2. Other biological/cellular fluids: centrifuge for 10 min at 1000*g* to remove insoluble particulate and cellular debris.
3. Sample preparation: most samples can be injected directly onto the capillary, although biological and cellular samples often require ultrafiltering (*see* **Note 13**).
4. In order to ultrafilter the samples, place 200 µL of each sample in a 30 kDa ultrafiltration device. Centrifuge the sample for 30 min at 9000*g*. Remove the ultrafiltrate for analysis.
5. Place 40 µL of either the filtered or unfiltered sample into a vial for analysis. Analyze the samples as described in **Subheading 3.1.**
6. **Figure 3** shows a typical electropherogram of a human plasma sample from a healthy volunteer.

3.3.1. Cytokine-Induced NO Production in Cultured Cells

During the inflammatory response in the human joint, cytokines such as IL-1, IL-6, and TNF-α are generated by macrophages and/or fibroblasts *(32–34)*. Some of these cytokines are known to induce iNOS thereby upregulating NO· production. For example, Sakurai et al. *(35)* has shown that NO· production, measured as nitrite levels in the cell supernatant, from freshly isolated synoviocytes can be upregulated by in vitro stimulation with a combination of IL-1, TNF-α, tumor necrosis factor beta (TNF-β), and LPS. Here, a similar system is described using synovial fibroblast-like cells isolated from OA synovial tissue. The cells are stimulated with TNF-α before the cell supernatant is analysed to determine the nitrite and nitrate levels.

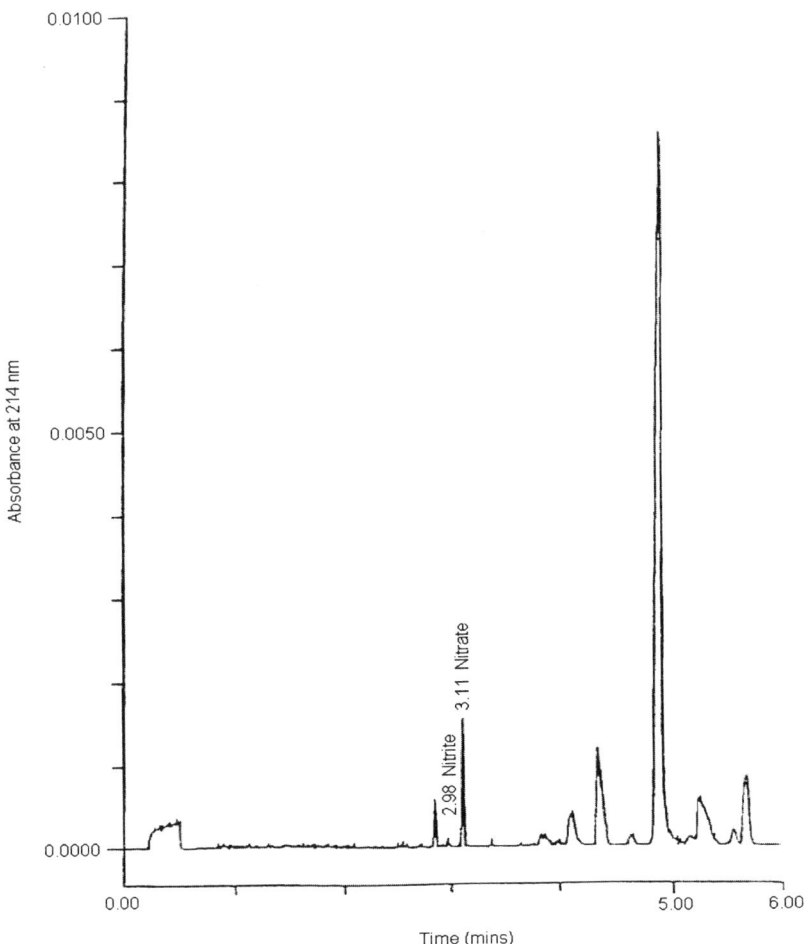

Fig. 3. Typical electropherogram of a human plasma sample from a healthy volunteer. Migration times for nitrite and nitrate were 2.98 and 3.11 min, respectively. Reproduced from *(30)* with permission.

3.3.1.1. Preparation of Synovial Fibroblast-Like Cells

1. To prepare DNase/collagenase solution, add 100 mg collagenase and 3 mg DNase to 20 mL of DMEM, inverse tube until collagenase has dissolved and filter sterilize through a 0.2-μm pore filter.
2. Wash synovial tissue in warm (37°C) DMEM containing 100 U/mL penicillin, 100 μg/mL streptomycin, without FCS (*see* **Note 14**).
3. Mince synovial tissue using sterile scissors.
4. Add the synovial tissue to the DNase/collagenase solution.
5. Incubate at 37°C in shaker for 90 min.

Analysis of Nitrite and Nitrate

6. At the end of this incubation period, add 20 to 30 mL of DMEM containing 10% foetal calf serum, 2 mM L-glutamine, 100 U/mL penicillin, 100 µg/mL streptomycin.
7. Pass the solution through a sterile cell sieve.
8. If the sieve becomes blocked, use the plunger of a 20-mL syringe to remove any undigested tissue.
9. Wash the sieve with DMEM containing 10% FCS, 2 mM L-glutamine, 100 U/mL penicillin, 100 µg/mL streptomycin.
10. Spin solution at 1000g for 10 min at room temperature.
11. Pour off supernatant.
12. Resuspend cell pellet in DMEM containing 10% FCS, 2 mM L-glutamine, 100 U/mL penicillin, 100 µg/mL streptomycin and leave in culture for 2 to 3 d to adhere to flask/plate.

3.3.1.2. STIMULATION OF SYNOVIAL FIBROBLAST-LIKE CELLS

1. Seed synovial fibroblasts-like cells in 24-well plates (1.5-cm diameter) at 10,000 cells/well in DMEM containing 10% FCS, 2 mM L-glutamine, 100 U/mL penicillin, 100 µg/mL streptomycin and leave to adhere overnight.
2. In order for cells to become quiescent, place cells in DMEM containing 0.1% FCS, 2 mM L-glutamine, 100 U/mL penicillin, 100 µg/mL streptomycin for 48 h.
3. Stimulate cells with TNF-α (10 ng/mL to 25 ng/mL) for 24 h in DMEM containing 2 mM L-glutamine, 100 U/mL penicillin, 100 µg/mL streptomycin, without FCS.
4. Remove supernatant, freeze in liquid nitrogen immediately, and store at –70°C until use. Treat the samples as described in **Subheading 3.1**.
5. **Figure 4** shows a typical electropherogram of fibroblast-like cells stimulated with 20 ng/mL TNF-α (*see* **Notes 15** and **16**).

3.3.2. NO• Generation in Hypoxic Inflammatory Tissues by Xanthine Oxidase

Inflamed tissues often become hypoxic reducing the amount of oxygen available to be used by iNOS in the formation of NO•. Instead, Zhang et al. *(19)* and Millar et al. *(20)* have suggested that NO• can be produced by xanthine oxidase via an oxygen independent mechanism. In ischaemic conditions, xanthine oxidase uses NADH to convert nitrite or nitrate to NO•. The CE method described in this chapter is also capable of simultaneously measuring nitrite, nitrate, NAD$^+$ and NADH. In this section we show how this assay has been used to monitor the nitrite, nitrate, NAD$^+$ and NADH levels during the formation of NO• by xanthine oxidase in vitro.

1. Dilute the stock solutions of nitrite, NADH and xanthine oxidase prepared according to **Subheading 2**. Mix together 8.5 µL xanthine oxidase, 100 µL NADH, 40 µL nitrite and 851.5 µL 0.01M PBS solution.
2. Incubate for 20 h at 37°C.

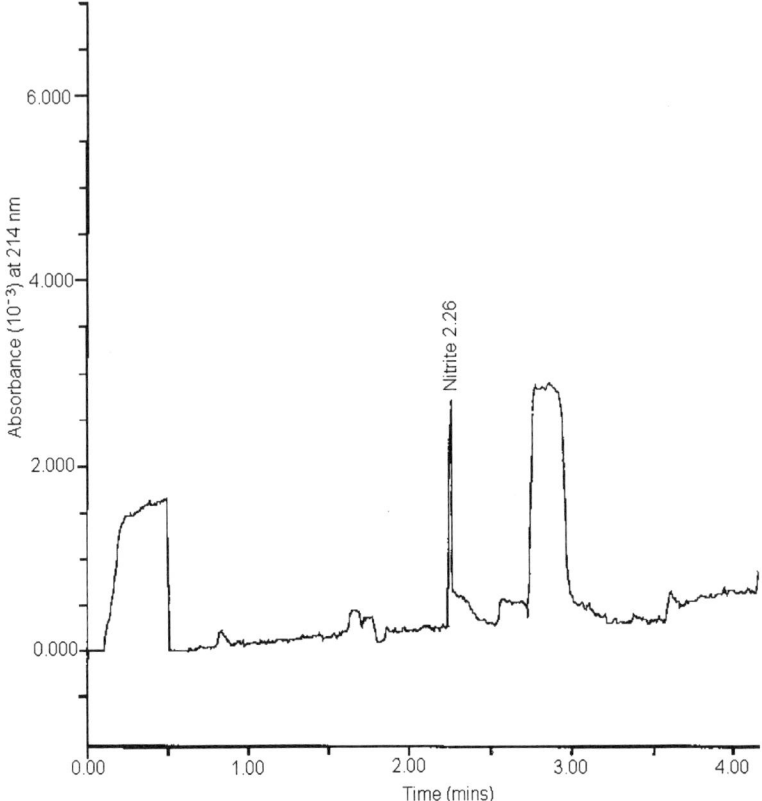

Fig. 4. A typical electropherogram of supernatant from fibroblast-like cells stimulated with 20 ng/mL TNF-α. Migration time for nitrite was 2.26 min.

3. Analyze the samples and controls using the method described in **Subheading 3.1.**, except that a 2-s hydrodynamic injection should be used instead of a 15-s injection (see **Note 17**).
4. Analyze each solution separately to determine the migration time of all the components including nitrate and NAD^+. Prepare a 4-mM nitrate solution by diluting 40 µL of the nitrite stock solution in 1 mL deionized water (see **Fig. 5A**). For 1 mL NAD^+ solution (100 µM) dilute 100 µL in 1 mL 0.01 M PBS solution.
5. In addition to these standards, analyze a solution containing 4 mM nitrite, 4 mM nitrate, 0.115 U xanthine oxidase, 100 µM NAD^+ and 100 µM NADH to determine whether all the components are adequately resolved (see **Fig. 5B**).
6. In order to determine the concentration of NAD^+ and NADH construct a calibration curve by analyzing standard solutions containing 0, 10, 50, 75, 100, 150 µM NAD^+ and NADH (see **Subheading 1.3.**).

Analysis of Nitrite and Nitrate

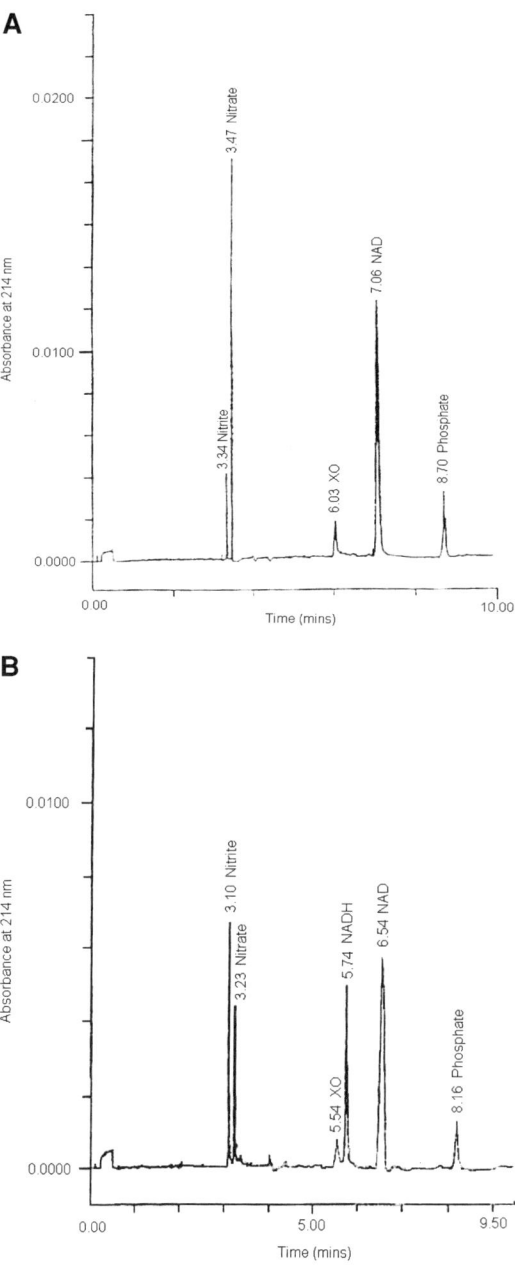

Fig. 5. **(A)** Electropherogram showing the separation between nitrite, nitrate, xanthine oxidase, and NAD$^+$ in one of the samples. Migration times for nitrite, nitrate, xanthine oxidase and NAD$^+$ were 3.34, 3.47, 6.03, and 7.08 mins, respectively. **(B)** Electropherogram showing the separation between nitrite, nitrate, xanthine oxidase,

4. Notes

1. Normally, the negatively charged surface of the fused silica capillaries used in CE attracts positively charged ions, forming a double layer. The cations in the outer layer migrate in the direction of the cathode, carrying water /buffer solution with them. The net flow of the buffer solution in the direction of the negative electrode is known as the electrosomotic flow (EOF). In this method, the EOF is reversed by the addition of TTAB; hence, the anions migrate toward the anode instead of the cathode. The polarity of the electrodes is also reversed so that the positive electrode is connected to the inlet side of the capillary and the negative electrode is connected to the capillary outlet. In combination with TTAB, the reversed polarity causes the migration of the ions to change so that anions are eluted first followed by neutral molecules and cations, respectively.
2. TTAB is an irritant. Care should be taken when handling this chemical and protective clothing should be worn.
3. The TTAB solution is placed through a cation exchange SPE cartridge to exchange the bromide ions present in the TTAB solution for hydroxide ions. In turn, this eliminates a baseline dip seen in the electropherogram, which is caused by the bromide ions present in the CE buffer solution. If this negative peak is not removed, it can interfere with the integration of the nitrite peak in the samples.
4. All the solutions/buffers should be prepared in double deionized water to ensure that background signals from ions in the reagents do not interfere with the assay.
5. Sodium nitrite and sodium nitrate are both flammable. Care should be taken not to expose them to naked flames and they should be stored in a "flammables" cupboard below 40°C, according to the manufacturer's guidelines. They are both harmful if inhaled or swallowed, so care should be taken during handling and protective clothing should be worn.
6. Concentrated sodium hydroxide causes severe burns. Care should be taken at all times and protective clothing should be worn.
7. The PBS tablets used were obtained from Sigma Chemicals Company (Dorset, UK). These tablets gave a solution of 0.01 M phosphate buffer, 0.0027 M potassium chloride, and 0.137 M sodium chloride when dissolved in water according to the manufacturer's instructions.
8. A P/ACE system 5500 equipped with a P/ACE diode array detector was used in combination with a System Gold data station (Beckman Instruments, Beaconsfield, UK). However, the use of a fixed wavelength UV detector would increase the sensitivity of the method.
9. Capillary used was obtained from Beckman Instruments, Beaconsfield, UK or Composite Metals Services, Worcestershire, UK. However, untreated fused silica capillaries from other manufacturers can be used.

Fig. 5 (*continued*) and NAD^+ and NADH in a sample spiked with 2 mM NADH. Migration times for nitrite, nitrate, xanthine oxidase, NAD^+, and NADH were 3.10, 3.23, 5.54, 5.74, and 6.54 min, respectively. Reproduced from *(30)* with permission.

10. It is important to analyze the nitrite and nitrate standard solutions separately so that the migration times of nitrite and nitrate can be determined. Additionally, it is also advisable to analyze a standard solution containing both nitrite and nitrate to confirm that these anions are sufficiently resolved.
11. The method was shown to be precise by the injection of a spiked plasma sample and a standard solution five times. The % relative standard deviation (%RSD) for the spiked plasma and the aqueous standard solutions for nitrite and nitrate were less than 3.0%. The linear regression coefficients for nitrite and nitrate were shown to be above 0.995 demonstrating that the assay was linear. Finally, the limit of detection for nitrite and nitrate was calculated to be 251 nM and 10 nM, respectively, (the limit of detection is generally defined as the concentration at which the signal obtained is three times the height of the noise level).
12. The proportion of nitrite present in a plasma or serum sample is very dependent on the length of time the red blood cells (RBCs) are left in contact with the plasma/serum *(31)*. Oxyhemoglobin present in the RBCs will oxidise nitrite to nitrate (*see* **Subheading 1.**), decreasing the nitrite level and increasing the nitrate concentration. Generally, it is advisable to use plasma and centrifuge the sample immediately after collection to limit the oxidation of nitrite. If collecting serum, the time taken to coagulate the sample before centrifugation should be kept constant between samples, in an attempt to standardize the amount of nitrite oxidized to nitrate. It also should be stressed that comparing nitrite and nitrate concentrations in serum and plasma should be avoided due to the differences in the sampling procedures, and, hence, the nitrite and nitrate levels *(30)*.

    The instability of nitrite in whole blood may explain the differences in the nitrite concentration in healthy human plasma and serum reported in the literature. Some publications have only used nitrite as a marker of NO$^{\bullet}$ production, overlooking its lack of stability in whole blood *(23,24)*. Nitrate measurement may have been avoided in these studies, as dietary intake is known to affect the nitrate concentration to a great extent than nitrite concentration in biological fluids. It is advisable to use both nitrite and nitrate as markers of NO$^{\bullet}$ production.
13. Ultrafiltration of biological and cellular samples is often required to remove proteins, which bind to the capillary. Coating of the capillary in this way causes the migration times to increase gradually. The capillary can be regenerated by rinsing the capillary with 0.1 M sodium hydroxide for 20 min. However, eventually it will be necessary to replace the capillary. In the case of viscous samples, such as synovial fluid, ultrafiltration is highly recommended. Highly viscous samples can affect the injection volume introduced onto the capillary and in some cases they can block the capillary.
14. It is important to prepare DNase/collagenase without FCS, as FCS will inhibit collagenase activity.
15. TNF-α stimulated synovial fibroblast-like cells from OA patients were found to give higher amounts of nitrite when compared to unstimulated cells. In this experiment our data showed that stimulated and unstimulated cells produced 35–40 μM and 20–23 μM, respectively. These levels of nitrite production are also similar

to those reported by Sakurai et al. *(35)* in TNF-α stimulated and unstimulated synoviocytes.
16. Nitrate was not detected in the cell supernatant from the unstimulated or stimulated OA fibroblast-like cells. The lack of haemoglobin in the cell supernatant would prevent NO• or nitrite being converted to nitrate. In this case, nitrate could be generated if the cells also produced superoxide. Under the correct conditions, superoxide could react with the NO• to form peroxynitrite, which would decompose to nitrate.
17. In some systems, it may be necessary to reduce the amount of sample injected onto the capillary, preventing capillary overload, and poor peak shapes. This is important if the concentration of the analytes is known to be well above the limit of detection. For instance, in the in vitro system described in **Subheading 3.3.2.**, a 2-s hydrodynamic injection is used as high concentrations of nitrite and NADH are used.

References

1. Underwood, J. C. E. (1992) *Pathology*. 1st ed. Churchill Livingstone, Edinburgh.
2. Hibbs, Jr, J. B., Taintor, R. R., Vavrin, Z., Rachlin, E. M. (1988) Nitric oxide: a cytotoxic activated macrophage effector molecule. *Biochem. Biophy. Res. Commun.* **157**, 87–94.
3. Nathan, C. F. and Hibbs, Jr., J. B. (1991) Role of nitric oxide synthesis in macrophage antimicrobial activity. *Curr. Opin. Immunol.* **3**, 65–70.
4. Frears, E. R., Zhang, Z., Blake, D. R., O'Connell, J. P., and Winyard, P. G. (1996) Inactivation of tissue inhibitor of metalloproteinase-1 by peroxynitrite. *FEBS Lett.* **381**, 21–24.
5. Rubbo, H., Parthasarathy, S., Barnes, S., Kirk, M., Kalyanaraman, B., and Freeman, B. A. (1995) Nitric oxide inhibition of lipoxygenase-dependent liposome and low-density lipoprotein oxidation: termination of radical chain propagation reactions and formation of nitrogen-containing oxidized lipid derivatives. *Arch. Biochem. Biophys.* **324**, 15–25.
6. Salvemini, D. and Masferrer, J. L. (1996) Interactions of nitric oxide with cyclooxygenase: in vitro, ex vivo, and in vivo studies. *Methods Enzymol.* **269**, 12–25.
7. Maccarrone, M., Corasaniti, M. T., Guerrieri, P., Nistico, G., and Finazzi, A.A. (1996) Nitric oxide-donor compounds inhibit lipoxygenase activity. *Biochem. Biophys. Res. Commun.* **219**, 128–133.
8. McInnes, I. B., Leung, B. P., Field, M., Wei, X. Q., Huang, F. P., Sturrock, R.D., et al. (1996) Production of nitric oxide in the synovial membrane of rheumatoid and osteoarthritis patients. *J. Exp. Med.* **184**, 1519–1524.
9. Connelly, L., Palacios-Callender, M., Ameixa, C., Moncada, S., and Hobbs, A. J. (2001) Biphasic regulation of NF-kappa B activity underlies the pro- and anti-inflammatory actions of nitric oxide. *J. Immunol.* **166**, 3873–3881.
10. Kuo, H. P., Wang, C. H., Huang, K. S., Lin, H. C., Yu, C. T., Liu, C. Y., et al. (2000) Nitric oxide modulates interleukin-1beta and tumor necrosis factor-alpha

synthesis by alveolar macrophages in pulmonary tuberculosis. *Am. J. Respirat. Crit. Care Med.* **161,** 192–199.
11. Katsuyama, K., Shichiri, M., Marumo, F., and Hirata, Y. (1998) NO• inhibits cytokine-induced iNOS expression and NF-kappaB activation by interfering with phosphorylation and degradation of I kappaB-alpha. *Arterioscler. Thromb. Vas. Biol.* **18,** 1796–1802.
12. Peng, H. B., Libby, P., and Liao, J. K. (1995) Induction and stabilization of I kappa B alpha by nitric oxide mediates inhibition of NF-kappa B. *J. Biol. Chem.* **270,** 14,214–14,219.
13. Spiecker, M., Darius, H., Kaboth, K., Hubner, F., and Liao, J. K. (1998) Differential regulation of endothelial cell adhesion molecule expression by nitric oxide donors and antioxidants. *J. Leuko. Biol.* **63,** 732–739.
14. Arnal, J. F., Dinh-Xuan, A. T., Pueyo, M., Darblade, B., and Rami, J. (1999) Endothelium-derived nitric oxide and vascular physiology and pathology. *Cell Mol. Life Sci.* **55,** 1078–1087.
15. Groves, J. T. (1999) Peroxynitrite: reactive, invasive and enigmatic. *Curr. Opin. Chem. Biol.* **3,** 226–235.
16. Feelisch, M. and Stamler, J. S. (1996) *Methods in Nitric Oxide Research.* Wiley, UK.
17. Vallance, P. and Chan, N. (2001) Endothelial function and nitric oxide: clinical relevance. *Heart* **85,** 342–350.
18. Prast, H. and Philippu, A. (2001) Nitric oxide as modulator of neuronal function. *Progress Neurobiol.* **64,** 51–68.
19. Zhang, Z., Naughton, D., Winyard, P. G., Benjamin, N., Blake, D. R., and Symons M. C. (1998) Generation of nitric oxide by a nitrite reductase activity of xanthine oxidase: a potential pathway for nitric oxide formation in the absence of nitric oxide synthase activity. *Biochem. Biophys. Res. Commun.* **249,** 767–772.
20. Millar, T. M., Stevens, C. R., Benjamin, N., Eisenthal, R., Harrison, R., and Blake, D. R. (1998) Xanthine oxidoreductase catalyses the reduction of nitrates and nitrite to nitric oxide under hypoxic conditions. *FEBS Letts.* **427,** 225–228.
21. Halliwell, B. and Gutteridge, J. M. C. (1999) Free radicals in biology and medicine. 3rd ed. Oxford University Press, Oxford.
22. Nazhat, N. B., Saadalla-Nazhat, R. A., Fairburn, K., Jones, P., Blake, D. R., Nielsen, B. R., et al. (1999) Nitrite determination in human plasma and synovial fluid using reation of nitric oxide with 3,5-dibromo-4-nitrosbenzene sulfonate (DBNBS). *Biochim. Biophys. Acta* **1427,** 276–286.
23. Ueki, Y., Miyake, S., Tominaga, Y., and Eguchi, K. (1996) Increased nitric oxide levels in patients with rheumatoid arthritis. *J. Rheumatol.* **23,** 230–236.
24. Farrell, A. J., Blake, D. R., Palmer, R. M., and Moncada, S. (1992) Increased concentrations of nitrite in synovial fluid and serum samples suggest increased nitric oxide synthesis in rheumatic diseases. *Ann. Rheum. Dis.* **51,** 1219–1222.
25. Brundin L., Svenungsson E., Morcos E., Andersson M., Olsson T., Lundberg I., et al. (1998) Central nervous system nitric oxide formation in cerebral systemic lupus erythematosus. *Ann. Neurol.* **44,** 704–706.

26. Giovannoni, G., Land, J. M., Keir, G., Thompson, E. J., and Heales, S. J. (1997) Adaptation of the nitrate reductase and Griess reaction methods for the measurement of serum nitrate plus nitrite levels. *Ann. Clin. Biochem.* **34,** 193–198.
27. El Menyawi, I., Looareesuwan, S., Knapp, S., Thalhammer, F., Stoiser, B., and Burgmann, H. (1998) Measurement of serum nitrite/nitrate concentrations using high-performance liquid chromatography. *J. Chromatog. B., Biomed. Sci. Appl.* **706,** 347–351.
28. Tsikas, D., Gutzki, F. M., Rossa, S., Bauer, H., Neumann, C., Dockendorff, K., et al. (1997) Measurement of nitrite and nitrate in biological fluids by gas chromatography-mass spectrometry and by the Griess assay: problems with the Griess assay-solutions by gas chromatography-mass spectrometry. *Anal. Biochem.* **244,** 208–220.
29. Chung, S. J. and Fung, H. L. (1992) Removal of ammonia interference in the redox chemiluminescence assay of nitric-oxide. *Anal. Lett.* **25,** 2021–2036.
30. Davies, C. A., Perrett, D., Zhang, Z., Nielsen, B. R., Blake, D. R., and Winyard, P. G. (1999) Simultaneous analysis of nitrite, nitrate and the nicotinamide nucleotides by capillary electrophoresis: Application to biochemical studies and human extracellular fluids. *Electrophoresis* **20,** 2111–2117.
31. Moshage, H., Kok, B., Huizenga, J. R., and Jansen, P. L. (1995) Nitrite and nitrate determinations in plasma: a critical evaluation. *Clin. Chem.* **41,** 892–896.
32. Hirano, T., Matsuda, T., Turner, M., Miyasaka, N., Buchan, G., Tang, B., et al. (1988) Excessive production of interleukin 6/B cell stimulatory factor-2 in rheumatoid arthritis. *Eur. J. Immunol.* **18,** 1797–1801.
33. Bergroth, V., Zvanifler, N. J., and Firestein, G. S. (1990) Cytokines in chronic inflammatory arthritis. III. Rheumatoid arthritis monocytes are not usually sensitive to γ-interferon, but have defective γ-interferon-mediated HA-DQ and HLA-DR induction. *Arthr. Rheum.* **32,** 1074–1079.
34. Firestein, G. S., Alvaro-Gracia, J. M., and Maki, M. (1990) Quantitative analysis of cytokine gene expression in rheumatoid arthritis. *J Immunol.* **144,** 3347–3353.
35. Sakurai, H., Kohsaka, H., Liu, M. F, Higashiyama, H., Hirata, Y., Kanno, K., et al. (1995) Nitric oxide production and inducible nitric oxide synthase expression in inflammatory arthritis. *J. Clin. Invest.* **96,** 2357–2363.

33

In Vivo Assays for COX-2

Chi-Chung Chan

1. Introduction

The discovery of two isoforms of the cyclooxygenase (COX) enzyme, COX-1 and COX-2, has provided the rationale for development of selective COX-2 inhibitors as a class of safer drugs for the treatment of pain, symptoms of osteoarthritis and rheumatoid arthritis (*see* reviews *1,2*). Broadly speaking, COX-1 is the constitutive "house-keeping" enzyme responsible for production of prostaglandins (PG) involved in physiological functions such as gastrointestinal cytoprotection and platelet functions. In contrast, COX-2 is rapidly and strongly upregulated upon inflammatory stimuli. COX-2 is the predominant isoform responsible for production of PGs involved in pain, inflammation, and fever. Thus, the therapeutic actions of conventional nonsteroidal antiinflammatory drugs (NSAIDs), which inhibit both COX-1 and COX-2, can be attributed to their inhibition of PG production during inflammation. On the other hand, the dose-limiting gastrointestinal toxicity of NSAIDs can be explained by their inhibitory action on COX-1. It is hypothesized that a selective COX-2 inhibitor will achieve therapeutic efficacy in osteoarthritis, rheumatoid arthritis, and pain management while substantially improved gastrointestinal toxicity profile owing to its COX-2 selectivity. This hypothesis is now supported by an extensive amount of data from preclinical and clinical studies with approved COX-2 inhibitors, such as rofecoxib *(3)* and celecoxib *(4)*, and COX-2 inhibitors currently in development, such as etoricoxib *(5)* and valdecoxib *(6)*. This chapter will describe the in vivo pharmacological assays used in the development of COX-2 inhibitors in general terms, with specific reference to rofecoxib and etoricoxib where applicable.

One of the key objectives in the development of COX-2 inhibitors was to show that these inhibitors have similar efficacy compared to nonselective NSAIDs. In this case, one can use existing NSAID-sensitive models of inflammation, pain, and pyresis. This would include carrageenan-induced paw edema, carrageenan-induced paw hyperalgesia, endotoxin-induced pyresis, and adjuvant-induced arthritis in rats. In the development of rofecoxib and etoricoxib, a nonprimate model of pyresis was developed to examine its efficacy in a nonrodent species *(7)*.

On the gastrointestinal toxicity side, a more rigorous requirement would apply because the goal was to show that COX-2 inhibitors have a significant margin of safety over nonselective NSAIDs. Traditionally, the gastrointestinal effects of NSAIDs were tested in rats by scoring the stomach lesions following acute or chronic dosing. This is sufficient for testing NSAIDs because they induce gastric lesions at efficacious doses. However, this type of measurement proves to be less useful for evaluation of COX-2 inhibitors, which do not induce stomach lesions in rats after chronic dosing for 2–3 wk even at high multiples of their efficacious dose *(3)*. Monitoring the absence of an endpoint would only give a qualitative measure. Thus, a more sensitive assay is needed to distinguish the COX-2 selectivity between COX-2 inhibitors, which can be subtle in some instances. In the development of rofecoxib and etoricoxib, a gastrointestinal permeability assay using ^{51}Cr as a permeability marker was established. Disruption of gastrointestinal integrity, manifested as enhanced gastrointestinal permeability, is amongst the earliest pathological events leading to the development of gastrointestinal lesions. An advantage of the noninvasive ^{51}Cr excretion assay is that it can be adapted to studies in large species such as nonhuman primates, in which case a practical method to monitor the presence of stomach lesions is often limited to gastric endoscopy. Two versions of this assay were developed. Urinary excretion of ^{51}Cr following oral dosing of ^{51}Cr-EDTA was used in rats. ^{51}Cr-EDTA is a complex which is excreted exclusively via the urine after oral dosing. Thus, urinary excretion of ^{51}Cr can be used as an index for gastrointestinal permeability. Alternatively, fecal excretion of ^{51}Cr after intravenous injection of ^{51}CrCl$_3$, which labels plasma proteins, was used in nonhuman primates to measure leakage of protein into the gastrointestinal tract. It should be noted that this type of assay has been used in human subjects to examine the effects of NSAIDs *(8)* and, in fact, rofecoxib *(9)* and etoricoxib *(10)*.

2. Materials
2.1. Models of Inflammation, Pain, and Pyrexia
2.1.1. Carrageenan-Induced Paw Edema in Rats
1. Male Sprague-Dawley rats, 150–200 g
2. Lambda carrageenan type IV (Sigma-Aldrich, catalog # C-3889, Oakville, Ontario) (*see* **Note 1**). A 1% solution in saline is prepared at least 1 wk before use and stored at 4°C.
3. Water displacement plethysmometer (Stoelting, Wood Dale, IL).

2.1.2. Carrageenan-Induced Paw Hyperalgesia in Rats

1. Male Sprague-Dawley rats, 90–110 g (*see* **Note 2**).
2. Lambda carrageenan type IV (Sigma Chem, catalog # C-3889, Oakville, Ontario) (*see* **Note 1**). A 2 % solution in saline is prepared at least 1 wk before use and stored at 4°C.
3. Paw pressure algesiometer (Stoelting).

2.1.3. Endotoxin-Induced Pyrexia in Rats

1. Male Sprague-Dawley rats, 150–200 g.
2. Lipopolysaccharide (LPS) from *Escherichia coli*, (Sigma Chem, catalog # L-2880). A working stock solution (0.9 mg/mL in saline) is prepared fresh on the day of experiment.
3. Thermistor thermometer (Cole-Parmer Labcor, model 8502-12, Anjou, Quebec).

2.1.4. Adjuvant-Induced Arthritis in Rats

1. Female Lewis rats, 150–170 g.
2. *Mycobacterium butyricum* (Fisher, catalog # DF0640-337, Montreal, Quebec). A working stock solution (5 mg/mL) is prepared fresh by grinding the powder in light mineral oil (Sigma Chem, catalog # M-3516) using a mortar and pestle on the day of experiment (*see* **Note 3**)
3. 1 cm^3 Glaspak syringes; 26-gauge precision Glide needles (Becton Dickinson, Franklin Lakes, NJ) (*see* **Note 4**).
4. Ketamine (Ketaset, Ayerst, Guelph, Ontario). Xylazine (Rompun, Bayer, Toronto, Ontario).
5. Mercury displacement plethysmometer (Stoelting).

2.1.5. Endotoxin-Induced Pyrexia in Squirrel Monkeys

1. Squirrel monkeys (*Saimiri sciureus*), 0.8–1.4 kg.
2. LPS from *Salmonella typhosa*, (Sigma Chem, catalog # L-6386). A working stock solution (3 µg/mL) is prepared by serial diluting a stock solution of 1 mg/mL using sterile saline on the day of experiment.
3. Telemetry equipment (all from Data Sciences, St. Paul, MN): temperature probe implants (TA10TA-F40); signal receiver (RLA2000); consolidation matrix (BCM-100); DataQuest Labpro software package.

2.2. Models of Gastrointestinal Permeability

2.2.1. Urinary Excretion of ^{51}Cr-EDTA in Rats

1. Male Sprague-Dawley rats, 300–360 g.
2. ^{51}Cr-EDTA (Draxis Pharmaceutical, Kirkland, Quebec); activity on calibration date: 1 mCi/mL.

2.2.2. Fecal Excretion of ^{51}CrCl$_3$ in Squirrel Monkeys

1. Squirrel monkeys (*Saimiri sciureus*), 0.8–1.4 kg.
2. ^{51}CrCl$_3$ (Draxis Pharmaceutical); activity on calibration date: 1 mCi/mL.

3. Methods
3.1. Models of Inflammation, Pain, and Pyrexia
3.1.1. Carrageenan-Induced Paw Edema in Rats (for additional details, see **Chapter 13**)

1. Rats are housed in a temperature and humidity controlled facility with 12-h light–dark cycle; they are fasted for 16–18 h before use.
2. A test compound or its vehicle are administered to rats at a dosing volume of 10 mL/kg at approx 9:00 AM The treatment groups are then coded to prevent observer bias.
3. One hour later, the paw volume (V_0) of a hind paw is measured using a water-displacement plethysmometer.
4. The hind paw is injected intraplantarly with 50 µL of a 1% carrageenan solution in saline using a 25-gauge needle.
5. Three hours later, the paw volume (V_3) is measured again and the increases in paw volume (V_3–V_0) are calculated. Percentage of inhibition in the treated group is calculated using the volume in the vehicle group as 0% inhibition.

3.1.2. Carrageenan-Induced Paw Hyperalgesia in Rats

1. Rats are housed in a temperature and humidity controlled facility with a 12-h light–dark cycle; they are fasted for 16–18 h before use (*see* **Note 5**).
2. At approx 9:00 AM on the day of the experiment, the response to mechanical compression (R_0) on one hind paw is monitored using an algesiometer. The rats are held such that the hind paw is positioned between a small surface and a blunt pointer on the algesiometer, which applies a force at a constant rate on the paw. Vocalization or paw withdrawal is taken as an end point and the force is noted.
3. Rats are then injected with 4.5 mg (150 µL of a 2% solution) carrageenan intraplantarly using a 25-gauge needle into the hind paw. A group of control rats receive an equivalent volume of saline injection.
4. Two h later, the saline-injected rats are dosed orally with a vehicle at a dosing volume of 10 mL/kg. The carrageenan-injected rats are dosed orally with either a test compound or its vehicle. The treatment groups are then coded to prevent observer bias.
5. One h later (i.e., 3 h after injection of carrageenan), another response to mechanical compression (R_3) on the injected paw was obtained using the procedure described in **step 2**. The difference between R_0 and R_3 is calculated and % hyperalgesia is determined using the value in the vehicle treated group as 0% hyperalgesia.

3.1.3. Endotoxin-Induced Pyrexia in Rats

1. Rats are housed in a temperature and humidity controlled facility with 12-h light–dark cycle; they are fasted for 16–18 h before use.
2. At approx 9:00 AM on the day of the experiment, the rats are placed temporarily in Plexiglas restrainers and their baseline rectal temperature is recorded using a

flexible temperature probe connected a digital thermometer. The same probe and thermometer are used for all animals to reduce experimental error. The rats are returned to their home cages after they are injected intraperitoneally with 2 mL/kg of saline or a 0.9 mg/mL LPS solution (1.8 mg/kg).
3. Five hours after LPS injection, another rectal temperature measurement is taken, followed by oral administration of a test compound or a vehicle. The saline injected rats receive vehicle only. Another temperature measurement is taken 2 h after administration of the test compound. Differences in rectal temperature between the compound-treated or the vehicle-treated group and the saline-injected group are computed. Percentage of inhibition in the compound-treated group is calculated using the value in the vehicle group as 0% inhibition.

3.1.4. Adjuvant-Induced Arthritis in Rats

1. Rats are anesthetized with intramuscular injection of ketamine (30 mg/kg) and xylazine (2 mg/kg). After a state of anesthesia is achieved, a hind paw is injected with 0.1 mL suspension containing 0.5 mg of *Mycobacterium butyricum* in light mineral oil. A group of mice is not injected with adjuvant as negative control.
2. Body weights, paw volume of the injected (primary paw), and the contralateral noninjected (secondary paw) and lateral radiographs under methoxyflurane anesthesia are measured on days 0, 14, and 21 following adjuvant injections. The radiographs are scored in a blinded fashion using a scoring system (*see* **Note 6**).
3. A test compound or a vehicle is given orally everyday throughout the course of the study starting from day 0 post-adjuvant injection (prophylactic protocol). In some cases, the test compound can also be given starting from day 14 post-adjuvant injection, when edema is evident in the secondary paw (therapeutic protocol).
4. All rats are euthanized on day 21 post-adjuvant injection. The end points are paw volumes of the primary and secondary paws, body weight changes, radiographic scores of the secondary paws, thymus, and spleen weights. Percentage of inhibition is calculated comparing the values in the compound-treated group and the vehicle treated group. In general, dose-response curves for % inhibition in paw volume of the primary and secondary paws on days 14 and 21 are constructed and ID_{50} values calculated.

3.1.5. Endotoxin-Induced Pyrexia in Squirrel Monkeys

1. Squirrel monkeys (*Saimiri sciureus*, 0.8–1.2 kg) are surgically implanted with sterilized temperature probes into the peritoneum using standard surgical procedures. These probes can be activated and deactivated by passing a magnet over the abdomen of the animals. The monkeys are allowed to recover from surgery for a minimum of 3 wk before being used for pyrexia studies.
2. On the evening before each experiment, the monkeys are placed individually in cages (24 × 24 × 33 in) in a room with controlled temperature and humidity (*see* **Note 5**). Each cage is equipped with a signal receiver which picks up a radio

signal from the temperature probe. The signal receiver is connected to a microcomputer via a consolidation matrix and the signals from the probe are processed using a software package. This system is able to continuously monitor core temperature in conscious, unrestrained monkeys.

3. At approx 9:00 AM on the day of the experiment, fasted monkeys are restrained temporarily in restraint chairs and are given a bolus injection of LPS at 6 µg/kg via a femoral vein (injection volume: 2 mL/kg). The monkeys are then returned to their cages and body temperature is recorded at regular intervals.
4. Two h after LPS injection, when the body temperature usually raises by 1.5–2°C, a test compound or a vehicle is given orally to the monkeys. Body temperature is monitored for additionally 2 h. Differences in body temperature from pre-LPS injection baseline are calculated at each time-point. Percentage inhibition is computed comparing the vehicle-treated and the compound-treated groups at defined time-points postdosing (*see* **Note 7**).

3.2. Models of Gastrointestinal Permeability

3.2.1. Urinary Excretion of ^{51}Cr-ETDA in rats

1. Rats are fasted for 16–18 h for acute single dose studies and given food *ad libitum* for chronic dosing studies. Immediately after the administration of the last dose of a test compound, each rat is given orally 2 mL of 1% methocel containing 10 µCi of ^{51}Cr-EDTA. The ^{51}Cr-EDTA solution is prepared by adding 10 µL of a stock solution (1 mCi/mL) per 2 mL of the dosing vehicle methocel (1%). Radioactivity of the ^{51}Cr-EDTA solution is determined by counting 100 µL-aliquot samples in quadruplicates.
2. The rats are placed individually in metabolism chambers with food and water *ad libitum*. Urine is collected for a 24-h period (*see* **Note 8**). At the end of the 24-h collection period, the urine volume is recorded and the radioactivity in the urine is determined by counting a 1-mL aliquot (in duplicates). The rats are either euthanised, or returned to their home cages if chronic dosing is continued. In the latter case, another ^{51}Cr-EDTA urinary excretion measurement will be performed after at least a 5-d washout period (*see* **Note 9**).
3. Urinary ^{51}Cr-EDTA excretion during the 24-h collection period is calculated as a percent of total administered ^{51}Cr-EDTA radioactivities.

3.2.2. Fecal Excretion of ^{51}CrCl3 in Squirrel Monkeys

1. Squirrel monkeys are dosed orally with a test compound or a vehicle at a dosing volume of 1 mL/kg for 1 to 5 d. Food and water are allowed *ad libitum*. One hour after administration of the last dose the monkeys are retrained using retrain chairs and ^{51}CrCl$_3$ in sterile saline (1 mL/kg, equivalent to 4–5 µCi per animal) is injected via a saphenous vein. The ^{51}CrCl$_3$ injection solution is prepared by diluting the stock solution (1 mCi/mL) 1:200 using sterile saline. Radioactivity in the ^{51}CrCl$_3$ solution is determined by counting 100 µL-aliquot samples in quadruplicates.

2. The monkeys are then housed individually in metabolism cages and food and water are allowed *ad libitum*. The feces are collected for a 24-hr period and the total radioactivities are determined (all feces are counted) (*see* **Note 9**).
3. ^{51}Cr fecal excretion is calculated as a percent of total injected dose.

4. Notes

1. Carrageenan is a family of linear sulfated polysaccharides obtained from the red seaweed (Irish moss). There are three main branches, named kappa, iota, and lambda carrageenan, which have different gelling properties and protein reactivity. Kappa and iota carrageenan form gels with water whereas lambda does not. Lambda carrageenan is used as a food additive because it interacts with proteins to stabilize a wide range of dairy products. When injected into soft tissues in rodents, lambda, carrageenan induces acute inflammation. It is important to use a preparation rich in lambda carrageenan (but not the other types) in the rat paw edema and hyperalgesia assay.
2. Smaller rats usually have better hyperalgesic responses.
3. Use caution and weigh out *M. butyricum* in a ventilated hood for safety reasons. Prepare the suspension in a safety hood.
4. Unlike the carrageenan assays, plastic syringes cannot be used because the adjuvant suspension (in mineral oil) is very viscous. Use caution during injection.
5. For acclimatization to a new environment (rats and monkeys) and to being housed alone (monkeys), it is preferable to deliver the animals to the laboratory from their home cages the evening before the experiment. The laboratory needs to be put on the same light-dark cycle as the animal housing facilities for that evening.
6. Classification of radiographic scores varies from laboratory to laboratory. The same principle, however, should apply. The scores should reflect the extent of damage to the soft tissues, erosion, osteolysis, periostitis, and alignment.
7. Monkeys are rested for at least 4 wk before use for another study.
8. A layer of mineral oil (0.2 mL) is added to the urine collecting tubes to prevent evaporation.
9. Residual ^{51}Cr levels is completely washed out after 5 d.

Acknowledgment

I thank R. Gordon, L. Xu, M. Panneton, and S. Solyom for their excellent technical assistance; Drs. S. Boyce and D. Visco for their help in the rat paw hyperalgesia assay and rat adjuvant-induced arthritis assay.

References

1. Vane, J. R., Bakhle, Y. S., and Botting, R. M. (1998) Cyclooxygenases 1 and 2. *Ann. Rev. Pharmacol. Toxicol.* **38,** 97–120.
2. Smith, W. L., DeWitt, D. L., and Garavito, R. M. (2000) Cyclooxygenases: structural, cellular and molecular biology. *Ann. Rev. Biochem.* **69,** 145–182.
3. Chan, C.-C., Boyce, S., Brideau, C., Charleson, S., Cromlish, W., Ethier, D., et al.

(1999) (Vioxx™), MK-0966, 4-(4'-methylsulfonyl)-3-phenyl-2-(5H)-furanone): a potent and orally active cyclooxygenase-2 inhibitor - pharmacological and biochemical profiles. *J. Pharmacol. Exp. Ther.* **290**, 551–560.
4. Pennning, T. D., Talley, J. J., Bertenshaw, S. R., Carter, J. S., Collins, P. W., Docter, S., et al. (1997) Synthesis and biological evaluation of the 1, 5-diarylpyrazole class of cyclooxygenase-2 inhibitors: identification of 4-[5-(4-methylphenyl)-3-(trifluoromethyl)-1H-pyrazole-1-yl]benzenesulfonamide (SC-58635, celecoxib). *J. Med. Chem.* **40**, 1347–1365.
5. Riendeau, D., Percival, M. D., Brideau, C., Charleson, S., Dube, D., Ethier, D., et al. (2001) Etoricoxib (MK-0663): Preclinical profile and comparison with other agents that selectively inhibit cyclooxygenase-2. *J. Pharmacol. Expt. Ther.* **296**, 563–571.
6. Talley, J. J., Brown, D.L., Carter, J. S., Graneto, M. J., Koboldt, C. M., Masferrer, J. L., et al. (2000) 4-[5-Methyl-3-phenylisoxazol-4-yl]- benzenesulfonamide, valdecoxib: a potent and selective inhibitor of COX-2. *J. Med. Chem.* **43**, 775–777.
7. Chan, C.-C., Panneton, M., Taylor, A. M., Therien, M., and Rodgers, I. W. (1997) A selective inhibitor of cyclooxygenase-2 reverses endotoxin-induced pyretic responses in non-human primates. *Eur. J. Pharmacol.* **327**, 221–225.
8. Warrington, S. J. Debbas, N. M., Farthing, M., Horton, M., Johnston, A., Thillainayagam, A., et al. (1990) Lornoxicam, indomethacin and placebo: comparison of effects on faecal blood loss and upper gastrointestinal endoscopic appearances in healthy men. *Postgrad. Med. J.* **66**, 622–626.
9. Sigthorsson, G., Crane, R., Simon, T., Hoover, M., Quan, H., Bolognese, J., et al. (2000) Cox-2 inhibition with rofecoxib does not increase intestinal permeability in healthy subjects: a double blind crossover study comparing rofecoxib with placebo and indomethacin. *Gut* **47**, 527–532.
10. Data presented at 2001 Eular conference.

34

Measurement of 8-epi-PGF$_{2\alpha}$ as a Marker of Lipid Peroxidation In Vivo by Immunoaffinity Extraction and Gas Chromatography-Mass Spectrometry

Nitin K. Gopaul and Erik E. Änggård

1. Introduction

Isoprostanes (IPs) are a recently discovered complex group of stable prostaglandin-like molecules formed by the free radical-catalyzed peroxidation of polyunsaturated fatty acids *(1)*. F$_2$-isoprostanes (F$_2$-IPs) are formed by the oxidation of arachidonic acid and can be classified into four major regioisomeric groups, and characterized by a *cis*-oriented side chain *(2)*. Because the majority of arachidonic acid is currently esterified in phospholipids, F$_2$-IPs are initially formed esterified and are subsequently released in the free form following cleavage by phospholipase A$_2$ *(3)*. The presence of F$_2$-IPs in vivo was initially reported by Morrow et al. *(1)*. The levels of one of the abundant isomers, 8-epi-PGF$_{2\alpha}$, was shown to increase by up to 200-fold in established animal models of oxidative injury *(4)*. High levels of F$_2$-IPs can disrupt the physicochemical integrity of cell membranes *(3)*, but more importantly can exert significant pharmacological activity. 8-epi-PGF$_{2\alpha}$ is a potent vasoconstrictor acting on the renal, pulmonary, and retinal vasculatures *(1,5,6)*, modulates platelet aggregation *(7)*, and is involved in the activation of intracellular signaling *(8)*. Isoprostanes can also be formed enzymatically by the cyclooxygenase pathway in platelets, monocytes and vascular smooth muscle *(9–11)*.

The measurement of 8-epi-PGF$_{2\alpha}$ is now recognized as a sensitive and reliable index of lipid peroxidation in vivo. Subjects with Type II diabetes have higher plasma levels of 8-epi-PGF$_{2\alpha}$ compared to healthy controls *(12,13)*. Several studies have reported elevated 8-epi-PGF$_{2\alpha}$ in human diseases associated with increased oxidative stress, including diabetes *(14)*, hypercholesterolemia *(15)*, hepatic cirrhosis *(16)*, Alzheimer's disease *(17)*, and cardiovascular *(18)* and respiratory *(19)* diseases. Dietary supplementation with antioxidants decreases plasma and tissue levels of 8-epi-PGF$_{2\alpha}$ in animal models of diabetes (streptozotocin-diabetic and Zucker obese rats) *(20,21)* and atherosclerosis *(22)*. Similar observations have been made in human studies *(14,15,23)*, which suggests that the measurement of 8-epi-PGF$_{2\alpha}$ can be used for monitoring the effects of antioxidant supplementation.

Existing techniques for the measurement of F$_2$-IPs in biological material include solid-phase extraction (SPE) on octadecylsilane (C$_{18}$), aminopropyl (NH$_2$) and silica cartridges, followed by thin-layer chromatography (TLC) and derivatization, prior to analysis by gas chromatography-mass spectrometry (GC-MS). Although this approach is relatively straightforward, it is time-consuming and the recovery of F$_2$-IPs (normally present in picomolar concentrations) tends to be low, especially when TLC is used. Attempts to increase the recovery of F$_2$-IPs using this technique generally result in the appearance of close-eluting contaminating peaks in the GC-MS chromatograms, because selectivity is usually based on the presence of terminal carboxyl groups. For quantitative determinations, multiple isomers are sometimes measured by comparing the area under several overlapping peaks to that of a single peak derived from a stable isotope-labeled internal standard *(24)*. On the other hand, selective measurement of specific F$_2$-IPs requires a high degree of sample purification (including HPLC) to isolate them from several isomers and endogenous prostaglandins *(25–27)*, and limits the application to small sample numbers.

In this chapter, we describe the use of a rapid semiautomated method based on immunoaffinity extraction and GC-MS for the measurement of 8-epi-PGF$_{2\alpha}$ in plasma, urine, and tissue. Samples are isolated under conditions that minimize the risk for ex vivo oxidation. The isolation of 8-epi-PGF$_{2\alpha}$ from biological material by immunoaffinity extraction is based on the specific interaction between 8-epi-PGF$_{2\alpha}$ and polyclonal anti-8-epi-PGF$_{2\alpha}$ antibodies, prepared by raising antisera against 8-epi-PGF$_{2\alpha}$ *(28)*. Following derivatisation of the immunoextracted material, quantitation of 8-epi-PGF$_{2\alpha}$ is carried out by stable-isotope dilution gas chromatography/negative ion chemical ionisation mass spectrometry, with selected ion recording. Because of its relative simplicity, coupled with automation of the immunoaffinity extraction process and GC-MS, this method can be easily adapted to small experimental setups as well as large-scale clinical intervention trials.

2. Materials
2.1. Blood Collection

1. Trisodium citrate (3.8%, w/v) solution in water. Stored at 4°C for up to 3 mo.
2. Indomethacin (2 m*M*) in 5% (w/v) NaHCO$_3$. Prepare fresh solutions prior to blood collection.
3. Butylated hydroxytoluene (BHT) 5 m*M* in ethanol. Stored at 4°C for up to 1 wk.

2.2. Urine Collection

1. BHT 5 mM in ethanol. Stored at 4°C for up to 1 wk.

2.3. Tissue Collection

1. Chloroform/methanol (2/1, v/v) mixture containing 0.005% (w/v) BHT. Stored at 4°C for up to 3 mo.
2. Sodium chloride solution (0.9%, w/v). Stored at room temperature for up to 3 months.
3. Ethanol containing 0.005% (w/v) BHT. Stored at 4°C for up to 3 months.

2.4. Extraction of 8-epi-PGF$_{2\alpha}$ in Plasma

1. 8-epi-PGF$_{2\alpha}$ and tetradeuterated 3,3',4,4'-[^{2}H$_4$]-8-epi-PGF$_{2\alpha}$ (8-epi-PGF$_{2\alpha}$-d$_4$) (Cayman Chemical Company, Ann Arbor, MI). Dilute each standard separately to 100 pg/µL in ethanol. Stable at –30°C for up to 6 mo.
2. Aqueous potassium hydroxide (1.0 M). Stored at room temperature.
3. Hydrochloric acid (0.1 M). Stored at room temperature.
4. 0.05 M sodium phosphate buffer, pH 7.4: 54 mM Na$_2$HPO$_4$, 13 mM NaH$_2$PO$_4$. Stored at 4°C for up to 3 mo.
5. Immunoaffinity cartridge prepared with an anti-8-epi-PGF$_{2\alpha}$ antiserum as described earlier *(28)*.
6. Acetone/water mixture (95/5, v/v). Stored at room temperature.

2.5. Extraction of 8-epi-PGF$_{2\alpha}$ in Urine

1. 8-epi-PGF$_{2\alpha}$ and tetradeuterated 3,3',4,4'-[^{2}H$_4$]-8-epi-PGF$_{2\alpha}$ (8-epi-PGF$_{2\alpha}$-d$_4$) (Cayman Chemical Company). Dilute each standard separately to 100 pg/µL in ethanol. Stable at –30°C for up to 6 mo.
2. Sodium phosphate buffer (0.05 M, pH 7.4): 54 mM Na$_2$HPO$_4$, 13 mM NaH$_2$PO$_4$. Stored at 4°C for up to 3 months.
3. Immunoaffinity cartridge prepared with an anti-8-epi-PGF$_{2\alpha}$ antiserum as described earlier *(28)*.
4. Acetone/water mixture (95/5, v/v). Stored at room temperature.

2.6. Extraction of 8-epi-PGF$_{2\alpha}$ in Tissue

1. 8-epi-PGF$_{2\alpha}$ and tetradeuterated 3,3',4,4'-[^{2}H$_4$]-8-epi-PGF$_{2\alpha}$ (8-epi-PGF$_{2\alpha}$-d4) (Cayman Chemical Company, Ann Arbor, MI, USA). Dilute each standard separately to 100 pg/µL in ethanol. Stable at –30°C for up to 6 months.
2. Aqueous potassium hydroxide (1.0 M). Stored at room temperature.
3. Hydrochloric acid solutions of 1.0 M and 0.1 M, water with pH adjusted to 2.0 using hydrochloric acid. Stored at room temperature.
4. Sep-Pak octadecylsilane (C$_{18}$, 500 mg) cartridges (Waters, Watford, UK).
5. Methanol, acetonitrile/water (15/85, v/v), hexane/ethyl acetate/propan-2-ol(30/65/5, v/v/v), acetone/water mixture (95/5, v/v). Stored at room temperature.
6. Sodium phosphate buffer (0.05 M, pH 7.4): 54 mM Na$_2$HPO$_4$, 13 mM NaH$_2$PO$_4$. Stored at 4°C for up to 3 mo.

7. Immunoaffinity cartridge prepared with an anti-8-epi-PGF$_{2\alpha}$ antiserum as described earlier *(28)*.

2.7. Derivatization and GC-MS of Extracted 8-epi-PGF$_{2\alpha}$

1. Extracted samples.
2. Pentafluorobenzyl bromide (PFB, 10% in acetone) and *N,N*-di-*iso*propylethylamine (DIPEA, 10% in acetone) (Sigma-Aldrich, Gillingham, UK). Stored at 4°C. PFB is a powerful lachrymator. All manipulations involving this compound should be carried out in a fume hood.
3. *N,O-bis*(trimethylsilyl)-trifluoroacetamide (BSTFA) (Pierce Chemical Company, Rockford, IL). Stored at 4°C.
4. Iso-octane containing 1% BSTFA. Prepare a fresh solution prior to use.

3. Methods
3.1. Sample Collection
3.1.1. Blood Collection and Plasma Preparation

1. Collect blood (5 mL) from the brachial vein in a 10-mL polyethylene tube containing a 3.8% trisodium citrate solution (blood/anticoagulant ratio of 9/1), indomethacin (as cyclooxygenase inhibitor) and BHT (as free radical scavenger) at final concentrations of 14 and 20 µM, respectively.
2. Allow the sample to stand for 30 min at 4°C to enable complete inhibition of cyclooxygenase enzymes.
3. Centrifuge the sample at 1120g for 15 min at 4°C to obtain platelet-poor plasma.
4. Transfer the plasma to a 5-mL polypropylene screw-cap tube and add BHT at a final concentration of 20 µM. Store the sample at −80°C until analysis (*see* **Note 1**).

3.1.2. Urine Collection

1. Collect urine (20 mL) into a graduated conical screw-cap polypropylene tube (50 mL).
2. Add BHT at a final concentration of 20 µM, divide into 4-mL aliquots and store these aliquots in 5-mL polypropylene screw-cap tubes at −80°C until analysis.

3.1.3. Tissue Collection and Preparation

1. Following anesthesia and sacrifice, carefully remove the tissue sample (0.1–0.5 g), quickly dry surfaces on filter paper and record the weight. Immediately immerse in liquid nitrogen for 3–4 min (*see* **Notes 2** and **3**).
2. Transfer the sample to a stainless steel percussion mortar (Biomedix, Pinner, UK) held on dry ice and pulverise rapidly.
3. Transfer the pulverised sample into a 50-mL conical polypropylene screw-cap tube (*see* **Note 4**) and homogenize with a polytron at a medium speed setting for 1–2 min in an ice-cold solution (20 mL) of chloroform/methanol (2/1), containing BHT (0.005%).

Measurement of 8-epi-PGF$_2\alpha$

4. Seal the homogenate under nitrogen and allow to stand for 1 h at room temperature.
5. Add 4 mL of sodium chloride (0.9%) to the homogenate and vortex for 15 s. Stand at room temperature for 5 min.
6. Centrifuge the solution at 1120g for 5 min at room temperature and isolate the chloroform layer (*see* **Note 5**).
7. Evaporate the chloroform under nitrogen at room temperature. Reconstitute the residue in ethanol (1 mL) containing BHT (0.005%) and store at −80°C until analysis. Use an aliquot (0.5 mL) of this reconstituted solution for solid-phase extraction and immunoaffinity extraction of 8-epi-PGF$_{2\alpha}$.

3.2. Extraction of 8-epi-PGF$_{2\alpha}$

3.2.1. Plasma

Plasma samples are subjected to alkaline hydrolysis for the measurement of total (sum of free plus esterified) 8-epi-PGF$_{2\alpha}$.

1. Transfer plasma (0.5 mL) to a glass tube followed by the addition of 8-epi-PGF$_{2\alpha}$-d$_4$ as an internal standard (1 ng in 10 µL of ethanol). Mix gently and stand for 10 min at 4°C to allow complete distribution.
2. Hydrolyze the sample with 1.0 M aqueous potassium hydroxide (0.5 mL) for 30 min at 40°C.
3. Terminate the hydrolysis by addition of 0.1 M hydrochloric acid (4.25 mL) and adjust the pH of the sample to 7.4 using 0.05 M sodium phosphate buffer (4.5 mL) (*see* **Note 6**).
4. Load the sample at 0.5 mL/min on the immunoaffinity cartridge (prepared with an anti-8-epi-PGF$_{2\alpha}$ antiserum), preconditioned with 8 mL sodium phosphate buffer (0.05 M, pH 7.4) (*see* **Note 7**).
5. Wash the cartridge with water (20 mL) to remove nonretained components and elute 8-epi-PGF$_{2\alpha}$ using 5.5 mL acetone/water (95/5) (*see* **Note 8**). Dry the sample under a slow stream of nitrogen at room temperature (*see* **Note 9**).
 For the measurement of free 8-epi-PGF$_{2\alpha}$, hydrolysis of plasma is not required. Plasma (0.5 mL) containing the internal standard 8-epi-PGF$_{2\alpha}$-d$_4$ (1 ng in 10 µL ethanol) is diluted with 0.05 M sodium phosphate buffer (1 mL) and loaded directly on the immunoaffinity cartridge, as in **step 4**.

3.2.2. Urine

1. Transfer urine (4 mL) to a glass tube followed by the addition of 8-epi-PGF$_{2\alpha}$-d$_4$ (1 ng in 10 µL ethanol) as an internal standard, and dilute with 0.05 M sodium phosphate buffer (16 mL) (*see* **Note 10**).
2. Load the sample at 0.5 mL/min on the immunoaffinity cartridge (prepared with an anti-8-epi-PGF$_{2\alpha}$ antiserum), preconditioned with 8 mL sodium phosphate buffer (0.05 M, pH 7.4) (*see* **Note 7**).
3. Wash the cartridge with water (20 mL) to remove nonretained components and elute 8-epi-PGF$_{2\alpha}$ using 5.5 mL acetone/water (95/5) (*see* **Note 8**). Dry the sample under a slow stream of nitrogen at room temperature (*see* **Note 9**).

3.2.3. Tissue

The tissue extract is hydrolyzed and 8-epi-PGF$_{2\alpha}$ is isolated by sequential solid-phase extraction of the hydrolysed sample using i) a commercially available C$_{18}$ cartridge and ii) an immunoaffinity cartridge specific for 8-epi-PGF$_{2\alpha}$.

1. Transfer an aliquot (0.5 mL) of the reconstituted solution into a glass tube and evaporate the solvent under nitrogen at room temperature.
2. Reconstitute the dried residue in ethanol (25 µL) containing BHT (0.005%), followed by the addition of 8-epi-PGF$_{2\alpha}$-d$_4$ (1 ng in 10 µL ethanol) as an internal standard.
3. Hydrolyze the sample with 1.0 M aqueous potassium hydroxide (0.5 mL) for 30 min at 40°C.
4. Terminate the hydrolysis by addition of 1.0 M hydrochloric acid (0.5 mL) and adjust the pH of the sample to 1.5 using 0.1 M hydrochloric acid (2 mL) (*see* **Note 6**).
5. Load the sample at 1.0 mL/min on a Sep-Pak C$_{18}$ cartridge primed with methanol (5 mL), water (5 mL, pH adjusted to 2.0 with hydrochloric acid).
6. Sequentially wash the C$_{18}$ cartridge with 10 mL each, of water (pH 2.0) and acetonitrile/water (15/85).
7. Elute lipids with 5 mL of hexane/ethyl acetate/propan-2-ol (30/65/5) and dry the eluate under nitrogen at room temperature.
8. Reconstitute the dried residue in ethanol (25 µL) containing BHT (0.005%), and dilute to 5 mL with sodium phosphate buffer (0.05 M, pH 7.4).
9. Load the sample at 0.5 mL/min on the immunoaffinity cartridge (prepared with an anti-8-epi-PGF$_{2\alpha}$ antiserum), preconditioned with 8 mL sodium phosphate buffer (0.05 M, pH 7.4) (*see* **Note 7**).
10. Wash the cartridge with water (20 mL) to remove nonretained components and elute 8-epi-PGF$_{2\alpha}$ using 5.5 mL acetone/water (95/5) (*see* **Note 8**). Dry the sample under a slow stream of nitrogen at room temperature (*see* **Note 9**).

3.3. Derivatization

Following immunoaffinity extraction, the sample is first derivatized to a pentafluorobenzyl bromide ester (PFB-ester), then to a trimethylsilyl ether (TMS-ether) before analysis by GC-MS (*see* **Fig. 1**). Formation of the PFB-ester increases the effective surface area for electron capture and chemical ionisation whereas TMS-ether formation increases volatility in the GC (*see* **Note 11**).

1. Add 40 µL of PFB (10% in acetone) and 20 µL of DIPEA (10% in acetone) to the dried sample in a screw-cap vial.
2. Seal the vial with a PTFE-lined cap and incubate at 45°C for 20 min.
3. Stand the sample at room temperature for 5 min then remove the solvent under a gentle stream of nitrogen (*see* **Note 12**).

4. Add BSTFA (50 µL) followed by 5 µL of DIPEA (10% in acetone) to the dried sample.
5. Seal the vial with a PTFE-lined cap and incubate at 45°C for 20 min.
6. Stand the sample at room temperature for 5 min then remove the solvent under a gentle stream of nitrogen (see **Note 12**).
7. Reconstitute the derivatized sample in 20 µL of iso-octane (containing 1% BSTFA) (see **Note 13**).

3.4. GC-MS

GC-MS is carried out in negative ion chemical ionisation (NICI) mode with ammonia as reagent gas, using single ion recording (SIR). The carboxylate anions of the PFB/TMS derivatives of 8-epi-PGF$_{2\alpha}$ and 8-epi-PGF$_{2\alpha}$-d$_4$ (which represent the [M-181]$^-$ species generated by the loss of the PFB group) are monitored at m/z 569 and 573, respectively. The following description applies to the use of a benchtop GC-MS consisting of the Autosystem XL GC (with an autosampler) coupled to a TurboMass MS (Perkin-Elmer, Beaconsfield, UK). Isoprostanes are separated on an SPB-1701 glass capillary column (30 m X 0.25 mm id, 0.25-µm film thickness, Supelco Inc., Bellefonte, PA).

1. Set up the carrier gas (helium) flow to 1.0 mL/min, and the ammonia pressure to 12 psi.
2. Program the GC oven to an initial temperature of 190°C (hold for 1 min following injection), increasing to 300°C at a rate of 15°C/min, with a final hold at 300°C for 5.7 min. The total GC run time is 14 min. The injector (250 °C) is vented 2 min after sample injection. The GC-MS interface is set at 275°C.
3. Set up the MS tuning parameters in negative CI mode as follows. Source page: electron energy, 70 eV; emission current, 503 µA; repeller, 0.7 V; lens 1, 143 V; lens 2, 13 V; source temperature, 150°C. MS: ion energy, 3.3 V; ion energy ramp, 1.0 V; LM resolution, 11.0; HM resolution, 10.4; multiplier, 441 V. Pressures: Pirani, < 1.7e-4 Torr; Penning, 1.4e-4 to 6.0e-4 Torr (see **Note 14**).
4. Programme the MS to operate a solvent delay of 3 min following sample injection, to activate the filament between 9 and 12 min into the run and to operate in SIR mode over this time, using the following settings: function type, SIR of 2 channels; channel mass 1 at 569.20, dwell 0.05 s; channel mass 2 at 573.20, dwell 0.05 s.
5. Inject a derivatised standard solution (4 µL) containing 8-epi-PGF$_{2\alpha}$ (100 pg/µL) and 8-epi-PGF$_{2\alpha}$-d$_4$ (250 pg/µL) to monitor peak retention times and the response (see **Fig. 2**).
6. Inject a solvent blank (4 µL) to remove traces of the standard solution that may have remained.
7. Inject the derivatized sample (4 µL) and record the peak responses. Quantitative determination of 8-epi-PGF$_{2\alpha}$ can be determined by the peak height ratio of 8-epi-PGF$_{2\alpha}$ against the internal standard 8-epi-PGF$_{2\alpha}$-d$_4$ (see **Fig. 3**) (see **Note 15**).

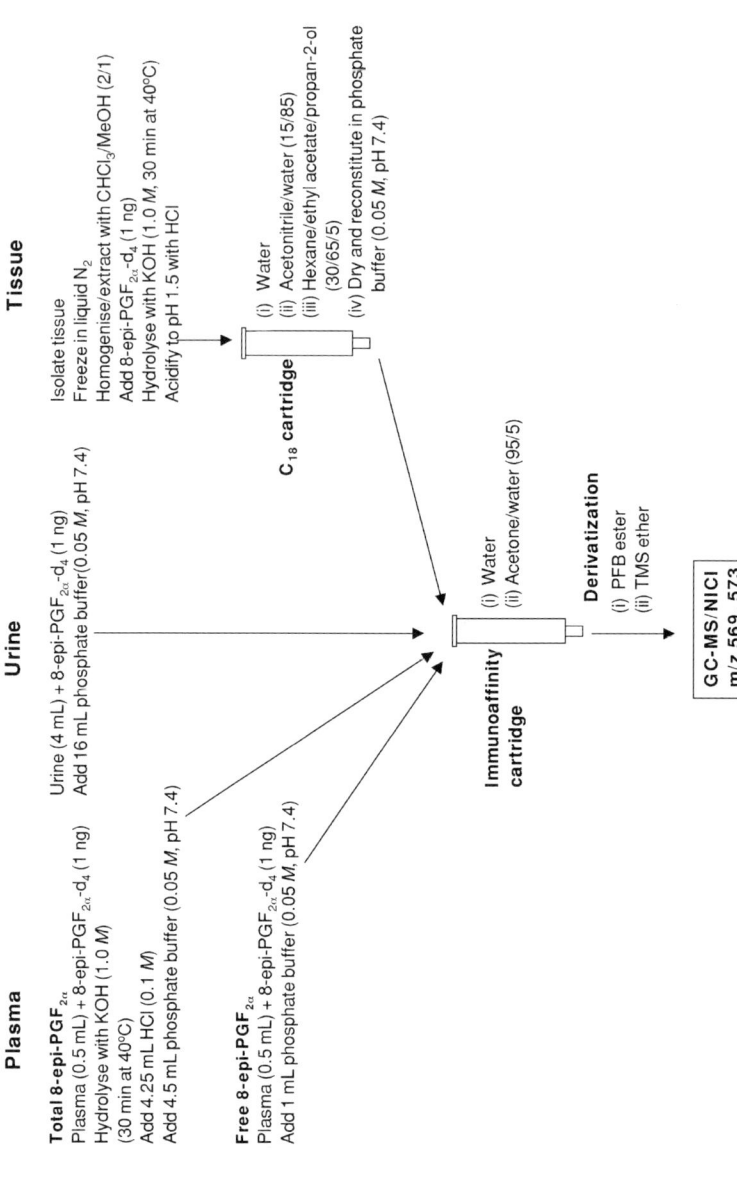

Fig. 1. Sample preparation and immunoaffinity extraction of plasma, urine and tissue for the measurement of 8-epi-PGF$_{2\alpha}$ by GC-MS.

4. Notes

1. Although extended storage of plasma can lead to increased levels of 8-epi-PGF$_{2\alpha}$ as a result of autoxidation *(2)*, the presence of BHT (final concentration in plasma 20 µM) in the sample and storage at –80°C largely minimises this process. In earlier experiments carried out to examine sample collection procedures, we found that the concentrations of 8-epi-PGF$_{2\alpha}$ in plasma processed immediately after blood collection were essentially the same as the levels determined after storage for 6 wk at –70°C *(12)*. It is advisable, however, to analyze plasma samples as soon as possible after collection. The same principle applies to the lipid extracts obtained from tissue following homogenisation and extraction with chloroform/methanol (2/1).
2. In situations where immediate sample analysis is not possible, tissue samples frozen in liquid nitrogen can be transferred to a –80°C freezer for storage.
3. The same approach has been used for the measurement of 8-epi-PGF$_{2\alpha}$ in food samples (vegetables, chicken, meat, and fish). In this case, sample weights ranging between 0.5–2.0 g can be used *(29)*.
4. It is helpful to keep a small spatula (used to transfer the pulverised sample from the mortar to the 50-mL conical tube) on dry ice, because this minimizes adhesion and potential loss of the sample on the surface of the spatula during transfer.
5. The chloroform is present as the lower layer and is separated from the top aqueous layer by a thin disk of undissolved material. The aqueous layer can first be removed by aspirating with a Pasteur pipet. To remove the layer of undissolved material, tilt the conical tube and aspirate carefully. The chloroform can then be transferred to a glass tube with a minimum of contamination from the aqueous phase.
6. The pH of the sample can be verified by using paper pH strips (BDH, Poole, UK) covering a pH range of 1 to 14 and 6–14. If precipitation is observed during modification of the pH, centrifuge the sample at 1000g for 5 min at room temperature and transfer the supernatant to another glass tube before the next step.
7. The immunosorbent, which consists of the purified immunoglobulin G (IgG) fraction from the antiserum coupled to sepharose gel, is suspended in sodium phosphate buffer (0.05 M, pH 7.4) and is placed in an empty standard 1.5-mL column (Varian, Harbor City, CA) fitted with a polyethylene frit at the lower end. The quantity of purified IgG obtained per mL of antiserum generates sufficient immunosorbent for the preparation of about 40 immunoaffinity cartridges.
8. The immunoaffinity steps can be programmed into an ASPEC XL sample processor (Gilson Medical Electronics, Villiers-le-Bel, France) and run automatically. A slow flow rate (0.5 mL/min) is used during loading to allow maximum interaction between 8-epi-PGF$_{2\alpha}$ and the immunosorbent material. Washing and elution steps can be set at higher flow rates (1.0 mL/min).
9. A slow stream of nitrogen at room temperature is sufficient to evaporate the acetone/water (95/5) mixture within half an hour. Increasing the flow of nitrogen causes cooling of the sample and may delay evaporation of the water present. Although slight warming (up to 30°C) can help speed up this step, it is preferable

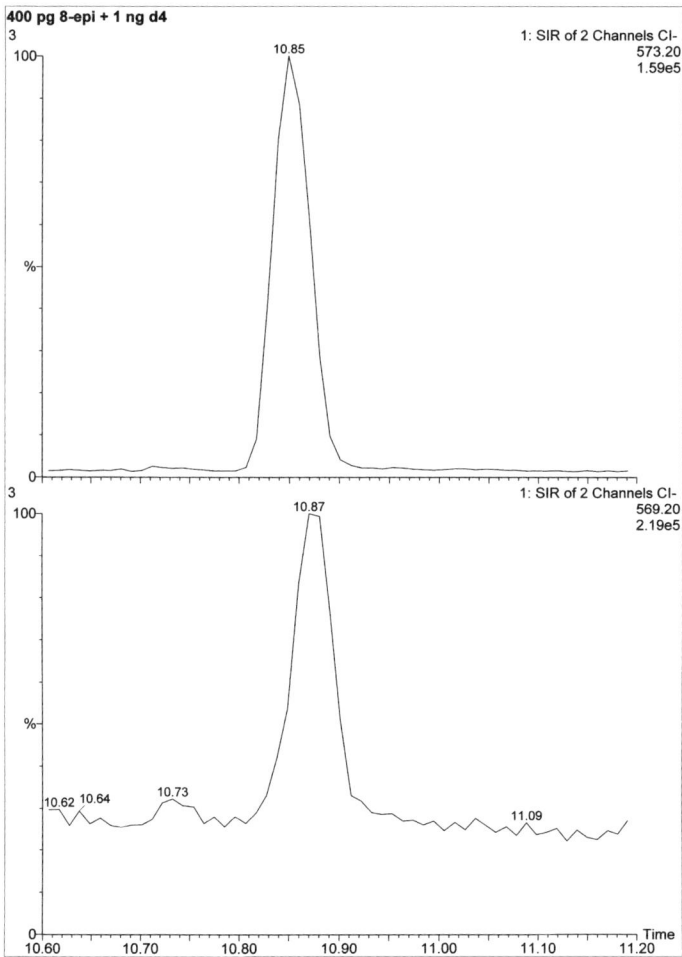

Fig. 2. GC-MS/NICI chromatogram in SIR mode of a standard mixture (injection volume 4 µL) containing 8-epi-PGF$_{2\alpha}$ (100 pg/µL) and 8-epi-PGF$_{2\alpha}$-d$_4$ (250 pg/µL) extracted on an immunoaffinity cartridge and converted to the PFB-ester/TMS-ether derivative. SIR was carried out at m/z 569 for 8-epi-PGF$_{2\alpha}$ (lower chromatogram) and m/z 573 for 8-epi-PGF$_{2\alpha}$-d4 (top chromatogram).

   to avoid heating the sample to minimise the risk of autoxidation. When approx 150–200 µL of sample is left in the glass tube, transfer to a screw-cap vial and continue evaporation until complete dryness.
10. Urine does not normally contain esterified lipids and it is not necessary to hydrolyze the sample prior to extraction of 8-epi-PGF$_{2\alpha}$.
11. It is essential that the sample is completely dry before derivatization, since the presence of moisture will prevent completion of the reactions involved.

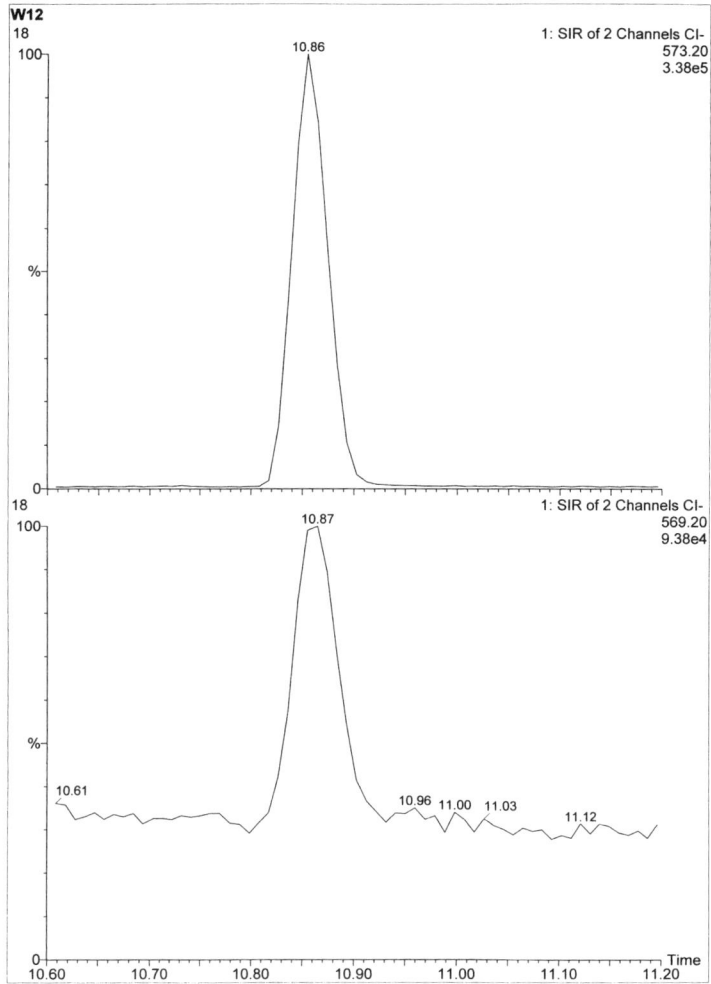

Fig. 3. GC-MS/NICI chromatogram in SIR mode of a plasma sample. Plasma (0.5 mL), to which 8-epi-PGF$_{2\alpha}$-d$_4$ (1 ng) was added, was extracted on an immunoaffinity cartridge and the final eluate converted to the PFB-ester/TMS-ether derivative. SIR was carried out at m/z 569 for 8-epi-PGF$_{2\alpha}$ (lower chromatogram) and m/z 573 for 8-epi-PGF$_{2\alpha}$-d$_4$ (top chromatogram). Quantitative determination of 8-epi-PGF$_{2\alpha}$ is determined by the peak height ratio of 8-epi-PGF$_{2\alpha}$ against the internal standard.

12. Heating of the sealed vial during the derivatization step causes the solvent pressure inside the vial to increase. Although the 5-min cooling period is intended to reduce the pressure, it is still advisable to turn the vial opening away from the operator while removing the screw-cap. Lowering the fume hood sash provides additional protection during this step.

13. Although derivatized standards (8-epi-PGF$_{2\alpha}$ and 8-epi-PGF$_{2\alpha}$-d$_4$) can be stored at –20°C for up to 2 mo without any significant degradation, derivatized extracts of biological sources are less stable and it is advisable to analyse the samples as soon as possible.
14. It is important to adjust the ammonia pressure (using the needle valve) to give a reading on the Penning gauge between 1.4e-4 and 6.0e-4 Torr. Ammonia pressures below or above this range decrease the efficiency of the chemical ionisation and result in a loss of signal at both m/z 569 and 573.
15. The recovery of 8-epi-PGF$_{2\alpha}$ using the immunoaffinity extraction procedure is 90–95%. The GC-MS assay has a limit of detection of about 10 pg/mL in plasma, with intra- and interassay coefficients of variation of 4.4 and 7.6%, respectively (determined at 50 pg/mL of 8-epi-PGF$_{2\alpha}$). Normal plasma concentrations of total 8-epi-PGF$_{2\alpha}$ from healthy individuals ($n = 9$) have been found in the range of 276–375 pg/mL (310 ± 9 pg/mL, mean ± SD; CV 2.9%) *(30)*. Five samples (4 mL, each) from the same human urine pool (without addition of 8-epi-PGF$_{2\alpha}$) were extracted, giving an average concentration of 125 ± 5 pg/mL (CV 4%).
16. Plasma 8-epi-PGF$_{2\alpha}$ concentration is normally expressed in pg/mL or p*M*. Alternatively, this can be normalized to the plasma arachidonic acid concentration, which is the precursor of 8-epi-PGF$_{2\alpha}$ *(30)*. Urinary 8-epi-PGF$_{2\alpha}$ concentration can be expressed in pg/mL or pg/mg creatinine (urinary creatinine is measured by a standard colorimetric method). Tissue 8-epi-PGF$_{2\alpha}$ is expressed in pg/g tissue and can be normalized to the tissue arachidonic acid.
17. The immunoaffinity cartridge can be regenerated following elution of the sample, by washing sequentially with 5 mL acetone/water (95/5), water (10 mL), and 10 mL sodium phosphate buffer (0.05 *M*, pH 7.4). This procedure enables the cartridge to be used approx 5 times.

References

1. Morrow, J. D., Hill, K. E., Burk, R. E., Nammour, T. M., Badr, K. F., and Roberts, L. J. II (1990) A series of prostaglandin F$_2$-like compounds are produced in vivo in humans by a non-cyclooxygenase, free radical-catalysed mechanism. *Proc. Natl. Acad. Sci. USA* **87,** 9383–9387.
2. Morrow, J. D., Harris, T. M., and Roberts, L. J. II (1990) Noncyclooxygenase oxidative formation of a series of novel prostaglandins: analytical ramifications for measurement of eicosanoids. *Anal. Biochem.* **184,** 1–10.
3. Morrow, J. D., Awad, J. A., Boss, H. J., Blair, I. A., and Roberts, L. J. II (1992) Noncyclooxygenase-derived prostanoids (F$_2$-isoprostanes) are formed in situ on phospholipids. *Proc. Natl. Acad. Sci. USA* **89,** 10,721–10,725.
4. Awad, J. A., Morrow, J. D., Hill, K. E., Roberts, L. J. II, and Burk, R. F. (1994) Detection and localization of lipid peroxidation in selenium and vitamin E-deficient rats using F$_2$-isoprostanes. *J. Nutr.* **124,** 810–816.
5. Banerjee, M., Kang, K. H., Morrow, J. D., Roberts, L. J. II, and Newman, J. H. (1992) Effects of a novel prostaglandin, 8-epi-PGF$_{2\alpha}$, in rabbit lung in situ. *Am. J. Physiol.* **263,** H660–H663.

6. Lahaie, I., Hardy, P., Hou, X., Hassessian, H., Asselin, P., Lachapelle, P., et al. (1998) A novel mechanism for vasoconstrictor action of 8-isoprostaglandin-$F_{2\alpha}$ on retinal vessels. *Am. J. Physiol.* **274**, R1406–R1416.
7. Pratico, D., Smyth, E. M., Violi, F., and FitzGerald, G. A. (1996) Local amplification of platelet function by 8-epi-$PGF_{2\alpha}$ is not mediated by thromboxane receptor isoforms. *J. Biol. Chem.* **271**, 14,916–14,924.
8. Kunapuli, P., Lawson, J. A., Rokach, J. A., Meinkoth, J. L., and FitzGerald, G. A. (1998) Prostaglandin $F_{2\alpha}$ and the isoprostane 8,12-iso-isoprostane $F_{2\alpha}$-III, induce cardiomyocyte hypertrophy: differential activation of downstream signaling pathways. *J. Biol. Chem.* **273**, 22,442–22,452.
9. Pratico, D., Lawson, J. A., and FitzGerald, G. A. (1995) Cyclooxygenase-dependent formation of the isoprostane, 8-epi prostaglandin $F_{2\alpha}$. *J. Biol. Chem.* **270**, 9800–9808.
10. Pratico, D. and FitzGerald, G. A. (1996) Generation of 8-epiprostaglandin $F_{2\alpha}$ by human monocytes: discriminate production by reactive oxygen species and prostaglandin endoperoxide synthase-2. *J. Biol. Chem.* **271**, 8919–8934.
11. Jourdan, K. B., Mitchell, J. A., and Evans, T. W. (1997) Release of isoprostanes by human pulmonary artery in organ culture: a cyclo-oxygenase and nitric oxide dependent pathway. *Biochem. Biophys. Res. Commun.* **233**, 668–672.
12. Gopaul, N. K., Änggård, E. E., Mallet, A. I., Betteridge, D. J., Wolff, S. P., and Nourooz-Zadeh, J. (1995) Plasma 8-epi-$PGF_{2\alpha}$ levels are elevated in individuals with non-insulin dependent diabetes mellitus. *FEBS Lett.* **368**, 225–229.
13. Gopaul, N. K., Manraj, M. D., Hébé, A., Lee Kwai Yan, S., Johnston, A., Carrier, M. J., et al. (2001) Oxidative stress could precede endothelial dysfunction and insulin resistance in Indian Mauritians with impaired glucose metabolism. *Diabetologia* **44**, 706–712.
14. Davi, G., Ciabattoni, G., Consoli, A., Mezzetti, A., Falco, A., Santarone, S., et al. (1999) In vivo formation of 8-iso-prostaglandin $F_{2\alpha}$ and platelet activation in diabetes mellitus: effects of improved metabolic control and vitamin E supplementation. *Circulation* **99**, 224–229.
15. Davi, G., Alessandrini, P., Mezzetti, A., Minotti, G., Bucciarelli, T., Constantini, F., et al. (1997) In vivo formation of 8-epi-prostaglandin $F_{2\alpha}$ is increased in hypercholesterolemia. *Arterioscler. Thromb. Vasc. Biol.* **17**, 3230–3235.
16. Pratico, D., Iuliano, L., Basili, S., Ferro, D., Camastra, C., Cordova, C., et al. (1998) Enhanced lipid peroxidation in hepatic cirrhosis. *J. Invest. Med.* **46**, 51–57.
17. Pratico, D., Lee, V. M. Y., Trojanowski, J. Q., Rokach, J., and FitzGerald, G. A. (1998) Increased F_2-isoprostanes in Alzheimer's disease: Evidence of enhanced lipid peroxidation *in vivo*. *FASEB J.* **12**, 1777–1783.
18. Delanty, N., Reilly, M., Pratico, D., Lawson, J. A., McCarthy, J. F., Wood, A. E., et al. (1997) 8-epi-$PGF_{2\alpha}$ generation during coronary reperfusion: A potential quantitative marker of oxidant stress *in vivo*. *Circulation* **95**, 2492–2499.
19. Reilly, M., Pratico, D., Lanken, P., Delanty, N., Rokach, J., Lawson, J. A., et al. (1998) Isoprostanes in the assessment of oxidant stress in vivo, in *Molecular and Cellular Basis of Inflammation* (Serhan, C. N. and Ward, P. A., eds.), Humana, Totowa, NJ, pp. 127–139.

20. Palmer, A. M., Thomas, C. R., Gopaul, N. K., Dhir, S., Änggård, E. E., Poston, L., et al. (1998) Dietary antioxidant supplementation reduces lipid peroxidation but impairs vascular function in small mesenteric arteries of the streptozotocin-diabetic rat. *Diabetologia* **41,** 148–156.
21. Laight, D. W., Desai, K. M., Gopaul, N. K., Änggård, E. E., and Carrier, M. J. (1999) F_2-isoprostane evidence of oxidant stress in the insulin resistant, obese Zucker rat: effects of vitamin E. *Eur. J. Pharmacol.* **377,** 89–92.
22. Kengatharan, M., Gopaul, N. K., Dhir, S., Pettersson, K., Carrier, M., and Änggård, E. E. (1997) Inhibition of 8-epi-prostaglandin $F_{2\alpha}$ production by vitamin E is associated with the reversal of endothelial dysfunction in the cholesterol-fed rabbit. *Br. J. Pharmacol.* **122(SS),** P155.
23. Chowienczyk, P. J., Brett, S. E., Gopaul, N. K., Meeking, D., Marchetti, M., Russell-Jones, D. L., et al. (2000) Oral treatment with an antioxidant (raxofelast) reduces oxidative stress and improves endothelial function in men with Type II diabetes. *Diabetologia* **43,** 974–977.
24. Morrow, J. D., Frei, B., Longmire, A. W., Gaziano, J. M., Lynch, S. M., Stauss, W. E., et al. (1995) Increase in circulating products of lipid peroxidation (F_2-isoprostanes) in smokers. Smoking as a cause of oxidative damage. *N. Engl. J. Med.* **332,** 1198–1203.
25. Wendelborn, D. F., Morrow, J. D., and Roberts, L. J. II (1990) Quantification of $9\alpha,11\beta$-prostaglandin F_2 by stable isotope dilution mass spectrometric assay. *Methods. Enzymol.* **187,** 51–62.
26. Li, W., Lawson, J. A., Reilly, M., Rokach, J., and FitzGerald, G. A. (1999) Quantitative analysis of F_2-isoprostanes by HPLC/tandem mass spectrometry. *Proc. Natl. Acad. Sci. USA* **96,** 13,381–13,386.
27. Mori, T. A., Croft, K. D., Puddey, I. B., and Beilin, L. J. (1999) An improved method for the measurement of urinary and plasma F_2-isoprostanes using gas chromatography mass spectrometry. *Anal. Biochem.* **268,** 117–125.
28. Bachi, A., Zuccato, E., Baraldi, M., Fanelli, R., and Chiabrando, C. (1996) Measurement of urinary 8-epi-prostaglandin $F_{2\alpha}$, a novel index of lipid peroxidation in vivo, by immunoaffinity extraction/gas chromatography - mass spectrometry. Basal levels in smokers and nonsmokers. *Free Rad. Biol. Med.* **20,** 619–624.
29. Gopaul, N. K., Halliwell, B., and Änggård, E. E. (2000) Measurement of plasma F_2-isoprostanes as an index of lipid peroxidation does not appear to be confounded by diet. *Free Rad. Res.* **33,** 115–127.
30. Gopaul, N. K., Zacharowski, K., Halliwell, B., and Änggård, E. E. (2000) Evaluation of the postprandial effects of a fast-food meal on human plasma F_2-isoprostane levels. *Free Rad. Biol. Med.* **28,** 806–814.

35

Laboratory Assessment of the Acute Phase Response

Using CRP as a Model

Robert F. Ritchie and Thomas B. Ledue

1. Introduction

Assessing whether an acute phase response (APR) is present or not presents a complex problem to clinicians and researchers. Part of this complexity is the nature of the process itself. As a result, choosing what method to use is crucial and fraught with pitfalls. Increasingly evident is the fact that the APR is constantly present in all creatures. The problem then is, what level of the APR are we proposing to investigate? The answer to this, a decade or so ago, was easily decided by the relative insensitivity of the assays then available; we simply could not detect low levels of the markers of inflammation. In the last few years, however, C-reactive protein (CRP) assays of increasing sensitivity have shown that, in fact, the continuum of CRP values extends essentially to zero and we are able to assay down to these extremely low levels with assurance. As a result, we again have to face the decision of what constitutes a significant level of inflammation; what is the clinical cut-point? Recent information indicates that even low levels of inflammation, as assessed by sensitive assays, can provide information relevant to specific and serious disease. In other words, there would appear that there is no level of APR which does not place us at some risk for illness. Although this represents a major contribution to our level of understanding, remaining is our inability to specify where this low level process exists; cystitis, gingivitis, bronchitis, post-exercise inflammation, early malignancy, or evolving coronary artery disease.

Part of the search for evidence of an APR includes the question of which assay should be used and for which analyte. Complexity once more appears. Many, if not most serum proteins, are upregulated and/or downregulated by a variety of often coincident physiologic processes. For example, the drive that increases acute phase protein synthesis, the family of cytokines, can also be blunted by a variety of therapeutic agents as are the protein levels themselves. As noted, both increases and decreases can, and often do, occur coincidentally. An inflammatory response fortunately can be modified by antiinflammatory medication. Further complication arises when we realize that each acute phase protein responds differently in time; some rapidly and to a marked degree, others slowly and much less dramatically. Although this appears to be confusing, it also provides a mechanism to evaluate the timing of an APR. Frequently, the onset of an APR is unknown to the patient or the physician. Such information is of immediate interest in medical care. For example, the rapid and dramatic response of CRP (3 log) within hours will fade to low levels after 2 or 3 d, unless the process becomes chronic. Another protein, α_1-antitrypsin, rises during the first to second day and remains two- to fivefold increased for several more days. Still others are delayed in response for several more days and remain elevated longer. Careful evaluation of the results of acute phase protein measurements can, as a result, provide information on the timing of a strong APR. For low level responses, many confounding factors make this unrealistic.

The decision of which analyte to measure is critical whatever the basic question. Furthermore, the cost and ease of testing becomes an issue. And finally, what is the level of knowledge in the user population; the care-givers? Traditionally, and without highly skilled laboratory expertise, the simple, office run, little equipment needed, erythrocyte sedimentation rate (ESR) answered the bill. It has gone out of vogue replaced by simple assays for the most classical of acute phase proteins, CRP. Initially, CRP was measured in a glass capillary tube where agglutination with antisera coated latex particles produced a visible precipitate. This procedure, like the ESR, was inexpensive, but unfortunately was also imprecise and insensitive. Immunoprecipitin tests performed in optical instruments followed. At first these were apparently ideal, but limited to serum concentrations above 20 mg/L (*see* **Fig. 1**). Below this, results were essentially meaningless. Pressure to provide accuracy below 20 mg/L provided incentive to design more sensitive assays. Ultimately the particle enhanced, high sensitivity CRP assay (hs-CRP) came onto the market. Measured levels to tenths of a mg/L are commonplace, but as careful examination has shown, these assays are not without problems.

Once an analyte has been selected, a reference preparation found, and a satisfactory assay chosen that meets rigorous scrutiny, the user is faced with the task of understanding what the results will mean when applied to the study

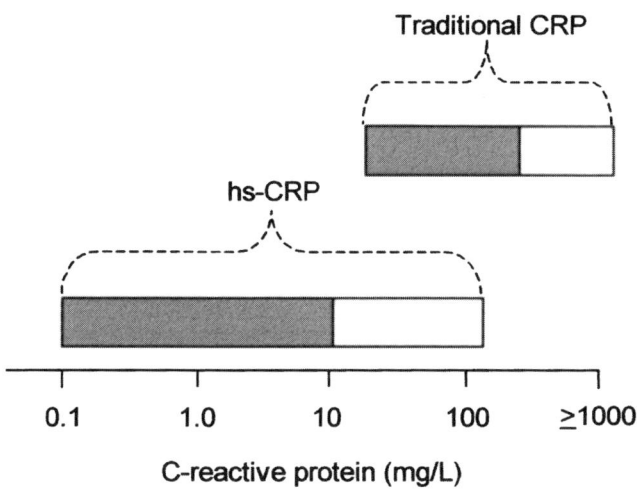

Fig. 1. Representative comparison of dynamic ranges for high sensitivity CRP (particle-enhanced) with a traditional (non-enhanced) light-scattering immunoassay. The shaded zone represents the assay's default measurement range and the clear zone corresponds to the extended assay range achieved by additional dilution(s).

cohort. Part of this understanding addresses what is considered normal ranges for our population, male or female, and over a lifetime. This becomes particularly important to a high sensitivity assay for CRP, which is affected by ubiquitous circumstances. The recent information that CRP levels in obese individuals are significantly higher than in persons of normal weight casts a shadow over this assay. It suggests that in addition to the age and sex being recorded, the height and weight becomes a factor in deciding what a value means.

The basic reason for performing a test for an acute phase protein such as CRP is to discover if an infection or inflammatory reaction exists, where, and if so, to what extent. Furthermore, clinical issues such as fever, swelling, localized pain, shortness of breath, delirium in the elderly, poor condition of a newborn, premature rupture of the membranes and following surgery, trauma or invasive procedures simplify the process by providing a focus. Several classical hallmarks that describe the APR may be completely absent. The need for sensitive assays is simply based on the fact that the absence of characteristic features gives the false impression than an infection does not exist. The elderly and the newborn are especially unresponsive and the laboratory can often provide the only evidence of an APR.

Understanding what the results will mean requires knowledge of what medications the subject is taking and detailed knowledge of the patient's general health status.

1.1. Methodology

Selecting a method for CRP analysis is not an easy task. Numerous assays are available including latex agglutination, radial immunodiffusion, electroimmunodiffusion, radioimmunoassay, enzyme immunoassay, fluorescent immunoassay, immunonephelometry, and immunoturbidimetry. Presently, there are more than 30 qualitative and 12 quantitative immunoassays that are approved for in vitro diagnostic use. Among the quantitative techniques, nephelometry and turbidimetry are the most commonly employed and account for nearly 97% of laboratories participating in the 2000 College of American Pathologists (CAP) proficiency program. However, because each laboratory, whether hospital, commercial, or physician office has different needs, the final choice of an instrument will undoubtedly reflect technical, clinical, environmental, and financial considerations. Fortunately, there are numerous resources available to assist one in the selection process. Annual publications such as *CAP Today* provide comparative summaries in tabular format of current instrument systems and is an excellent starting point. Additional resources include journal articles, talking with other laboratorians, as well as reviewing results from external quality assurance programs.

Despite their popularity, most (non-enhanced) nephelometric and turbidimetric immunoassays for CRP suffer from poor precision at low concentrations. Data from CAP survey respondents reveal that among-manufacturer CVs ranged from 30–60% at CRP concentrations <6 mg/L *(1)*. At CRP concentrations >20 mg/L, among-manufacturer CVs were generally <20%. Similar findings have been observed in external quality assurance schemes in the United Kingdom and Belgium *(2,3)*. In addition, most of these assays have a practical lower detection limit around 10 mg/L—a level that has been widely used as an indicator of a subclinical infection or inflammation *(4–6)* and one that is well above the normal adult reference range. Poor sensitivity notwithstanding, most of these assays are sufficient for traditional applications as a marker of occult infection, inflammation, or tissue necrosis (*see* **Table 1**).

There is substantial evidence in the literature that CRP concentration within the reference range can provide valuable information of existing inflammation. In neonates, for example, baseline CRP values are typically very low, and even significant increases as a result of infection may not be detectable with traditional assays *(7,8)*. More recently, numerous prospective risk studies have demonstrated that baseline CRP, at concentrations in the normal reference range, is an independent predictor of future cardiovascular disease in apparently healthy men and women *(9–13)*. In direct comparisons with traditional and novel biomarkers of coronary heart disease risk, CRP was the single strongest predictor of future coronary events. As aforementioned, however, the lack

Table 1
Conditions Associated with Modulating CRP Concentration

Increased levels
    Acute phase response   Malignancies with widespread metastases
    Bacterial and fungal infections   Crohn's disease
    Rheumatic fever   Ulcerative colitis
    Active rheumatoid arthritis   Renal transplant failure
    Vascular disorders   Early pregnancy
    Myocardial infarction   Intrauterine devices
Decreased levels
    Infancy
    Antiinflammatory therapy
    No known deficiency states described

Table 2
Physiologic Factors Known to Influence CRP Concentration

Race
Age and gender
Time of year
Lifestyle (smoking, obesity, alcohol, rigorous exercise)
Medications (oral contraceptives, hormone replacement
therapy, statins, aspirin, antibiotics)

of adequate precision and sensitivity at low levels of CRP (10 mg/L), virtually preclude the use of traditional (non-enhanced) assays for atherosclerotic cardiovascular disease risk assessment *(1)*. Consequently, more than half a dozen manufacturers have recently introduced hs-CRP assays *(14,15)*. Despite the improved sensitivity of these new tests, numerous clinical and laboratory issues need to be confirmed or clarified before widespread screening of the general population can be recommended *(15–17)*.

Preanalytical considerations. As with most laboratory tests, multiple variables may affect the results for a patient from whom a specimen has been collected for CRP measurement (*see* **Table 2**). Indeed, the subject of preanalytic effects on laboratory results has been the focus of two widely referenced books *(18,19)*. Aside from some of the non-modifiable variables (e.g., age, gender, race, and so on) are issues related to specimen collection (fasting vs non-fasting, specimen type, sample handling, and biological variability). For additional information the reader is referred elsewhere *(17,20)*. The protocol described later is for the measurement of non-enhanced C-reactive protein by immunoturbidimetry.

Table 3
Preparation of the CRP Calibration Curve

	Standard 6 120 mg/L	Standard 5 90 mg/L	Standard 4 60 mg/L	Standard 3 30 mg/L	Standard 2 15 mg/L	Standard 1 7.5 mg/L
4% PEG-PBS (mL)	1.000	1.000	1.000	1.000	2.000	1.000
Calibrator 7 (mL)	0.250	0.176	0.111	0.052	0.052	Add 1.00 mL of Standard 2

2. Materials

1. Goat antihuman CRP-IgG fraction from DiaSorin (Stillwater, MN) (*see* **Note 1**).
2. Diluent: 0.01 M phosphate-buffered saline (PBS), consisting of 8 g/L sodium chloride, 1.39 g/L sodium dibasic anhydrous, 0.24 g/L sodium monobasic, adjusted to pH 7.4 with 1 M NaOH or 1 M HCl.
3. Buffer: PBS containing 40 g/L polyethylene glycol (PEG 8000) (*see* **Note 2**).
4. Calibrator 7 and Controls from DiaSorin. Values ascribed to these materials are traceable to the Certified Reference Material 470 (*see* **Note 3**).
5. Patient samples: Serum should be obtained aseptically by venipuncture. Allow blood to clot at room temperature; rim clot with an applicator stick, if necessary, and centrifuge for at least 10 min at approx 3000 rpm. Aspirate at least 0.5 mL of cell-free serum promptly to avoid excess hemolysis.
6. Variable pipets (5 to 1000 µL) and associated tips.
7. Spectrophotometer or a programmable turbidimeter.

3. Methods

1. Dilute the CRP antiserum 1:31 in 4% PEG-PBS buffer (1 mL of antiserum is sufficient for 155 determinations). Allow the reagent to incubate at room temperature for 1 h, then filter through a 0.22-µm filter.
2. Prepare a 6-point CRP calibration curve according to **Table 3**.
3. Dilute patient samples and controls 1:5 in 4% PEG-PBS buffer, mix thoroughly and incubate for 15 min at room temperature. Centrifuge the standards, controls, and patient samples for 5 min at a minimum of 3000 rpm. Transfer the supernatant to the analyzer and assay within 2 h (*see* **Note 4**).
4. Assays are performed in accordance with the manufacturer's instrument guidelines. Assay-specific parameters are listed in **Table 4** (*see* **Note 5**).
5. In one tube, substitute deionized H2O for the stated sample volume in order to obtain a reagent blank.
6. Calculate the change in absorbance ($T_{final}-T_{initial}$) for each of the standards, controls, and samples. Next, subtract the change in absorbance for the reagent blank from each of the standards, controls and samples to derive the final absorbance reading (*see* **Table 5**).
7. Plot the change in absorbance values for each of the standards on the y-axis

Table 4
CRP Assay Parameters

Parameter	Setting
Temperature (C)	25
Wavelength (nm)	340
Sample volume (µL)	20
Diluent volume, dH$_2$0 (µL)	5
Time of initial reading (s)	0.5
Time of final reading (s)	300

Table 5
Laboratory Data for the Described CRP Assay

	$T_{initial\ (0.5\ s)}$	$T_{final\ (300\ s)}$	Absorbance (340 nm) △ Absorbance ($T_{final} - T_{initial}$)	△ Absorbance adjusted for Reagent blank	Interpolated value (mg/L)
Reagent blank	−0.0021	−0.0024	−0.0003	—	
Standard 1 (7.5 mg/L)	−0.0011	0.0043	0.0054	0.0057	
Standard 2 (15 mg/L)	−0.0013	0.0147	0.0160	0.0163	
Standard 3 (30 mg/L)	0.0008	0.0326	0.0318	0.0321	
Standard 4 (60 mg/L)	0.0055	0.0607	0.0552	0.0555	
Standard 5 (90 mg/L)	0.0098	0.0805	0.0707	0.0710	
Standard 6 (120 mg/L)	0.0168	0.1004	0.0836	0.0839	
Control 1	0.0111	0.0632	0.0521	0.0524	54
Control 2	0.0116	0.0315	0.0199	0.0202	18
Patient sample 1	0.0187	0.0557	0.0370	0.0373	34
Patient sample 2	0.0228	0.0915	0.0687	0.0690	82

against the value of the calibration curve on the *x*-axis. These points are used to draw a curve that optimally fits the data (*see* **Fig. 2**). Alternatively, one may use curve-fitting algorithms available on most laboratory analyzers or computers.
8. The change in absorbance values for the controls and test samples are interpolated from the drawn curve to obtain the final concentration.
Samples which yield absorbance changes above the highest calibrator are further diluted in PBS and reassayed with subsequent correction for dilution (*see* **Note 6**). Samples that yield absorbance changes below the lowest calibrator are either reported as "< 7.5 mg/L" or reassayed using a more sensitive test (e.g., hs-CRP).

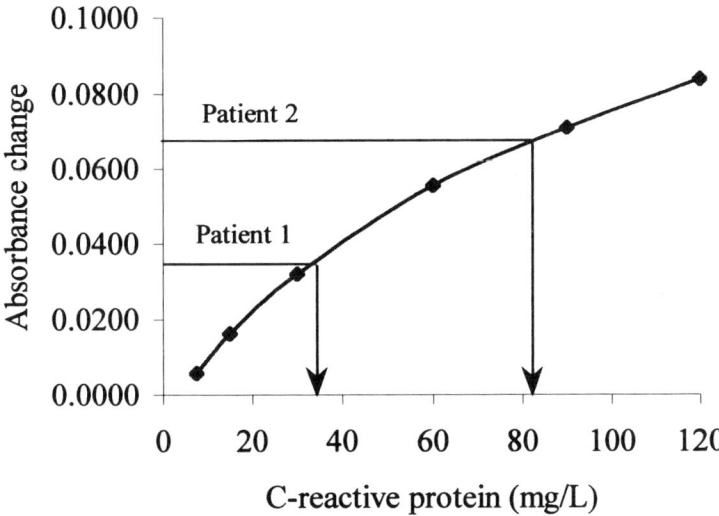

Fig. 2. Calibration curve for the described CRP assay. Absorbance data for the calibrators are plotted on the y-axis against the assigned concentrations on the *x*-axis. Concentrations for the patient samples are then interpolated from the fitted curve.

4. Notes

1. In general, monospecific antiserum with high titer is preferred and is available from various vendors. In order to minimize background signal from the reagent the antiserum is usually an IgG fraction or processed (i.e., water dialyzed) to remove nonspecific and unstable protein. Titer between lots of antiserum should remain relatively constant.
2. The inclusion of PEG in the reaction buffer results in a shortened reaction time, increased sensitivity, and a widening of the calibration range by driving the point of equivalence towards higher antigen concentrations. In practice, most CRP assays work well with a final reaction cell concentration of 40 g/L. It should be noted that the quality of PEG may vary by manufacturer and lot and should be carefully evaluated prior to implementation.
3. There are two widely recognized lyophilized standards for CRP: the WHO 1st International Reference Preparation (IRP) for C-reactive Protein Immunoassay (85/506) *(21)*, introduced in 1986 and Certified Reference Material 470 (CRM 470), referred to in the U.S. as the Reference Preparation for Proteins in Human Serum (RPPHS) and introduced in 1993–94 *(22)*. Both preparations have values provided in both mass/volume and international units. The value in CRM 470/ RPPHS was assigned from WHO IRP 85/506.
4. Serum may contain light-scattering particles such as immune complexes, immunoglobulin aggregates or lipoproteins, which in turn increase the sample blank. Similarly, samples that are icteric or hemolyzed may also adversely affect the

initial absorbance readings. In general, increasing the sample dilution or reducing the amount of serum delivered to the reaction cell may be sufficient to overcome these concerns. Clarification of lipemic samples by delipidation or high speed centrifugation to minimize background "noise" is also possible provided the process does not result in a loss of specific antigen. If serum is grossly lipemic, it should be assayed by an alternative method, such as enzyme immunoassay or a new sample obtained. Measurement of sample blanks should always be performed to minimize nonspecific signal interference.
5. Depending on the measuring device used the volume of antigen and antibody can be revised to minimize antiserum consumption while maintaining appropriate signal. Care should be exercised to maintain the required sensitivity without a corresponding loss of precision.
6. In light-scattering immunoassays as the antigen concentration increases beyond the equivalence point, smaller immune complexes are formed which result in diminished signal. This diminished signal may correspond to an antigen concentration in antibody excess or, beyond the equivalence point in antigen excess. This problem is common with analytes such as CRP where there is a wide pathological range of values. Indeed, among 9 hs-CRP immunoassays reviewed by Roberts et al. antigen excess was detected among three of the assays *(15)*.

References

1. Johnson, A. M., Whicher, J. T., Ledue, T. B., Carlström, A., Itoh, Y., and Petersen, P. H. (2000) Effect of a new international reference preparation for proteins in human serum (certified reference material 470) on results of the College of American Pathologists Surveys for Plasma Proteins. *Arch. Pathol. Lab. Med.* **124,** 1296–1501.
2. Lauder, I. (1991) *United Kingdom external quality assurance schemes, annual report 10th edition.* London, Department of Health.
3. Devleeschouwer, N., Libeer, J. C., Chapelle, J. P., Struway, C. L., Gyssels, C., L'hoir, A., et al. (1994) Factors influencing between-laboratory variability of C-reactive protein results as evidenced by the Belgian external quality assessment (EQA) scheme. *Scand. J. Clin. Lab. Invest.* **54,** 435–440.
4. Thompson, D., Milford-Ward, A., and Whicher, J. T. (1992) The value of acute phase protein measurements in clinical practice. *Ann. Clin. Biochem.* **29,** 123–131.
5. Wilkins, J., Gallimore, J. R., Moore, E. G., and Pepys, M. B. (1998) Rapid automated high sensitivity enzyme immunoassay of C-reactive protein. *Clin. Chem.* **6,** 1358–1361.
6. Price, C. P., Trull, A. K., Berry, D., and Gorman, E. G. (1987) Development and validation of a particle-enhanced turbidimetric immunoassay for C-reactive protein. *J. Imm. Meth.* **99,** 205–217.
7. Sable, K. G. and Wadsworth, C. H. (1979) C-reactive protein in early diagnosis of neonatal septicemia. *Scand. J. Clin. Lab. Invest.* **68,** 825–831.
8. Wasunna, A., Whitelaw, A., Gallimore, R., Hawkins, P. N., and Pepys, M. B. (1990) C-reactive protein and bacterial infection in preterm infants. *Eur. J. Pediatr.* **149,** 424–427.

9. Ridker, P. M., Hennekens, C. H., Burins, J. E., and Rifai, N. (2000) C-reactive protein and other markers of inflammation in the prediction of cardiovascular disease in women. *N. Engl. J. Med.* **342,** 836–843.
10. Ridker, P. M., Cushman, M., Stampfer, M. J., Tracy, R. P., and Hennekens, C. H. (1997) Inflammation, aspirin, and the risk of cardiovascular disease in apparently healthy men. *N. Engl. J. Med.* **336,** 973–979.
11. Köenig W., Sund, M., Fröhlich, M., Fischer, H.-G., Löwell, H., Döring, A., et al. (1999) C-reactive protein, a sensitive marker of inflammation, predicts future risk of coronary heart disease in initially healthy middle-aged men. Results from the MONICA (Monitoring trends and determinants in cardiovascular disease) Augsburg cohort study, 1984–1992. *Circulation* **99,** 237–242.
12. Kuller, L. H., Tracy, R. P., Shaten, J., and Meilahn, E. N. (1996) Relationship of C-reactive protein and coronary heart disease in the MRFIT nested case-control study: Multiple risk factor intervention trial. *Am. J. Epidemiol.* **144,** 537–547.
13. Danesh J., Whincup, P., Walker, M., Lennon, L., Thompson A., Appleby, P., et al. (2000) Low grade inflammation and coronary heart disease: prospective study and updated meta-analyses. *Brit. Med. J.* **321,** 199–204.
14. Roberts, W. L., Sedrick, R., Moulton, L., Spencer, A., and Rifai, N. (2000) Evaluation of four automated high-sensitivity C-reactive protein methods: implications for clinical and epidemiological applications. *Clin. Chem.* **46,** 461–468.
15. Roberts, W. L., Moulton, L., Law, T. C., Farrow, G., Cooper-Anderson, M., Savory, J., et al. (2000) Evaluation of nine automated high-sensitivity C-reactive protein methods: implications for clinical and epidemiological applications. Part 2. *Clin. Chem.* **47,** 418–425.
16. Köening, W. (2001) C-reactive protein and cardiovascular risk: Has the time come for screening the general population? *Clin. Chem.* **47,** 9–10.
17. Ledue, T. B. and Rifai, N. (2001) High sensitivity immunoassays for C-reactive protein: Promises and pitfalls. *Clin. Chem. Lab. Medicine* (In Press).
18. Young, D. S. (1997) *Effects of Preanalytical Variables on Clinical Laboratory Tests.* 2nd ed. (Young, D. S., ed.), AACC, Washington, DC.
19. Guder, W. G., Narayanan, S., Wisser, H., and Zawta, B. (1996) *Samples: From the patient to the laboratory: The Impact of Preanalytical variables on the quality of laboratory results.* (Guder W. G., ed.), GTI, Verlag Darmstadt, Germany.
20. Ledue, T. B. and Rifai, N. (2001) Pre-analytic and analytic sources of variations in C-reactive protein measurement. In *Cardiac Markers* (Wu, A., ed.), Humana, Totowa, NJ, 2nd ed. (In Press)
21. W.H.O. Expert Committee on Biological Standardization. (1987) W.H.O. Expert Committee on Biological Standardization 37th report. W.H.O. Tech. Rep. Ser. 760. Geneva: W.H.O., pp. 21–22.
22. Whicher, J. T., Ritchie, R. F., Johnson, A. M., Baudner, S., Bienvenu, J., Blirup-Jensen, S., et al. (1994) New international reference preparation for proteins in human serum (RPPHS). *Clin. Chem.* **40,** 934–938.

36

Assays of Matrix Metalloproteinases (MMPs) and MMP Inhibitors

Bioassays and Immunoassays Applicable to Cell Culture Medium, Serum, and Synovial Fluid

Jon B. Catterall and Tim E. Cawston

1. Introduction

The metalloproteinases (MMPs) are a diverse family of enzymes that, together, are capable of degrading all the constituents of the extracellular matrix (ECM). They are required for normal development and for general turnover of the ECM, but are elevated in many pathological conditions including inflammatory disease such as arthritis and many cancers *(1)*. These enzymes are tightly regulated at three main points, transcription, activation, and inhibition. All MMPs are secreted in a proform, which requires initial activation by another proteinase, and once activated, there are at least four specific MMP inhibitors (tissue inhibitors of metalloproteinases, or TIMPs) which can bind irreversibly *(2)*. MMPs such as MMP-1 (collagenase 1) are also susceptible to proteolytic cleavage (this can be autologus cleavage) in the hinge region producing N and C terminal fragments which lose there ability to degrade specific substrates, i.e., cleaved MMP-1 can no longer cut triple helical collagen. MMPs often have overlapping substrate specificities: there are at least five commonly found collagenases, MMP-1, MMP-2, MMP-8, MMP-13, and MMP-14 (MMP-18 is also a collagenase but has only been found so far in xenopus) which will all degrade triple helical collagen in a bioassay (*see* **Subheading 3.1.**).

MMP activity can be assayed directly using labelled substrates in bioassays or activity assays (*see* **Chapter 9**). As MMPs have overlapping substrate specificities these assays are unable to determine the activity of a specific MMP. These assays do, however, determine the actual level of enzymes available to degrade the substrate and can be modified to give an estimation of total MMP

From: *Methods in Molecular Biology, vol. 225: Inflammation Protocols*
Edited by: P. G. Winyard and D. A. Willoughby © Humana Press Inc., Totowa, NJ

present (both active and inactive). The total levels measured in a bioassay will not include MMP which has been inactivated by TIMP or has been cleaved. Immunoassays on the other hand usually measure the total level of a specific MMP, which often includes MMP/TIMP complexes, although this is dependent on the antibodies used. The immunoassays determine the level of a specific MMP but give no information about the activation state of the enzyme. An increase in a specific MMP may well not lead to a subsequent increase in the degradation of ECM as the MMP could all be in the pro-form or irreversibly inhibited by TIMPs.

From this brief introduction it is clear that neither the immunoassays nor the bioassays for metalloproteinases give the complete functional picture and so great care must be made in interpreting the results. Bioassays give information on the degradative pressure for a specific substrate but do not give complete information about which enzyme is causing the destruction, while immunoassays give detailed information on the amount of a specific enzyme but nothing about its functionalitity. This chapter describes some of the more commonly used bioassays and immunoassays used for MMP and TIMP research.

2. Materials

The following table gives some of the more commonly available commercial ELISA kits and substrates for the study of MMPs and TIMPs. The list below (see **Table 1**) is not meant to be definitive or a recommendation but is more a guide demonstrating the range of products available.

3. Methods
3.1. Bioassays

These assays all attempt to determine the amount of active MMP within a sample by measuring the degradation of specific substrates. In the most commonly used bioassays these substrates are labelled using [^{3}H] acetic anhydride for sensitivity and ease of detection. These simple enzyme activity assays can also easily be converted to determine TIMP concentrations by using a known amount of metalloproteinase and looking for reduced degradation. Most activity assays work well with biological fluids with the exception of serum. Serum samples give very poor activities as most MMPs in serum are tightly complexed with α_2-macroglobulin.

3.1.1. Preparation of Type I Collagen Substrate

1. Type I collagen is prepared from newborn calf skin. The skin (30 cm × 30 cm) is frozen and the hair removed. The skin is thawed to 4°C and all further steps are performed at this temperature using precooled buffers.

Table 1
Examples of Commercially Available Assays for MMPs and TIMPs

	Immunoassay	Activity assay
Amersham Pharmacia[a]		
MMP-1	Total MMP including complexed	Antibody capture system
MMP-2	Pro MMP only	Antibody capture system
MMP-3	Total MMP	—
MMP-7	Pro MMP only	—
MMP-8	Pro MMP and active, not complexed	Antibody capture system
MMP-9	Pro and complexed Pro-MMP	Antibody capture system
MMP-13	Pro MMP and active, not complexed	Antibody capture system
TIMP-1	Free and complexed	—
TIMP-2	Free and complexed	—
Calbiochem[b]		
MMP-1	Pro MMP only	Fluorescent substrate
MMP-2	—	Fluorescent substrate
MMP-3	—	Fluorescent substrate
MMP-7	—	Fluorescent substrate
MMP-8	—	Fluorescent substrate
MMP-9	Pro MMP only	—
MMP-13	—	Fluorescent substrate
R & D Systems[c]		
MMP-1	Pro-MMP only	—
MMP-3	Total MMP	—
MMP-8	Total MMP	Fluorokine E activity assay
MMP-9	Total MMP	—
TIMP-1	Total TIMP	—
Biosource International[d]		
TIMP-1	Total TIMP	—
TIMP-1	Matched antibody pairs for ELISA	—
The Binding Site[e]		
MMP-1	Pro-MMP-1	—
MMP-2	Pro-MMP-2	—
MMP-3	Pro-MMP-3	—

[a]Little Chalfont, Buckinghamshire, UK.
[b]CN Bioscience UK, Beeston, Nottingham, UK.
[c]Abingdon, Oxford, UK.
[d]Nivelles, Belgium.
[e]Birmingham, UK.

2. The skin is diced and ground in an electric mincer with dry ice to prevent the samples warming during the grinding process. In all the following stages the preservative toluene (0.03% v/v) is included.
3. The minced skin is washed three times with 1.5 L of 0.9% (w/v) NaCl for 30 min followed by two further washes in water. During the washes, the skin is stirred before filtering through cheese cloth. The wash supernatants are discarded.
4. The washed minced skin is resuspended in 1.5 L of 0.5 M acetic acid and stirred slowly overnight. The sample is filtered and the supernatant retained as it contains the collagen. A second overnight extraction in acetic acid is performed and combined with the first.
5. The acetic acid extracts are clarified by centrifugation (7500g, 2 h, 4°C) and the pellets discarded.
6. The collagen is precipitated by dialysis against 5% (w/v) NaCl in 0.1 M acetic acid (2 changes of 12 L). The precipitated collagen is pelleted by centrifugation (7500g, 2 h, 4°C).
7. Collagen pellets are gently resuspended in 2–3 L of 0.5 M acetic before dialysing against a further 5 L of 0.5 M acetic acid overnight (or until the pellet is dissolved).
8. Collagen is reprecipitated by dialysis against 20 mM disodium hydrogen phosphate (at least four changes of 20 L). Collagen is collected by centrifugation (7500g, 30 min, 4°C).
9. Collagen pellets are again gently resuspended in 2–3 L of 0.5 M acetic acid and stirred until dissolved. The collagen is precipitated by slowly adding 5% (w/v) NaCl and collected by centrifugation (7500g, 30 min, 4°C). Pellets are washed in 1 L of 20% (w/v) NaCl and the collagen collected by centrifugation (7500g, 30 min, 4°C).
10. Collagen pellets are dissolved in 0.5 M acetic acid overnight. The collagen solution is clarified by centrifugation (30,000g, 1 h, 4°C) and the supernatant dialyzed against 0.1 M acetic acid (10 L) before freeze drying. Collagen samples are stored desiccated at –20°C until required.

3.1.2. Preparation of Gelatin Substrate

Gelatin is denatured collagen and is prepared by heating collagen at 56°C for 30 min. Before denaturation, freshly prepared di-isopropyl-phosphofluoridate (DFP, from a 200 mM stock in dry isopropanol) is added, to give a final concentration of 2 mM. This inhibits any serine proteinases possibly produced by low level bacterial contamination.

3.1.3. Preparation of Casein Substrate

1. Casein (Hammerstein grade) is not particularly pure and so needs to be further purified before use. Casein is dissolved overnight at 4°C in 10 mM NaOH to a final concentration of 30 mg/mL.
2. The pH is lowered to 4.6 using glacial acetic acid and the casein precipitates. The casein is collected by centrifugation at 1000g for 15 min. Gentle centrifugation is

used otherwise the pellet is very difficult to redissolve.
3. Steps 1 and 2 are repeated.
4. Redissolve the pellet to 10 mg/mL in 10 mM NaOH and store at –20°C.

3.1.4. Labeling of Type I Collagen Substrate

1. All steps are carried out at 4°C. Dissolve 250 mg of collagen in 50 ml of 0.2 M acetic acid and dialyze against 2 L of 10 mM disodium tetraborate (pH 9.0), 0.2 M CaCl$_2$. The calcium is included in the dialysis to prevent the precipitation of the collagen. If the collagen precipitates it must be dialyzed back into 0.2 M acetic acid and the dialysis repeated. Some collagen preparations may require higher concentrations of CaCl$_2$.
2. Stir collagen solution very slowly in a large conical flask in preparation for the addition of the label.
3. Place the base of the tube containing [^{3}H]-acetic anhydride (25 mCi, TRK-2, Amersham Life Sciences Ltd.) in dry ice. Add 1 mL of dry dioxane to the acetic anhydride. The dioxane freezes at the bottom of the tube. The dioxane/acetic anhydride is thawed rapidly and added to the collagen solution. The acetic anhydride pot is washed with a further 1 mL of dioxane which is also added to the collagen solution. The collagen is stirred for a further 30 min.
4. Dialyze the collagen against 50 mM Tris-HCl (pH 7.6), 0.2 M NaCl, 5 mM calcium acetate, and 0.03% (v/v) toluene until the [^{3}H] activity of the diffusate is reduced to background. Labeled collagen is diluted to a final concentration of 1 mg/mL and further diluted with unlabeled collagen at 1 mg/mL to a final concentration of 200,000 dpm/mg of collagen. The collagen solution is dialysed into 0.2 M acetic acid and stored at –20°C.

3.1.5. Labeling of Gelatin Substrate

1. [^{3}H] labeled gelatin is prepared from labeled collagen as described in **Subheading 3.1.2.**

3.1.6. Labeling of Casein Substrate

Casein can be labelled using a similar protocol as described for collagen (*see* **Subheading 3.1.4.**). The casein is labelled at 10–20 mg/mL in borate buffer minus the calcium and once labelled is stored at –20°C.

3.1.7. Sample Preparation

MMPs are often secreted in an inactive proform and require activation for total MMP determination. This is done by either trypsin or amino-phenyl-mercuric acetate (APMA) treatment.

1. APMA activation: Buffer B (*see* **Subheading 3.1.8.**, paragraph 4) in either the collagenase, gelatinase, or caseinase assay is modified to four parts buffer B to 1 part 10 mM APMA. A 10 mM solution of APMA is prepared by dissolving 35.2 mg of APMA in 200 µL of dimethylsulfoxide before further diluting to 10 mL

with 20 m*M* Tris-HCl pH 8.0–9.5. The addition of this Tris/APMA buffer mix to the assay and incubation at 37°C is enough to activate any pro-MMP within the sample. If the length of the assay is less than 3 h, either trypsin activation or preincubation for 1 h at 37°C with APMA is required.

2. Trypsin activation: Add an equal volume of 20 μg/mL trypsin to each sample and incubate at room temperature for 15 min. Inhibit the trypsin by adding an equal volume of 100 μg/mL soybean trypsin inhibitor and make up to 100 μL with buffer A (*see* **Subheading 3.1.8.**, paragraph 2) ready for use in the bioassays. If the 96-well plate modification is used (*see* **Subheading 3.1.9.**), the samples are made up to 50 μL with buffer A.

3.1.8. Collagenase Assay

1. Thaw labeled collagen (1 mg/mL in 0.2 *M* acetic acid) and dialyze against 50 m*M* Tris-HCl buffer, pH 7.6, containing 0.2 *M* NaCl and 0.03% (v/v) toluene.
2. Prepare the following duplicated control samples in 400 μL tubes: 100 μL of buffer A (25 m*M* sodium cacodylate, pH 7.6, 0.05% (v/v) Brij 35, 0.02% NaN$_3$); 10 μL trypsin (100 μg/mL in 1 m*M* HCl) in 90 μL buffer A; 100 μL of buffer A containing 100 μg/mL of bacterial collagenase. If the sample contains high salt or serum then an equivalent blank needs to be included (*see* **Note 1**).
3. Prepare test samples in duplicate and make up to 100 μL in buffer A. Samples may require activation (*see* **Subheading 3.1.7.**).
4. Add 100 μL of buffer B (100 m*M* Tris-HCl, pH 7.6, 15 m*M* CaCl$_2$, 0.02% NaN3) to all tubes. Calcium is included in buffer B as it is required for the thermostability of MMPs.
5. Add 100 μL of the dialyzed [^{3}H]-labeled collagen at 1 mg/mL to all tubes. Incubate at 37°C for 1–20 h. Centrifuge tubes at 13,000*g* for 10 min to remove undigested collagen (collagen can be difficult to pellet in polypropylene tubes as the fibrils tend to adhere to the tube at the liquid surface interface). Collect 200 μL of supernatant, mix with scintillation fluid, and count in a scintillation counter.
6. Subtract the blank values (buffer A only controls) from all test results. If the trypsin digest results are high then the collagen is not in a fibrillar form and the assay should be discarded and fresh fibrillar collagen prepared (*see* **Note 2**). The bacterial collagenase tubes represent total lysis values for 100 μg of labelled collagen.
7. Results are expressed in units/mL where 1 U of activity is defined as the amount of enzyme required to degrade 1 μg of collagen/min at 37°C. This value can be obtained using the following :

$$\text{Units per mL} = \frac{\text{Test mean} \times 100 \, (\mu g/mL \text{ of collagen}) \times \text{dilution factor}}{\text{mean bacterial collagenase} \times \text{time (min)} \times \text{sample volume (mL)}}$$

3.1.9. 96-Well Plate Modification of the Collagenase Assay (5)

1. Thaw labeled collagen (1 mg/mL in 0.2 *M* acetic acid) and dialyze against 50 m*M* Tris-HCl buffer, pH 7.6, containing 0.2 *M* NaCl and 0.03% (v/v) toluene.
2. Duplicate control wells are prepared in a 96-well plate as follows: 50 μL buffer A

(see **Subheading 3.1.8.**, paragraph 2); 5 µL of trypsin (100 µg/mL in 1 mM HCl) and 45 µL of buffer A; 50 µL of bacterial collagenase (100 µg/mL) in buffer A. If samples contain appreciable amounts of salt or serum then a sample control should be included (see **Note 1**).
3. Add test samples in at least duplicate and make up to 50 µL with buffer A. Sample may require activation (see **Subheading 3.1.7.**).
4. Add 50 µL of buffer B to all wells (see **Subheading 3.1.8.**, paragraph 4).
5. Add 50 µL of the dialyzed [^{3}H]-labeled collagen at 1 mg/mL to all wells. Cover the plate and incubate at 37°C for 1–20 h. Pellet the undigested collagen by centrifugation of the plates at 1300g for 30 min (centrifugation speeds are lower for the 96 well plate assay as the collagen does not adhere to polystyrene—see **Subheading 3.1.8.**, paragraph 5).
6. Remove 50 µL of supernatant and combine with 200 µL of Supermix scintillation fluid (Wallac) in a 96-well low crosstalk plate before reading in a scintillation counter.
7. Subtract the blank values (buffer A only controls) from all test results. If the trypsin digest results are high, then the collagen is not in a fibrillar form and the assay should be discarded and fresh fibrillar collagen prepared (see **Note 2**). The bacterial collagenase tubes represent total lysis values for 100 µg of labeled collagen.
8. Results are expressed in units/mL where 1 U of activity is defined as the amount of enzyme required to degrade 1 µg of collagen/min at 37°C. This value can be obtained using the following:

$$\text{Units per mL} = \frac{\text{Test mean} \times 50 \text{ (µg/mL of collagen)} \times \text{dilution factor}}{\text{mean bacterial collagenase} \times \text{time (min)} \times \text{sample volume (mL)}}$$

3.1.10. Modification of the Collagenase Assay to Measure TIMP (see **Note 3**)

1. Collagenase assays are performed as described previously (see **Subheading 3.1.8.**).
2. Extra control samples containing active MMP-1 (bacterial collagenase is not suitable as it is not inhibited by TIMPs), circa 0.06 units for a 20 h assay, such that 70–80% of the total collagen included in the assay is degraded.
3. MMP-1 is added to all test tubes and the amount of TIMP present within the samples is determined by the reduction in the release of collagen fragments against the control.
4. The amount of TIMP present is determined using the following formula.

$$\text{U/mL} = \frac{(\text{active collagenase control mean} - \text{test mean}) \times 100 \text{ (µg of collagen)}}{\text{mean bacterial collagenase} \times \text{time (min)} \times \text{sample volume (mL)}}$$

3.1.11. Gelatinase Assay

1. [^{3}H]-labeled gelatin is treated with DFP (2 mM final concentration) (see **Subheading 3.1.2.**). The gelatin is heated to 55°C for 30 min before cooling to 4°C for immediate use.

2. The following controls are prepared: duplicate tubes containing 50 µL of buffer A (*see* **Subheading 3.1.8.**, paragraph 2); 5 µL trypsin (100 µg/mL in 1 mM HCl) in 45 µL buffer A to determine total lysis.
3. Samples are made up to 50 µL with buffer A in at least duplicate. Samples may require activation (*see* **Subheading 3.1.7.**).
4. Add 100 µL of buffer B (*see* **Subheading 3.1.8.**, paragraph 4) followed by 100 µL of [^{3}H] labeled gelatin.
5. Samples are incubated at 37°C for 1–20 h before the addition of 50 µL of 90% (w/v) trichloroactetic acid. Samples are left on ice for 20 min.
6. Pellet undigested gelatin by centrifugation at 13,000g for 10 min and count 200 µL of the supernatant in a scintillation counter for 1 min.
7. The mean blank values are subtracted from the test values and the results calculated in units per mL as for the collagenase assay (*see* **Subheading 3.1.8.**, paragraph 7). One unit is defined as the amount of gelatinase required to digest 1 µg of gelatin per min at 37°C.

3.1.12. Caseinase Assay

1. [^{3}H]-labeled casein is thawed and treated with fresh DFP (2 mM final concentration; *see* **Subheading 3.1.2.**). The casein is cooled to 4°C for use the same day.
2. Control samples are prepared as follows: duplicate tubes containing 50 µL of buffer A (*see* **Subheading 3.1.8.**, paragraph 2); 5 µL trypsin (100 µg/mL in 1 mM HCl) in 45 µL buffer A to determine total lysis.
3. Samples are made up to 50 µL with buffer A in duplicate tubes. Samples may require activating before testing (*see* **Subheading 3.1.7.**).
4. Add 100 µL of buffer B (*see* **Subheading 3.1.8.**, paragraph 4) followed by 100 µL of [^{3}H] labeled casein.
5. Samples are incubated at 37°C for 1–20 h before the addition of 50 µL of 18% (w/v) trichloroactetic acid. Samples are left on ice for 20 min.
6. Pellet undigested casein by centrifugation at 13,000g for 10 min and count 200 µL of the supernatant in a scintillation counter for 1 min.
7. The mean blank values are subtracted from the test values and the results calculated in U/mL as for the collagenase assay (*see* **Subheading 3.1.8.**, paragraph 7). One unit is defined as the amount of enzyme required to digest 1 µg of casein per min at 37°C.

3.1.13. Other Activity Assays for MMPs

1. Fluorogenic peptide substrate assays: In brief, these assays involve the use of quenched fluorescent substrates. The substrates are short peptide sequences which contain the known cleavage site for a particular MMP. At one end of the peptide is attached a fluorescent donor group, and to the other a quenching acceptor group which absorbs energy over the same wavelengths as the donor emits. While the peptide substrate is intact, then the close proximity of the quencher to the donor prevents any light emission. However, when an MMP

MMPs and MMP Inhibitors 361

cleaves the peptide, the donor and quencher become separated with a resulting increase in fluorescence which can be measured using a fluorimeter. Assays and fluorescent substrates have been reviewed *(6,7)*. A fluorescent substrates based activity assay *(8)* is at present the only reported activity assay to work successfully with serum samples. It is believed that the substrate used is small enough to gain access to the MMP while bound to α_2-macroglobulin. The assay also works successfully with other biological fluids including tissue culture medium and synovial fluid *(9)*.
2. Zymograms and reverse zymograms are electrophoretic techniques for visualising both active enzyme and inhibitors. These techniques are reviewed in detail in **Chapter 9** of this book.
3. Others substrates: Recently, succinylated gelatin has been described as novel substrate for gelatinases. The assay relies upon the exposure of primary amines after the substrate has been degraded by gelatinases *(10)*.
4. Immunocapture activity assays: These assays combine the sensitivity of monoclonal antibodies with a substrate to determine activity levels. As with an ELISA, a 96-well plate is coated with a primary capture antibody which is specific for the MMP of interest. Samples are incubated and any non-specific MMPs are removed by washing. Active MMP can be detected either using one of the fluorescent MMP substrates or using a modified substrate. Modified pro-urokinase with an MMP cleavage site replacing the plasmin activation site was used to determine MMP-9 activity in saliva *(11)*. This form of activity assay is marketed by Amersham Pharmacia Biotech.

3.2. Immunoassays

These assays address levels of particular MMPs within a biological fluid but usually do not address activation state. When using immunoassays it is particularly important to know exactly what the assay measures. For example, does it only measure pro-MMP or active MMP? If it measures total MMP, does that include MMP bound to TIMP? Another complication that can occur with some immunoassays is the presence of rheumatoid factor, which can interfere.

3.2.1. MMP-1 ELISA (see **Note 4**)

1. Immunosorp high-protein-binding 96-well ELISA plates (Nunc) are coated overnight at 4°C with the polyclonal antibody RRU CL-1. The primary antibody is added at a final concentration of 2 µg/mL in 100 µL of PBS containing 0.02% (w/v) sodium azide.
2. The plate is washed once with wash buffer (PBS, 0.1% (v/v) Tween-20, 0.25 mM thimerosal).
3. None specific protein binding is prevented by blocking each well with 200 µL of blocking buffer (PBS, 0.02% (w/v) sodium azide, 10 mg/mL BSA) at room temperature for at least 2 h. The plate can be stored in blocking buffer at 4°C for up to 1 mo.

4. The plate is washed once with wash buffer.
5. A standard curve of recombant MMP-1 in protein diluent (wash buffer containing 0.5 mg/mL BSA) is prepared in duplicate at between 5 and 50 ng/mL. Samples can be added either neat or diluted in protein diluent. Standard and sample are added at 100 µL/well and incubated at either room temperature for 2 h or overnight at 4°C.
6. The plate is washed three times with wash buffer.
7. Secondary antibody (biotinylated polyclonal CL-1 anti-MMP-1, 2 µg/mL) is added at 100 µL/well and incubated at room temperature for 2 h.
8. The plate is washed three times with wash buffer.
9. Streptavidin conjugated horseradish peroxidase (DAKO) is added at 100 µL per well and 1/5000 dilution in protein diluent. The streptavidin conjugate is incubated at room temperature for 30 min.
10. The plate is washed three times with wash buffer.
11. The ELISA is developed using orthophenylene diamine (OPD) as a substrate, which is prepared fresh in phosphate citrate buffer (1 tablet of OPG to 12 mL of citrate buffer). The OPD substrate is added at 100 µL/well at timed intervals across the plate and a yellow color develops after about 5 min, which becomes darker after the addition of 50 µL/well of stop solution (3 M sulfuric acid).
12. The absorbance at 490 nm is measured and the results for the test samples calculated by reference to the standard curve.

3.2.2. TIMP-1 ELISA

This ELISA uses a very similar protocol to that used for the MMP-1 ELISA (*see* **Subheading 3.2.1.**) with the following differences:

1. ELISA plates are coated with the polyclonal anti-TIMP-1 antibody RRU T5 at 4 µg/mL in PBS (*see* **Note 5**).
2. Duplicate standards are prepared between 5 and 50 ng/mL using recombinant TIMP-1.

3.2.3. One Step Immunoassays

These immunoassays are a variation upon the more common ELISA techniques. In a one step (EIA) immunoassay, the sample is incubated with both the immobilized primary antibody and the secondary antibody tagged with a detection enzyme such as alkaline phosphatase. After incubation, any unbound secondary antibody and contaminating protein is washed away. The MMP or TIMP is quantified by a secondary color reaction using the detection enzyme bound to the secondary antibody. These assays appear to work well with complex biological fluids including serum, saliva, and synovial fluids and descriptions of methods for the following enzymes can be found: MMP-1 *(12)*, MMP-2 *(13)*, MMP-3 *(14)*, MMP-7 *(15)*, and MMP-20 *(16)*.

3.2.4. Collagen Cleavage ELISA

This ELISA, unlike the previously described immunoassays, is an ELISA version of the activity assays. Antibodies are generated to the neoepitopes generated when a collagenase cleaves triple helical collagen to give the characteristic three-fourths and one-fourth digest pattern. Details for the preparation of neoepitope antibodies can be found in *(17)*. As each type of collagen contains a particular α chain, ELISA protocols can be developed that can distinguish between collagen types. This can be useful if trying to determine the breakdown of collagen in a mixed population such as cartilage (mainly type II) and synovial tissue (mainly type I). This method of detection of breakdown is also extremely useful for determining degradation which has occurred within an explant culture or extracted tissue, as the epitopes can be recovered by partial digestion of the tissue to liberate the epitopes *(18)*.

4. Notes

1. The blank values of the bioassay can be affected by high salt, high serum, high calcium, other chaotropic ions, and some metal ions. High background values can also be caused by preparations of collagen not forming a high percentage of fibrils and being susceptible to cleavage by other proteinases within the samples. Variation in the level of calcium ions can often correct the variability seen in fibril formation between preparations.
2. Trypsin blanks are higher in acetylated collagen as some labeled lysine groups are found within the telopeptide regions which are susceptible to trypsin cleavage. Also, excessive labeling with acetic anhydride can retard fibril formation leading to higher trypsin blanks *(4)*.
3. The TIMP assay can easily be adapted for the 96-well plate version of the collagenase assay (*see* **Subheading 3.1.9.**).
4. This assay is available from Amersham Pharmacia Biotech and the antibodies are available from Cambio, Cambridge, UK.
5. These antibodies are available from Cambio.

References

1. Nagase, H. and Woessner, J. F. (1999) Matrix metalloproteinases. *J. Biol. Chem.* **274,** 21,491–21,494.
2. Cawston, T. E. (1996) Metalloproteinase inhibitors and the prevention of connective tissue breakdown. *Pharmacol. Ther.* **70,** 163–182.
3. Shingleton, W. D., Hodges, D. J., Brick, P., and Cawston, T. E. (1996) Collagenase: A key enzyme in collagen turnover. *Biochem. Cell Biol.* **74,** 759–775.
4. Sellers A, Cartwright E, Murphy G, and Reynolds J. J. (1977) Evidence that latent collagenases are enzyme-inhibitor complexes. *Biochem. J.* **261,** 1031–1034.
5. Koshy, P. J. T., Rowan, A. D., Life, P. F., and Cawston, T. E. (1999) 96-well plate

assays for measuring collagenase activity using H-3-acetylated collagen. *Anal. Biochem.* **275,** 202–207.
6. Fields, G. B. (2001) Using fluorogenic peptide substrates to assay matrix metalloproteinases, in *Methods in Molecular Biology. Vol. 151. Matrix Metalloproteinase Protocols* (Clark, I. M., ed.), Humana, Totowa, NJ.
7. Knight, C. G. (1995) Fluorometric assays of proteolytic-enzymes. *Proteolytic Enzymes: Aspartic and Metallo Peptidases* **248,** 18–34.
8. Beekman, B., Drijfhout, J. W., Bloemhoff, W., Ronday, H. K., Tak, P. P., and Koppele, J. M. T. (1996) Convenient fluorometric assay for matrix metalloproteinase activity and its application in biological media. *FEBS Lett.* **390,** 221–225.
9. Beekman, B., Drijfhout, J. W., Ronday, H. K., and Koppele, J. M. T. (1999) Fluorogenic MMP activity assay for plasma including MMPs complexed to alpha(2)-macroglobulin. *Ann. NY Acad. Sci.* **878,** 150–158.
10. Baragi, V. M., Shaw, B. J., Renkiewicz, R. R., Kuipers, P. J., Welgus, H. G., Mathrubutham, M., et al. (2000) A versatile assay for gelatinases using succinylated gelatin. *Matrix Biol.* **19,** 267–273.
11. Hanemaaijer, R., Visser, H., Konttinen, Y. T., Koolwijk, P., and Verheijen, J. H. (1998) A novel and simple immunocapture assay for determination of gelatinase-B (MMP-9) activities in biological fluids: Saliva from patients with Sjogren's syndrome contain increased latent and active gelatinase-B levels. *Matrix Biol.* **17,** 657–665.
12. Zhang, J., Fujimoto, N., Iwata, K., Sakai, T., Okada, Y., and Hayakawa, T. (1993) A one-step sandwich enzyme-immunoassay for human matrix metalloproteinase-1 (interstitial collagenase) using monoclonal-antibodies. *Clin. Chim. Acta* **219,** 1–14.
13. Fujimoto, N., Mouri, N., Iwata, K., Ohuchi, E., Okada, Y., and Hayakawa, T. (1993) A one-step sandwich enzyme-immunoassay for human matrix metalloproteinase 2 (72-kDa gelatinase type-IV collagenase) using monoclonal-antibodies. *Clin. Chim. Acta* **221,** 91–103.
14. Obata, K., Iwata, K., Okada, Y., Kohrin, Y., Ohuchi, E., Yoshida, S., et al. (1992) A one-step sandwich enzyme-immunoassay for human matrix metalloproteinase-3 (stromelysin-1) using monoclonal-antibodies. *Clin. Chim. Acta* **211,** 59–72.
15. Ohuchi, E., Azumano, I., Yoshida, S., Iwata, K., and Okada, Y. (1996) A one-step sandwich enzyme immunoassay for human matrix metalloproteinase 7 (matrilysin) using monoclonal antibodies. *Clin. Chim. Acta* **244,** 181–198.
16. Wang, T., Aoki, T., Iwata, K., Takata, T., Uchida, T., Knauper, V., et al. (2000) One-step sandwich enzyme immunoassay using monoclonal antibodies for detection of human enamelysin (MMP-20). *Eur. J. Oral Sci.* **108,** 530–537.
17. Billinghurst, R. C., Ionescu, M, and Poole, A. R. (2001) Immunoassay for collagenase-mediated cleavage of Types I and II collagens, in *Methods in Molecular Biology. Vol.151. Matrix Metalloproteinase Protocols* (Clark, I. M., ed.), Humana, Totowa, NJ.
18. Hollander, A. P., Heathfield, T. F., Webber, C., Iwata, Y., Bourne, R., Rorabeck, C., et al. (1994) Increased damage to type-II collagen in osteoarthritic articular-cartilage detected by a new immunoassay. *J. Clin. Invest.* **93,** 1722–1732.

Index

A

Acute phase response (APR),
   analyte selection for assay, 343, 344
   C-reactive protein assay, *see* C-reactive protein
Adjuvant-induced arthritis, COX-2 inhibition evaluation, 323, 325, 327
Aggrecanase,
  cleavage, 89
  interglobular domain catabolite measurement,
    gel electrophoresis, 92, 97
    materials, 90, 91, 96
    neoepitope antibodies, 95, 96
    overview, 89, 90
    sample preparation, 91, 92, 96, 97
    standard curve,
      generation, 91, 96
      interpretation, 93, 95
    Western blot, 92, 93, 97
Air pouch models,
  applications, 182
  carrageenan air pouch,
    air injection, 183, 186
    inflammatory cell analysis, 183, 184, 187
    lavage, 183
    materials, 182, 186
  chronic granulomatous air pouch,
    air pouch formation, 184
    angiogenesis analysis,
      anesthesia, 193, 195
      applications, 194, 195
      digest analysis, 194, 195
      lavage, 194, 195
      materials, 192
      overview, 191
      vessel visualization, 194–196
    croton oil injection, 184, 187
    lavage and analysis, 184, 187
    materials, 182, 186
  granuloma-mediated articular cartilage degradation model,
    cartilage destruction assessment, 183, 185, 188
    implantation of cartilage, 183, 185, 188
    materials, 182, 183, 186
    rat femoral head cartilage isolation, 182, 184, 187, 188
    wrapping of cartilage, 182, 184
  history of study, 181
  leukocyte subset migration in response to chemokines and cytokines,
    air pouch formation, 141, 143
    calculations, 142
    cell counting, 142
    inflammation induction, 141
    lavage, 141, 142
    materials, 140, 141
    overview, 139, 140
    peritonitis model comparison, 143–145

Angiogenesis,
  chronic granulomatous air pouch
      model,
    air pouch formation, 184
    anesthesia, 193, 195
    applications, 194, 195
    digest analysis, 194, 195
    lavage, 194, 195
    materials, 192
    overview, 191
    vessel visualization, 194–196
  therapeutic targeting, 191
AP-1, inhibitor screening,
  cell treatment with inhibitors, 21, 22
  luciferase detection, 21, 22
  materials, 20, 21
  overview, 19, 20
  plasmids, 20
  transfection, 21, 22
APR, *see* Acute phase response
Arachidonic acid, ear inflammation
    model, 133
Arthritis,
  collagen induction, *see*
      Collagen-induced arthritis
  rat monoarticular arthritis model,
      see Methylated bovine
      serum albumin;
      *Mycobacterium
      tuberculosis*; Zymosan
  rheumatoid arthritis, *see*
      Rheumatoid arthritis
Arthus reaction, *see* Pleural
    inflammation models
Atherosclerosis, *see* Coronary artery
    occlusion and reperfusion

B–C

Bovine serum albumin, *see*
    Methylated bovine serum
    albumin
Calcium flux,
  fluorescence measurement
      and imaging,
    flow cytometry, 53, 54
    fluorometry, 52
    free cytosolic calcium
        calculation, 51, 52
    imaging,
      confocal imaging, 54, 55
      photobleaching, 58
      ratiometric imaging, 54, 57, 58
      time-resolved imaging, 55
    materials, 48
    microfluorometry, 52, 56, 57
    near plasma membrane
        calcium, 55, 56
    principles, 47, 48
    probes,
      calcium affinity, 48, 49
      loading of cells, 50, 51, 56
      single- versus
          dual-wavelength
          probes, 49, 50
      types, 49
  inflammation role, 47
  manipulation of cytosolic free
      calcium, 56, 57
Cantharidin, ear inflammation
    model,
  mouse, 132
  rat, 132
Capillary electrophoresis,
  nitrate/nitrite assays,
    calibration curve, 310, 311, 317

cytokine induction in synovial
    fibroblast-like cells,
    311–313, 317, 318
  materials, 307–309, 316
  running conditions, 309, 310
  sample preparation, 309, 311,
    316, 317
  xanthine oxidase nitric oxide
    generation in hypoxic
    inflammatory tissues,
    313, 314, 318
  principles, 307
Capsaicin, ear inflammation
  model, 133
Carrageenan air pouch, *see* Air
  pouch models
Carrageenan-induced ear
  inflammation, rodent model, 134
Carrageenan-induced paw edema,
  applications, 109, 110, 118, 119
  carrageenan types and features,
    115, 120
  COX-2 inhibition evaluation,
    322, 324
  croton oil ear edema
    combination, 135
  induction of inflammation, 117, 120
  inflammatory response, 115
  materials, 116, 120
  quantitative analysis, 117, 118, 120
  statistical analysis, 118
Carrageenan-induced paw
  hyperalgesia, COX-2 inhibition
  evaluation, 323, 324, 327
Carrageenan pleurisy, inflammation
  model, 125, 127
Cartilage degradation assays,
  articular cartilage structure, 99
  cartilage culture, 100–102, 104, 105

collagen degradation assay,
    101–105
  cytotoxicity assay, 101
  dissection of human specimens,
    appearance, 99
    sources of tissue, 99
    technique, 101, 102
  materials, 100, 101
  pig cartilage samples, 100, 104
  proteoglycan degradation,
    dimethylmethylene blue assay,
    101, 102, 105
  overview, 99
Caseinase, *see* Matrix
  metalloproteinases
CGD, *see* Chronic granulomatous
  disease
Chaos theory, specificity of drug
  action, 265–267
Chromium-51, gastrointestinal
  permeability assays,
  fecal excretion, 323, 326, 327
  materials, 323
  principles, 322
  urinary excretion, 323, 326, 327
Chronic granulomatous disease
  (CGD), oxidase defects, 61
CIA, *see* Collagen-induced arthritis
Collagen, degradation assay, 101–105
Collagenase, *see* Matrix
  metalloproteinases
Collagen-induced arthritis (CIA),
  immune response, 175
  materials, 176–178
  mouse model and quantification,
    176–178
  rat model, 176–178
  rheumatoid arthritis similarity, 175

Complement,
    activation assays,
        enzyme immunoassay, 72–74
        materials, 70–74
        neocpitopes in activation
            products, 70
        overview, 69, 70
        test samples, 72, 74
    inflammation role, 69
Confocal microscopy, calcium
    imaging, 54, 55
Coronary artery occlusion
    and reperfusion,
    animal models,
        materials, 201, 202
        overview, 200, 201
        pig, 205–207
        rabbit, 203–205, 207
        rat, 202, 203, 206, 207
    cardiac injury degree factors, 200
    cardiovascular disease burden, 199
    history of study, 199, 200
    reperfusion injury, 200
COX inhibitors, see
    Cyclooxygenase inhibitors
C-reactive protein (CRP),
    acute phase response, 343–345
    assays,
        absorbance measurement, 348,
            349, 351
        calibration curve, 348
        dilution, 348, 350, 351
        materials, 348, 350
        overview, 346, 347
        parameters, 348, 349, 351
    modulators, 347
    obesity levels, 345

Croton oil,
    chronic granulomatous air pouch,
        air pouch formation, 184
        croton oil injection, 184, 187
        lavage and analysis, 184, 187
        materials, 182, 186
    ear inflammation model,
        mouse, 131, 136
        rat, 131, 134–136
CRP, see C-reactive protein
Cyclooxygenase (COX) inhibitors,
    chaos theory and specificity,
        265–267
    COX-2 inhibition,
        gastrointestinal permeability
            assays using chromium-51
            fecal excretion, 323, 326, 327
            materials, 323
            principles, 322
            urinary excretion, 323,
                326, 327
        inflammation, pain,
            and pyresis models,
            adjuvant-induced arthritis,
                323, 325, 327
            carrageenan-induced paw
                edema, 322, 324
            carrageenan-induced paw
                hyperalgesia, 323,
                324, 327
            endotoxin-induced pyrexia,
                323–326
            materials, 322, 323, 327
        overview, 321, 322
        rationale, 321, 322
    development using carrageenan-
        induced paw edema assay,
        109, 110, 118, 119
    isoforms of enzyme, 321
    side effects, 270

specificity in inflammation
    models, 264, 265
  therapeutic index, 263, 264
Cytochrome c, oxidase assay, 64, 67

D–E

2,3-Diaminonaphthalene, *see* Nitrite
    assays
Dithranol, ear inflammation
    model, 133
Doctrine of Signatures, 264, 272
Ear inflammation models,
  advantages, 129, 130
  applications, 129
  arachididonic acid-induced
      inflammation, 133
  cantharidin-induced
      inflammation,
    mouse, 132
    rat, 132
  capsaicin-induced
      inflammation, 133
  carrageenan-induced
      inflammation, 134
  combined agents, 134, 135
  croton oil-induced inflammation,
    mouse, 131, 136
    rat, 131, 134–136
  dithranol-induced
      inflammation, 133
  ethyl phenylpropiolate-induced
      inflammation, 132, 136
  materials, 130, 131, 135
  mezerein-induced
      inflammation, 134
  mustard oil-induced inflammation
      in mouse ear skin, 132
  12–0-tetradecanoylphorbol
      13-acetate-induced
      inflammation, 131, 136
  zymosan-induced inflammation,
      133–135

Electrophoretic mobility shift assay
    (EMSA),
  nuclear factor-κB activation
      assay,
    gel electrophoresis, 15, 16
    materials, 10
    probe labeling, 15, 16
    SCW-arthritis analysis, 150, 151,
        156, 157
ELISA, *see* Enzyme-linked
    immunosorbent assay
EMSA, *see* Electrophoretic mobility
    shift assay
Endotoxin-induced pyrexia, COX-2
    inhibition evaluation, 323–326
End point, study design, 266
Enzyme-linked immunosorbent
    assay (ELISA),
  adhesion molecule expression
      assay on endothelial cells,
      27, 29, 30, 32
  complement activation assay,
      72–74
  matrix metalloproteinases and
      inhibitors,
    collagen cleavage assay, 363
    matrix metalloproteinase-1,
        361–363
    one step immunoassay, 362
    TIMP-1, 362, 363
Ethyl phenylpropiolate, ear
    inflammation model, 132, 136

F–G

Flow cytometry,
  adhesion molecule expression
      assay on endothelial cells,
      27
  calcium measurement, 53, 54
  oxidase assay, 65, 66
  phagocytosis assay, 41, 42, 44, 45

Gas chromatography-mass
spectrometry, *see*
Prostaglandin $F_{2\alpha}$, 8-epi isomer
Gelatinase, *see* Matrix
metalloproteinases
Group A streptococcus, *see*
SCW-arthritis

I

IBD, *see* Inflammatory bowel
disease
ICAM-1, *see* Intercellular adhesion
molecule-1
IL-1, *see* Interleukin-1
Immune rejection,
cellular response,
antigen-presenting cells, 240, 241
effector cells and tissue
damage, 241, 242
lymphocytes, 240, 241
histological features, 242, 243
skin transplant model,
anesthesia, 244
applications, 243
assessment,
macroscopy, 246
microscopy, 246
cellular response, 243
donor skin preparation, 244–247
materials, 244
recipient preparation, 245, 247
skin transplant, 245, 247
unbandaging and monitoring,
245–247
triggering, 239, 240
Immunohistochemistry, *see*
Rheumatoid arthritis; *specific
molecules*

Inflammatory bowel disease (IBD),
pathogenesis, 209
trinitrobenzene sulfonic acid rat
model,
anticolitic drug testing, 214, 215
inducible nitric oxide synthase,
activity assay, 210, 213, 217
expression, 209
Western blot, 211, 213
induction, 211, 215, 216
macroscopic assessment, 211
materials, 210, 211
myeloperoxidase,
activity assay, 212, 217
expression, 210
overview, 209, 210
statistical analysis, 215
Inflammatory response,
cell patterns in inflammatory
exudates, 110–113
key stages and targeting, 3–6
Intercellular adhesion molecule-1
(ICAM-1),
endothelial cell expression
assays,
cytokine stimulation of cells,
26, 27, 31
enzyme-linked immunosorbent
assay, 27, 29, 30, 32
flow cytometry, 27
materials, 26, 27, 31
overview, 25
reverse transcriptase-
polymerase chain
reaction, 26, 28, 29
RNA isolation, 26–28, 31
Western blot, 26, 27, 29, 32
inflammation role, 5, 273
radiolabeled antibody targeting,
see Radiolabeled antibodies

Index

Interleukin-1 (IL-1), inflammation role, 3, 6, 7
Ischemia/reperfusion injury, *see* Coronary artery occlusion and reperfusion; Kidney

K

Kidney,
  acute renal failure complications and etiology, 223
  chronic renal failure etiology and management, 223, 224
  inflammation,
    free radicals, 224, 225
    ischemia/reperfusion injury, 225
    mediators, 224
  rat ischemia/reperfusion injury model,
    anesthesia, 228, 231
    animals, 227, 230, 231
    biochemical analysis of serum and urine, 234
    bladder cannula, 229, 232
    blood collection, 229, 230, 232, 233
    ethics, 227, 231
    ischemia induction, 229, 230, 233
    kidney removal and storage, 230
    materials, 226, 227
    overview, 225, 226
    reperfusion, 230, 233
    sacrifice, 230, 234
    surgery, 228, 229, 231, 232
    temperature maintenance, 228, 231

L–M

Lipid peroxidation, *see* Prostaglandin $F_{2\alpha}$, 8-epi isomer

Luminol, oxidase assay, 64, 65, 67
Matrix metalloproteinases (MMPs), bioassays,
  casein substrate,
    caseinase assay, 360
    labeling, 357
    preparation, 356, 357
  fluorogenic peptide assays, 360, 361
  gelatin substrate,
    gelatinase assay, 359–361
    labeling, 357
    preparation, 356
  immunocapture activity assay, 361
  overview, 354
  sample preparation, 357, 358
  type I collagen substrate,
    collagenase assays, 358, 359, 363
    labeling, 357
    preparation, 354, 356
collagenases, 353
commercial assays, 354, 355
enzyme-linked immunosorbent assay,
  collagen cleavage assay, 363
  matrix metalloproteinase-1, 361–363
  one step immunoassay, 362
  TIMP-1, 362, 363
functions, 353
inflammation role, 6
rheumatoid arthritis role, 77
substrate specificity, 353, 354
tissue inhibitors, 353, 359, 362
zymography,
  developing and staining, 80
  electrophoresis, 80

gel casting, 79, 80, 86
materials, 78, 84–86
molecular species and interpretation, 81, 83
principles, 77
quantitative analysis, 84
Methylated bovine serum albumin, pleural inflammation model, 126, 127
rat monoarticular arthritis model,
animals, 164, 169
digestion of cartilage, 166, 167
end points, 167, 168, 171, 172
intra-articular injection, 167, 170, 171
overview, 161–163
patella analysis, 161, 162
sensitization and stimulus dose schedules, 167, 173
stimuli preparation, 165, 166, 169, 170
Mezerein-induced inflammation, 134
MMPs, see Matrix metalloproteinases
Mustard oil, inflammation induction in mouse ear skin, 132
Mycobacterium tuberculosis, rat monoarticular arthritis model,
animals, 164, 169
cyclosporin effects, 163
digestion of cartilage, 166, 167
end points, 167, 168, 171, 172
intra-articular injection, 167, 170, 171
methotrexate effects, 163
naproxen effects, 162, 163
overview, 161–163
patella analysis, 161, 162
sensitization and stimulus dose schedules, 167, 173
stimuli preparation, 165, 166, 169, 170
Myeloperoxidase,
assays, see Oxidase assays
inflammatory bowel disease, activity assay in trinitrobenzene sulfonic acid rat model, 212, 217
expression, 210

N

NBT, see Nitroblue tetrazolium
Neutrophil, see Oxidase assays; Phagocytosis
NF-κB, see Nuclear factor-kB
Nitrate assays,
capillary electrophoresis,
calibration curve, 310, 311, 317
cytokine induction in synovial fibroblast-like cells, 311–313, 317, 318
materials, 307–309, 316
principles, 307
running conditions, 309, 310
sample preparation, 309, 311, 316, 317
xanthine oxidase nitric oxide generation in hypoxic inflammatory tissues, 313, 314, 318
formation from nitric oxide, 306
overview, 306, 307
Nitric oxide (NO),
assays, see Nitric oxide synthase; Nitrate assays; Nitrite assays; Nitrotyrosine
inflammation role, 305
peroxynitrite formation, 292, 293
synthesis, 291

Nitric oxide synthase (NOS),
  arginine/citrulline activity assay,
    incubation conditions, 295
    materials, 293
    principles, 294
  induction, 306
  inflammatory bowel disease
      and inducible isoform,
    activity assay in
        trinitrobenzene sulfonic
        acid rat model, 210,
        213, 217
    expression, 210
    Western blot, 211, 213
  isoforms, 291, 306
Nitrite assays,
  capillary electrophoresis,
    calibration curve, 310, 311, 317
    cytokine induction in synovial
        fibroblast-like cells,
        311–313, 317, 318
    materials, 307–309, 316
    principles, 307
    running conditions, 309, 310
    sample preparation, 309, 311,
        316, 317
    xanthine oxidase nitric oxide
        generation in hypoxic
        inflammatory tissues,
        313, 314, 318
  2,3-diaminonaphthalene assay,
    fluorescence measurement, 296
    materials, 293
    sample preparation, 295, 296
    sensitivity, 295
  formation from nitric oxide, 306
  overview, 306, 307
Nitroblue tetrazolium (NBT),
    oxidase assay, 66

Nitrotyrosine,
  formation, 296, 297
  immunohistochemical
      localization,
    antibodies, 297
    color development, 298, 299
    controls, 297, 298
    incubations, 298, 299
    materials, 294
  Western blotting,
    blotting, 299, 301
    efficiency, 299–301
    immunoprecipitation, 299
    materials, 294
NO, see Nitric oxide
Nonsteroidal antiinflammatory
    drugs (NSAIDs), see
    Cyclooxygenase inhibitors
Northern blot, SCW-arthritis
    analysis, 149, 154, 155
NOS, see Nitric oxide synthase
Nuclear factor-kB (NF-κB),
  activation studies,
    cell culture and cytokine
        stimulation, 10, 11
    electrophoretic mobility shift
        assay,
      gel electrophoresis, 15, 16
      materials, 10
      probe labeling, 15, 16
    materials, 8–10
  inflammation role, 4, 5, 305
  inhibitor screening,
    cell treatment with inhibitors,
        21, 22
    luciferase detection, 21, 22
    materials, 20, 21
    overview, 19, 20
    plasmids, 20
    transfection, 21, 22

inhibitory protein,
  glutathione *S*-transferase fusion
    protein expression, 14
  kinase assay,
    immuno-complex kinase
      assay, 12, 14–16
    materials, 9
    phosphorous-32 metabolic
      labeling, 11, 12, 16
  kinase complex, 7, 8
  nitric oxide regulation, 305
  processing, 7

O

Oxidase assays,
  cytochrome *c* reduction, 64, 67
  flow cytometry assay, 65, 66
  luminescence assays, 64, 65, 67
  materials, 62
  microscopy,
    fluorescence microscopy, 66
    luminescence, 66
    nitroblue tetrazolium
      reduction, 66
  oxidases, 61, 62
  oxygen electrode assay, 62–64,
    66, 67

P

Paw edema, *see* Carrageenan-
  induced paw edema
Peritonitis, mouse model,
  inflammation induction, 142
  leukocyte subset migration in
    response to chemokines and
    cytokines,
    air pouch model comparison,
      143–145
    calculations, 143
    cell counting, 143

lavage, 143
overview, 139, 140
materials, 140, 141
Peroxidase, *see* Oxidase assays
Peroxynitrite, formation, 292, 293
Phagocytosis,
  assays,
    adherence versus
      internalization, 43, 44
    fixing and staining of cells, 42
    flow cytometry and
      parameters, 41, 42, 44, 45
    fluorescence microscopy, 41, 42
    fluorescent labeling, 38, 39, 45
    materials, 37, 45
    opsonization, 37, 38, 45
    overview, 36, 37
    phagocytosable particles, 37, 45
    stimuli presentation,
      micromanipulation, 40, 41
      sedimentation, 40
      suspensions, 39, 40
  inflammatory response, 35, 36
  neutrophils,
    mechanisms, 35
    receptors, 36
Pharmacodynamics,
  definition, 263
  iconoclastic approach, 263–267
Pharmacokinetics, definition, 263
Pleural inflammation models,
  advantages over carrageenan-
    induced paw edema, 123
  applications, 110
  carrageenan pleurisy, 125, 127
  crystal-induced pleurisy, 125–127
  materials, 124
  methylated bovine serum albumin
    pleurisy, 126, 127

pleurisy induction, 123–127
reverse passive Arthus reaction,
124, 126, 127
Polymerase chain reaction, *see*
Reverse transcriptase-
polymerase chain reaction
Prostaglandin $F_{2\alpha}$, 8-epi isomer
activity, 329
assays, overview, 330
formation, 329
immunoaffinity extraction and
gas chromatography-mass
spectrometry,
blood,
collection, 330, 332, 337
plasma extraction, 331, 333,
337, 338
derivatization, 332, 334, 335,
338–340
gas chromatography-mass
spectrometry, 335, 340
materials, 330–332
principles, 330
tissue,
collection, 331–333, 337
extraction, 331, 332, 334,
337, 338
urine,
collection, 331, 332
extraction, 331, 333, 337, 338
lipid peroxidation marker, 329, 330
Proteoglycan, degradation assay,
101, 102, 105

R

Radiolabeled antibodies,
adhesion molecule targeting,
273–276, 278–280
data handling, 278, 279, 281
preparation,
indium labeling, 277, 279
iodine labeling, 276, 277, 280
materials, 274, 275, 279
technetium labeling, 277, 280
Radiolabeled leukocytes,
applications, 274
data handling, 279, 281
injection, 276, 278, 280, 281
preparation,
indium labeling, 278
materials, 275
technetium labeling, 277
Renal failure, *see* Kidney
Reverse transcriptase-polymerase
chain reaction (RT-PCR),
adhesion molecule expression
assay on endothelial cells,
26, 28, 29
SCW-arthritis analysis, 149, 155
Rheumatoid arthritis,
aggrecanase-generated
interglobular domain
catabolites, *see* Aggrecanase
cartilage degradation, *see*
Cartilage degradation assays
collagen-induced arthritis model,
see Collagen-induced
arthritis
immunohistochemistry
of synovium,
hematoxylin eosin staining, 287
immunoperoxidase
histochemistry, 288, 289
materials, 284–286, 289
microscopic analysis, 289
sectioning of tissue, 287
synovial tissue processing
and freezing, 286
targets, 283, 284

Vectabond coating of slides, 286, 287
inadequacy of models, 270, 271
matrix metalloproteinase role, 77, 89
SCW-arthritis model, *see* SCW-arthritis
RNase protection assay (RPA), SCW-arthritis analysis, 150, 155, 156
RPA, *see* RNase protection assay
RT-PCR, *see* Reverse transcriptase-polymerase chain reaction

S

Scarring,
    evaluation in rodent models, 257
    transforming growth factor-β effects, 250, 251
SCW-arthritis,
    clinical evaluation, 148, 151, 157, 158
    genetic susceptibility, 157
    Group A streptococcus cell wall response, 147
    histological evaluation,
        fixation, 148, 153
        histological staining, 148, 153, 158
        immunohistochemical staining, 148, 153
    induction, 147, 148, 151
    materials for model formation, 147–151, 157
    protein analysis,
        electrophoretic mobility shift assay, 150, 151, 156, 157
        isolation of proteins, 150, 156
        Western blot, 150, 156
    transcript analysis,
        Northern blot, 149, 154, 155
        reverse transcriptase-polymerase chain reaction, 149, 155
        RNA isolation, 149, 154
        RNase protection assay, 150, 155, 156
        tissue collection and preparation, 154
Selectins,
    endothelial cell expression assays,
        cytokine stimulation of cells, 26, 27, 31
        enzyme-linked immunosorbent assay, 27, 29, 30, 32
        flow cytometry, 27
        materials, 26, 27, 31
        overview, 25
        reverse transcriptase-polymerase chain reaction, 26, 28, 29
        RNA isolation, 26–28, 31
        Western blot, 26, 27, 29, 32
    inflammation role, 273
    radiolabeled antibody targeting, *see* Radiolabeled antibodies
Skin transplant, *see* Immune rejection
Superoxide,
    inflammation role, 292
    peroxynitrite formation, 292, 293
    production, 291, 292

T

12–0-Tetradecanoylphorbol 13-acetate, ear inflammation model, 131, 136
TGF-β, *see* Transforming growth factor-β

Therapeutic index, definition, 263, 264
TNF-α, *see* Tumor necrosis factor-α
Transforming growth factor-β (TGF-β), wound healing effects, 250, 251
Trinitrobenzene sulfonic acid rat model. *see* Inflammatory bowel disease
Tumor necrosis factor-α (TNF-α), inflammation role, 3, 6, 7

V

Vascular cell adhesion molecule-1 (VCAM-1),
  endothelial cell expression assays,
    cytokine stimulation of cells, 26, 27, 31
    enzyme-linked immunosorbent assay, 27, 29, 30, 32
    flow cytometry, 27
    materials, 26, 27, 31
    overview, 25
    reverse transcriptase-polymerase chain reaction, 26, 28, 29
    RNA isolation, 26–28, 31
    Western blot, 26, 27, 29, 32
  inflammation role, 5, 273
  radiolabeled antibody targeting, *see* Radiolabeled antibodies
VCAM-1, *see* Vascular cell adhesion molecule-1

W

Western blot,
  adhesion molecule expression assay on endothelial cells, 26, 27, 29, 32

aggrecanase interglobular domain catabolites, 92, 93, 97
inducible nitric oxide synthase in inflammatory bowel disease, 211, 213
nitrotyrosine,
  blotting, 299, 301
  efficiency, 299–301
  immunoprecipitation, 299
  materials, 294
SCW-arthritis analysis, 150, 156
Wound healing,
  embryo versus adult, 250
  process, 249, 250
  rodent models,
    administration of agents, 256
    advantages, 251
    evaluation,
      inflammation, 256, 259
      reepithelialization, 256
      scarring, 257
      vascularization, 257
      wound strength, 257, 258
    excisional wounds, 255, 259
    harvesting of wounds, 255
    histology processing, 256
    incisional wounds, 253–255, 258
    materials, 251
    wound gape, 252
  transforming growth factor-β effects, 250, 251

Z

Zymography, matrix metalloproteinases,
  developing and staining, 80
  electrophoresis, 80
  gel casting, 79, 80, 86
  materials, 78, 84–86

molecular species
and interpretation, 81, 83
principles, 77
quantitative analysis, 84
Zymosan,
ear inflammation models, 133–135
rat monoarticular arthritis model,
animals, 164, 169
digestion of cartilage, 166, 167
end points, 167, 168, 171, 172
intra-articular injection, 167, 170, 171
overview, 161–163
patella analysis, 161, 162, 167–169, 171, 172
proteoglycan loss and assay, 163, 168, 169, 172
sensitization and stimulus dose schedules, 167, 173
statistical analysis, 169, 172
stimuli preparation, 165, 166, 169, 170